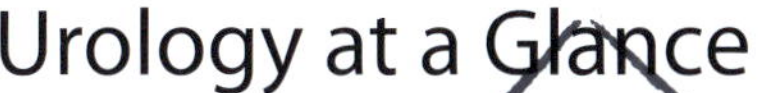

Urology at a Glance

Axel S. Merseburger • Markus A. Kuczyk
Judd W. Moul
Editors

Urology at a Glance

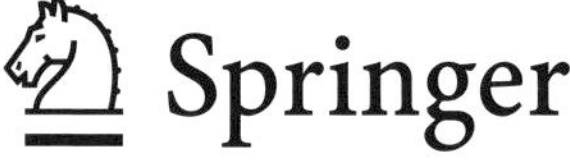

Editors
Axel S. Merseburger
Department of Urology and Urologic Oncology
Medical School of Hannover (MHH)
Hannover
Germany

Judd W. Moul, MD
Division of Urologic Surgery
Duke University Medical Center
Durham, NC
USA

Markus A. Kuczyk
Department of Urology and Urologic Oncology
Medical School of Hannover (MHH)
Hannover
Germany

ISBN 978-3-642-54858-1 ISBN 978-3-642-54859-8 (eBook)
DOI 10.1007/978-3-642-54859-8
Springer Heidelberg New York Dordrecht London

Library of Congress Control Number: 2014951199

Printed on acid-free paper

Springer is part of Springer Science+Business Media (www.springer.com)

Contents

Part I

From Symptoms to Diagnosis

Haematuria

1

Hannes Cash and Mario W. Kramer

1.1 Definition

Haematuria is the presence of red blood cells in the urine. Blood visible in the urine is called gross haematuria (Fig. 1.1). Microhaematuria is defined as ≥3 red blood cells (RBCs) per high-power field on microscopic examination. Chemical urine dipstick has a high sensitivity of up to 1–2 RBCs × 10^{12} per litre. In general >5,000 RBCs/µl urine or approx. 1-ml blood/urine is needed to achieve visibility. The causes of haematuria are either nephrologic or urologic.

1.2 Medical History

Medical history should include nephrologic and urologic diseases: previous systemic infections, pre-existing medical renal disease, systemic autoimmune disease, skin disease, haemoptysis, epistaxis, history of tuberculosis (sterile leucocyturia with microhaematuria), travel history (e.g. schistosomiasis), medication (i.e. anticoagulants), B symptoms, dysuria and fever, episodes of flank pain, renal colic, lower urinary tract symptoms, history of cancer and past or current smoking. Drug history is of importance since it can be a cause of haematuria (e.g. antibiotics or NSAIDs ⇒ interstitial nephritis). A concise family history may lead to causes of benign familial haematuria (thin basement membrane disease (TBMD), polycystic kidney disease or Alport syndrome). Of most importance is the history of risk factors for

H. Cash, MD (✉)
Department of Urology, Charité University Medicine Berlin,
Campus Benjamin Franklin, Hindenburgdamm 30, Berlin 12200, Germany
e-mail: hannes.cash@charite.de

M.W. Kramer, MD
Department of Urology and Urological Oncology, Hannover Medical School, Carl-Neuberg-Str. 1, Hannover 30625, Germany
e-mail: kramer.mario@mh-hannover.de

A.S. Merseburger et al. (eds.), *Urology at a Glance*,

DOI 10.1007/978-3-642-54859-8_1,

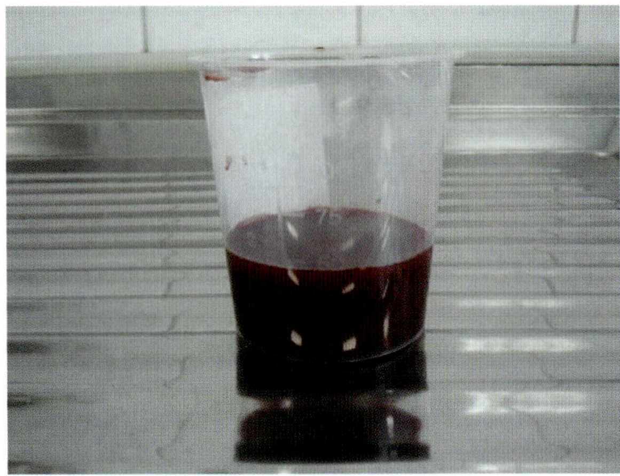

Fig. 1.1 Urine sample of a patient with gross haematuria

Table 1.1 Common risk factors for urinary tract malignancy in patients with asymptomatic haematuria

Risk factors
Male gender
Age (>35 years)
Past or current smoking
Occupational or other exposure to chemicals or dyes (benzenes or aromatic amines)
Analgesic abuse
History of gross haematuria
History of urologic disorder or disease
History of irritative voiding symptoms
History of pelvic irradiation
History of chronic urinary tract infection
History of exposure to known carcinogenic agents or chemotherapy such as alkylating agents
History of chronic indwelling foreign body

Reference: AUA Guidelines 2012

urinary tract malignancies in patients with asymptomatic haematuria, which are displayed in Table 1.1.

1.3 Diagnostics

The diagnostic workup should always include a physical examination with inspection and palpation of the abdomen and palpation of both flanks. In some cases a concise examination can indicate a diagnosis: flank pain in conjunction with cystitis (pyelonephritis); digital rectal examination (DRE) with suspect and/or painful prostate (prostate cancer, prostatitis); palpable kidney mass (kidney tumour or cystic kidney disease); and fever, tonsillitis and oedema (post-infectious glomerulonephritis after infection with *Streptococcus pyogenes*). In asymptomatic haematuria (AMH), the clinical examination alone will not be conclusive in most cases.

After excluding benign causes of haematuria (present or recent menstruation, trauma, viral infections, vigorous exercise, pre-existing medical renal disease, urinary tract infection or recent urologic procedures which do not require a full diagnostic workup), further diagnostic measures are prompted.

Laboratory test should include an initial urine dipstick analysis followed by urine microscopy as well as laboratory test of kidney function (serum creatinine, blood urea nitrogen) and infection parameters (white blood cell count, CRP).

Special attention should be given to the microscopic evaluation of the urine: acanthocytes (syn: spur cells) especially when found in combination with proteinuria and erythrocyte cylinders indicate glomerulonephritis; renal biopsy and nephrologic diagnostics may be indicated. In case of haematuria with normal-shaped cells, further urologic evaluation is necessary.

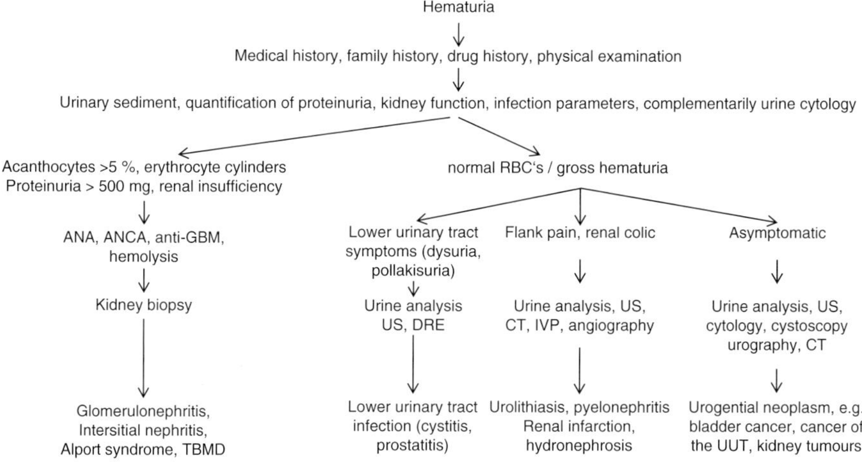

Ultrasonography (US) should be used to evaluate the urinary tract including the kidneys and bladder (kidney stones, hydronephrosis, renal tumours, tumours of the renal pelvis, larger bladder tumours). With the aid of duplex sonography, infarction of the renal parenchyma or thrombosis of the renal vein can be diagnosed. Possible malignant causes of haematuria are bladder cancer, cancer of the upper urinary tract (UTT) and renal cell carcinoma. In all patients with AMH and age ≥35 years, urologic evaluation including a cystoscopy is indicated. Urine cytology should be used complementarily. The initial evaluation of AMH should also include radiologic imaging with multiphasic computed tomography (CT) with an excretory phase. For patients with contraindications for a CT (renal insufficiency, contrast allergy, pregnancy), magnetic resonance urography or retrograde pyelogram (RPG) presents a diagnostic alternative.

1.4 Differential Diagnosis of Haematuria

Differential diagnosis	Frequency of haematuria	Diagnostics
Cystitis, pyelonephritis	+++	Urine dipstick, US, blood test
Bladder cancer and/or tumours of the UUT	+++	US, cystoscopy, cytology, multiphasic CT with urography alternatively MRU, RPG or IVP
Urolithiasis	+++	Urine dipstick, blood test, US, low-dose CT or IVP
Prostatitis	+/++	DRE, urine dipstick, transrectal US, blood test
Glomerulonephritis	++	Urinary sediment, proteinuria, serologic testing (i.e. ANCA), kidney biopsy
Interstitial nephritis	++	Urinary sediment, eosinophilia, kidney biopsy
Prostate cancer	(+)	DRE, PSA, transrectal US, ultrasound-guided transrectal biopsy
Kidney cancer	(+)	US, CT/MRI
Polycystic kidney disease	+	Family history, US
Renal infarction	+	Duplex US, angiography
Alport syndrome	+	Family history, amblyacousia, eye disorders, kidney biopsy
TBMD	+	Family history, kidney biopsy

Dysuria

2

Christoph A.J. von Klot

2.1 Definition

In the field of urology, dysuria is used in slightly varying ways and includes difficulties during urination up to a painful or burning sensation during voiding. Dysuria can have a variety of underlying medical conditions, the most common of which at young age is urinary tract infection that occurs mostly in adolescent women. Older patients mostly tend to have dysuria due to benign prostate hyperplasia; therefore, dysuria in the elderly population mostly occurs in the male population.

2.2 Medical History

The medical history should include the length of dysuric symptom as well as type of onset, i.e. sudden or gradual. Concomitant symptoms suggestive of infection, such as fever, flank pain, chills, burning sensation and urethral discharge, should be assessed. Patients with dysuria should be asked about the occurrence of gross haematuria. Voiding function should be evaluated with questions in accordance with the International Prostate Symptom Score (IPSS): feeling of incomplete bladder emptying, frequency, urgency, weak stream, straining, nocturia and intermittency. Also an orientation about the past medical history needs to be obtained focussing on trauma to the pelvis or urethra, previous infections especially urethritis and urinary tract infections in general and surgery of the lower urinary tract. The medical history should also include a thorough look on vegetative symptoms, signs of depression,

C.A.J. von Klot
Department of Urology and Urological Oncology, Hannover University Medical School, Carl-Neuberg-Str. 1, Hannover 30625, Germany
e-mail: klot.christoph@mh-hannover.de

A.S. Merseburger et al. (eds.), *Urology at a Glance*,
DOI 10.1007/978-3-642-54859-8_2, © Springer-Verlag Berlin Heidelberg 2014

bowel irregularities and the neurological status. Finally the complete list of current medication needs to be obtained and correlation of symptoms with food or medication intake tested.

2.3 Diagnostics

Since the symptom of dysuria is highly variable and unspecific, a vast selection of diagnostic tools may be applied depending on patient age, medical history and clinical findings.

Acute dysuria together with urgency and frequency hints towards a urinary tract infection. Diagnostics include urine dipstick testing and a physical examination with the focus on the suprapubic bladder and flank region. Further testing including urine sediment, urine culture or a sterile catheter specimen of urine may be warranted if diagnosis is unclear. Further workup for recurrent infections is advised.

Itching and tingling sensation with or without urethral discharge may be symptoms of urethritis. First morning urine shows at least ten white blood cells per high-power field in urine sediment. Diagnostic tools include physical examination for lymphadenopathy, ulcers and urethral discharge on palpation of the urethra. Urethral swabs should be subjected to a microbiological examination [1]. A lot of patients with negatively tested lab results respond to antibiotic treatment suggesting initial false-negative tests.

Dysuric symptoms, pain during defaecation and a painful digital rectal examination may be signs of prostatitis. Diagnosis of prostatitis may be challenging since symptoms are highly variable and range from severe febrile infection to a clinically completely asymptomatic course. Symptoms can be assessed using the validated Chronic Prostatitis Symptom Score (NIH-CPSI). When prostatitis is suspected, the workup includes the following: testing for post-void residual volume, digital rectal examination and ultrasound of the prostate, PSA measurement, urine sediment and urine microbiological testing, uroflowmetry and separate testing of initially voided urine, midstream urine, expressed prostatic secretion after prostatic massage and urine after prostatic massage. Testing may be reduced to midstream urine plus urine after prostatic massage as more cost-efficient test [2, 3].

Dysuria in conjunction with signs of voiding dysfunction in the absence of infection is indicative of lower urinary tract obstruction. Diagnostics include an IPSS Score, bladder diary, measurement of residual urine and uroflowmetry, bladder wall thickness and a digital rectal examination in men.

A variety of clinical causes of obstruction can be identified on physical examination such as meatal stenosis, lichen sclerosus, palpable prostate cancer phimosis and anatomical abnormalities. Filling cystometry and pressure-flow measurement are not mandatory. A urodynamic evaluation for benign prostatic hyperplasia should however be undertaken in a certain subset of patients: voided volume ≤150 ml, patient age <50 or >80 years, post-void residual volume

>300 ml, suspicion of neurological disease, previous pelvic surgery, patients with previous unsuccessful invasive treatment, bilateral hydronephrosis and patients with a maximum flow rate of more than 15 ml/s on uroflowmetry. Patients with suspicion of lower urinary tract obstruction should be checked for sequelae of bladder outlet obstruction including reduced renal function, hydronephrosis, infection, bladder diverticula and bladder calculus [4].

For bladder outlet obstruction, causes other than benign prostate enlargement have to be considered. A none bell-shaped plateau curve in uroflowmetry may hint towards meatal stenosis or urethral stricture. In this case, a retrograde urethrogram and urethrocystoscopy can be applied to clarify urethral anomalies and can also identify foreign bodies of the urethra and urinary bladder.

In dysuria especially in conjunction with gross haematuria or microhaematuria without infection, malignancy must be ruled out. In men > age 40 years, a digital rectal examination and PSA value are performed. Urethral and bladder cancer should be examined via urethrocystoscopy. If diagnosis is unclear, bladder washout cytology and biopsy may be performed [5–7].

Pathology of the upper urinary tract usually does not typically cause dysuria as a symptom. However, diagnostics of the upper urinary tract, i.e. retrograde or IV pyelography and upper urinary tract cytology, must be included when malignancy cannot be ruled out or the cause of haematuria is unclear. Imaging of the upper urinary tract may reveal a lower ureteric stone which can cause dysuric symptoms.

In women with dysuric symptoms, gynaecological workup may be necessary to reveal specific causes of dysuria in the female population. Vaginitis may be caused by bacterial infection and fungal infection, and allergic or atrophic vaginitis may be due to oestrogen deficiency. Patients need to be evaluated for vaginal discharge, vaginal irritation, itching, redness, dyspareunia and dysuria. Gynaecological workup includes pH testing, cytology and microscopic evaluation as well as a vaginal examination [8].

Endometriosis as the first clinical manifestation in the urinary tract is rare. If the urinary tract is involved, the most common site is the urinary bladder. Diagnostic workup is usually initiated due to dysuria and predominantly urgency and frequency with concomitant haematuria in premenopausal women. Endovesical endometriosis is confirmed by cystoscopic examination with histological confirmation of suspicious lesions of the bladder mucosa [9].

Another cause of dysuria may lie in the diagnosis of bladder pain syndrome/interstitial cystitis (BPS/IC). No specific test is able to reliably identify BPS/IC as such. The diagnosis of BPS/IC is therefore mainly one of exclusion. Hydrodistention of the bladder wall with occurrence of small petechial haemorrhages may be helpful but is not specific as are the so-called Hunner ulcers which can be found in less than 50 % of patients with BPS/IC. Today IC is referred to as the typical clinic entity with Hunner ulcers and inflammation while BPS includes a wider range of clinical findings. Diagnosis is based on the 'International Society for the Study of BPS' (ESSIC) [10] (Fig. 2.1).

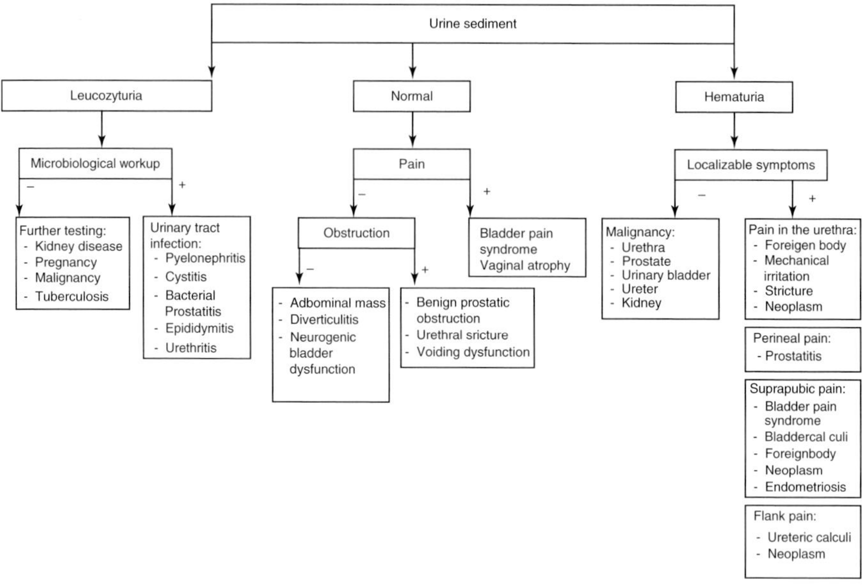

Fig. 2.1 Clinical decision making for diagnostic tests in patients with dysuric symptoms

2.4 Differential Diagnosis

Since dysuria is described as a symptom and not the underlying disease, we do not discuss the aspect of differential diagnoses; however, aside from the above-mentioned diagnostic considerations, a variety of secondary clinical conditions and rare conditions can cause dysuric symptoms. Among these are:

- Drugs and chemical irritants such as hygiene sprays, soaps, or even toilet paper
- Mass in the abdomen or diverticulitis
- Reactive arthritis with urethritis/Reiter's syndrome with urethritis as a sequela
- Psychogenic disorders and somatization disorders
- Mechanical irritation after physical activities: horseback riding and bicycling
- Adenovirus, herpesvirus and *Schistosoma haematobium*

References

1. Chute CG, Panser LA, Girman CJ, Oesterling JE, Guess HA, Jacobsen SJ, et al. The prevalence of prostatism: a population-based survey of urinary symptoms. J Urol. 1993;150(1):85–9.
2. Ludwig M, Schroeder-Printzen I, Lüdecke G, Weidner W. Comparison of expressed prostatic secretions with urine after prostatic massage–a means to diagnose chronic prostatitis/inflammatory chronic pelvic pain syndrome. Urology. 2000;55(2):175–7.
3. Brede CM, Shoskes DA. The etiology and management of acute prostatitis. Nat Rev Urol. 2011;8(4):207–12. Available from: http://dx.doi.org/10.1038/nrurol.2011.22.

4. Oelke M, Bachmann A, Descazeaud A, Emberton M, Gravas S, Michel MC, et al. EAU guidelines on the treatment and follow-up of non-neurogenic male lower urinary tract symptoms including benign prostatic obstruction. Eur Urol. 2013;64(1):118–40. Available from: http://dx.doi.org/10.1016/j.eururo.2013.03.004.
5. Babjuk M, Burger M, Zigeuner R, Shariat SF, van Rhijn BWG, Compérat E, et al. EAU guidelines on non-muscle-invasive urothelial carcinoma of the bladder: update 2013. Eur Urol. 2013;64(4):639–53. Available from: http://dx.doi.org/10.1016/j.eururo.2013.06.003.
6. Heidenreich A, Abrahamsson PA, Artibani W, Catto J, Montorsi F, Van Poppel H, et al. Early detection of prostate cancer: European Association of Urology recommendation. Eur Urol. 2013;64(3):347–54. Available from: http://dx.doi.org/10.1016/j.eururo.2013.06.051.
7. Tetu B. Diagnosis of urothelial carcinoma from urine. Mod Pathol. 2009;22 Suppl 2:S53–9. Available from: http://dx.doi.org/10.1038/modpathol.2008.193.
8. Pandit L, Ouslander JG. Postmenopausal vaginal atrophy and atrophic vaginitis. Am J Med Sci. 1997;314(4):228–31.
9. Perez-Utrilla Perez M, Aguilera Bazán A, Alonso Dorrego JM, Hernández A, de Francisco MG, Martín Hernández M, et al. Urinary tract endometriosis: clinical, diagnostic, and therapeutic aspects. Urology. 2009;73(1):47–51. Available from: http://dx.doi.org/10.1016/j.urology.2008.08.470.
10. van de Merwe JP, Nordling J, Bouchelouche P, Bouchelouche K, Cervigni M, Daha LK, et al. Diagnostic criteria, classification, and nomenclature for painful bladder syndrome/interstitial cystitis: an ESSIC proposal. Eur Urol. 2008;53(1):60–7. Available from: http://dx.doi.org/10.1016/j.eururo.2007.09.019.

3 Male Infertility

George Kedia

3.1 Definition

Infertility is a disease of the reproductive system defined by the failure to achieve a clinical pregnancy after 12 months or more of regular unprotected sexual intercourse [1]. Infertility affects both men and women. The components of the evaluation of the men include medical history, physical and ultrasound examination, semen analysis and endocrine and genetic tests.

3.2 Medical History

A detailed history of an infertile men should include family history, developmental history (descensus testis, pubertal/mental development, voice mutation, loss of body hair), systemic diseases (diabetes, renal and liver insufficiency, cancer, hemochromatosis), infections (mumps orchitis, sinopulmonary symptoms, sexually transmitted infection, genitourinary tract infections), surgical procedures (vasectomy, orchiectomy, herniorrhaphy), exogenous factors (medications, cytotoxic chemotherapy, radiation therapy) and lifestyle factors (alcohol, obesity, smoking, drugs, anabolic steroids). A detailed sexual history should also be obtained, including libido, frequency of intercourse and previous fertility assessments of the men and their partner.

G. Kedia
Department of Urology and Urological Oncology, Hannover Medical School, Carl-Neuberg-Str. 1, Hannover 30625, Germany
e-mail: kedia.george@mh-hannover.de

A.S. Merseburger et al. (eds.), *Urology at a Glance*,
DOI 10.1007/978-3-642-54859-8_3, © Springer-Verlag Berlin Heidelberg 2014

3.3 Diagnostics

The evaluation of an infertile men should begin with a physical examination that focuses on the secondary sex characteristics including general appearance (constitution type, eunuchoid features, body fat, muscle mass), breasts (gynecomastia), hair (pubic, axillary and facial), skin (sebum production, acne, pallor, skin wrinkling) and external genitalia (size of the penis, testicular volume, epididymis, vas deferens). Absence or partial atresia of the vas deferens, epididymal thickening and cysts, varicocele and scrotal hernia can be detected by inspection and digital or ultrasound examination of the scrotum. Ultrasound examination of the testis should be performed to measure the testicular volume and also to exclude tumours and microcalcifications, especially in men with a history of cryptorchidism. Transrectal ultrasound examination is recommended in men with a low volume of ejaculate (<1.5 mL) to exclude obstruction of the ejaculatory ducts caused by a prostatic cyst (Mullerian cyst) or stenosis of the ejaculatory ducts due to infection or surgery.

The semen analysis, standardised by the WHO [2], is essential for the evaluation of the male partner of an infertile couple. The standard semen analysis consists of the following: measurement of semen volume and pH, microscopy for debris and agglutination, assessment of sperm concentration, motility and morphology, sperm leukocyte count and search for immature germ cells [3]. More specialised semen analysis (e.g. detection of sperm autoantibodies, semen biochemistry) are optional. If the semen analysis and the investigation of the female partner are normal, then specialised tests of sperm function should be performed.

Microbiological investigation is indicated in men with abnormal urine or semen samples, urinary tract infections, male accessory gland infections and sexually transmitted diseases.

The endocrine tests include measurements of follicle-stimulating hormone (FHS), luteinizing hormone (LH), serum testosterone and sex hormone-binding globulin (SHBG). Serum prolactin should be measured in men with a low serum testosterone and normal to low serum LH.

Magnetic resonance imaging (MRI) of the pituitary gland should be performed in infertile men with unexplained hypogonadotropic hypogonadism or high serum prolactin.

In men with oligoasthenoteratozoospermia (OAT) or azoospermia, karyotyping and deletions in the azoospermic factor (AZFa, AZFb, AZFc) region of the Y-chromosome are recommended for diagnosis and for genetic counselling. The infertile men with absence of the vas deferens, low seminal fluid volume and acidic pH should be tested for mutations in the CFTR (cystic fibrosis transmembrane conductance regulator) gene.

Open biopsy of the testis should be performed to exclude tumour in infertile men with risk factors for testicular cancer (male infertility, cryptorchidism, history of a testicular tumour, testicular atrophy). In infertile men with azoospermia or extreme OAT, a normal testicular volume and normal FSH levels, a diagnostic testicular biopsy should be considered to differentiate between testicular insufficiency and obstruction of the male genital tract. Testicular fine-needle aspiration (TEFNA), testicular sperm extraction (TESE) or microsurgical epididymal sperm aspiration

(MESA) is usually performed as part of a therapeutic intervention for assisted reproduction in azoospermic men. The flow chart (Fig. 3.1) demonstrates the pathway from symptoms to diagnosis.

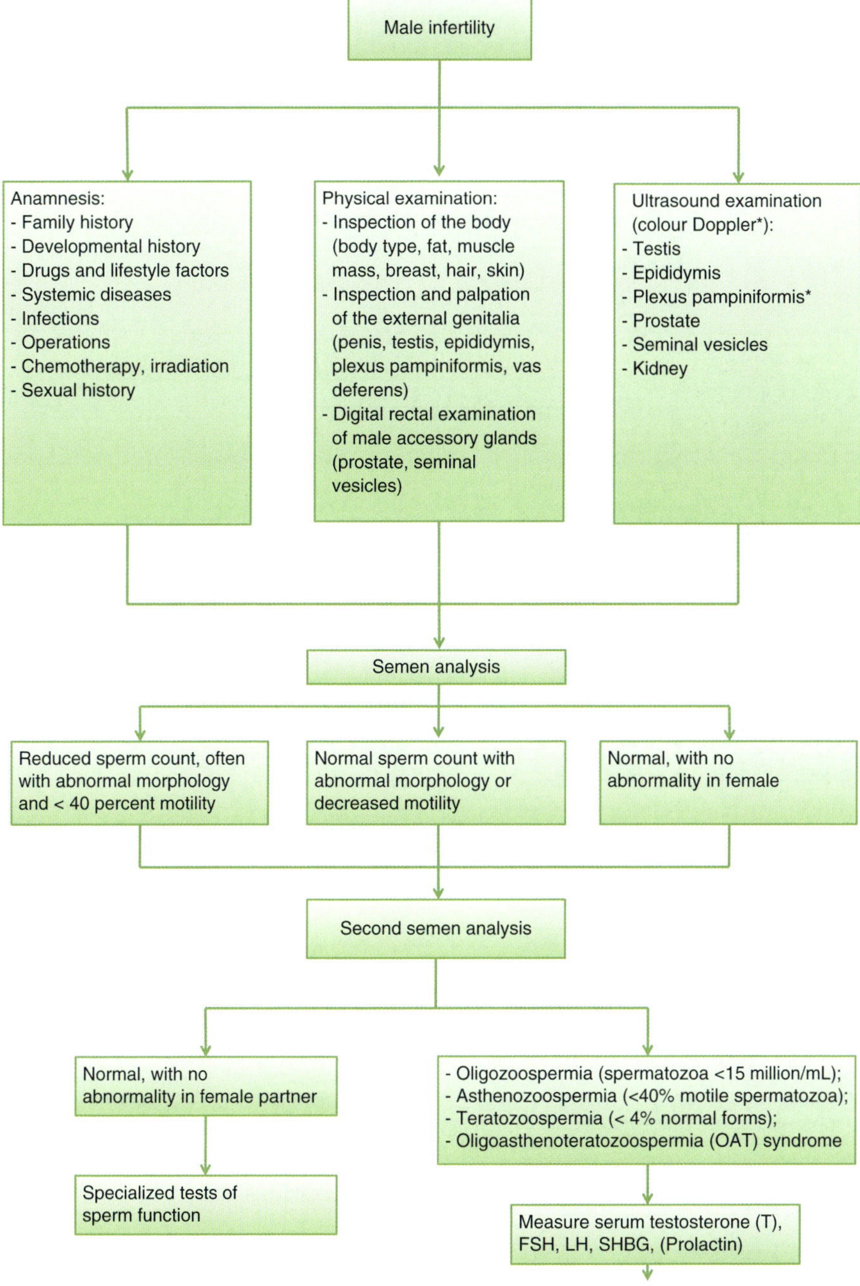

Fig. 3.1 Flow chart demonstrating the pathway from symptoms to diagnosis

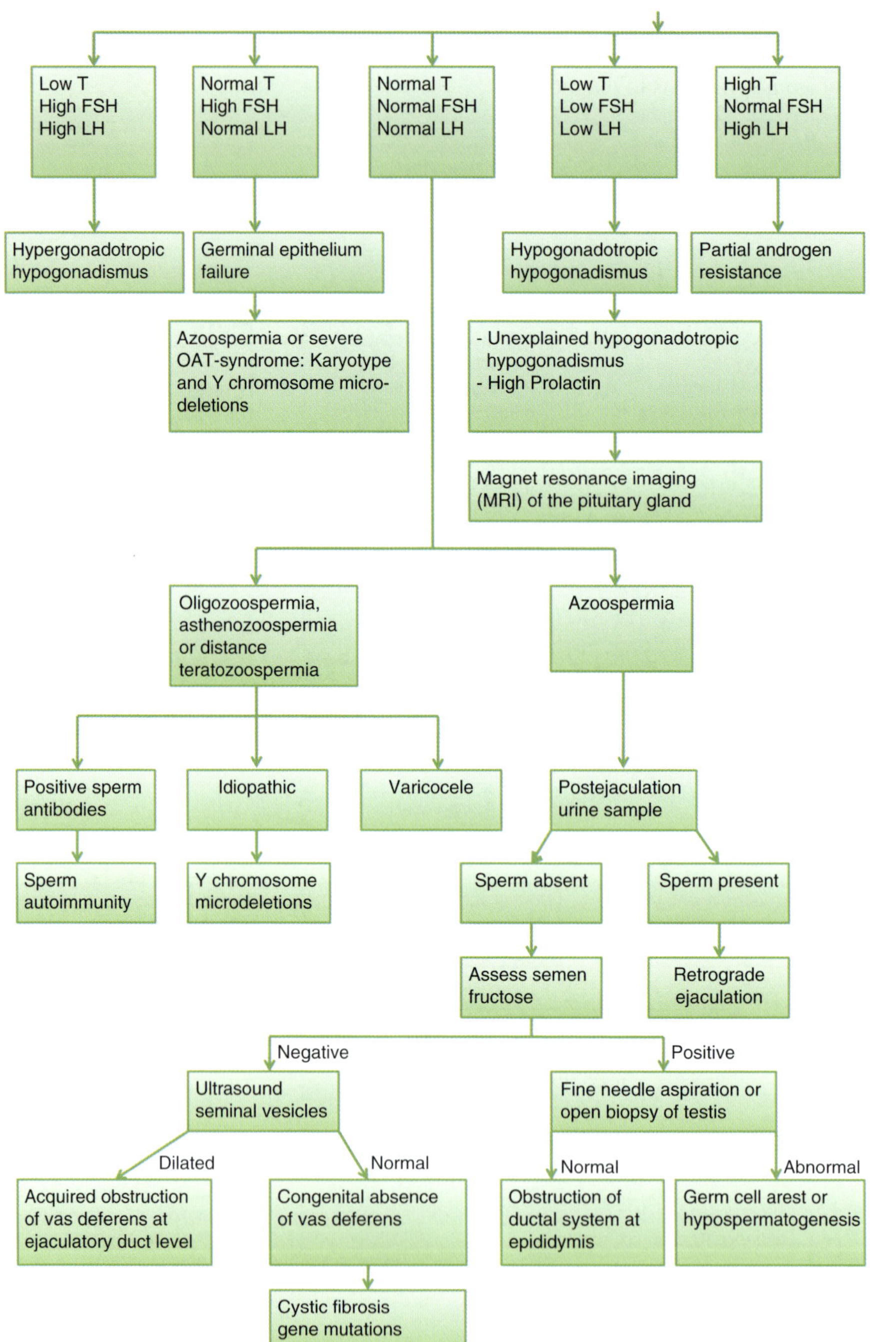

Fig. 3.1 (continued)

3.4 Differential Diagnosis

Reasons for male infertility

Differential diagnosis	Incidence	Diagnostics
Hypothalamic-pituitary disorders Kallmann's syndrome Idiopathic hypogonadotrophic hypogonadismus Multiorgan genetic disorders (e.g. Prader-Willi syndrome, Bardet-Biedl syndrome, familial cerebral ataxia) Malignant CNS tumours Pituitary adenoma Empty sella Hyperprolactinaemia Surgery, trauma Granulomatous illness Hemochromatosis Drugs, anabolic steroids Irradiation Vascular disorders (infarction, aneurysm) Obesity Nutritional defeciencies	++++	Medical/clinical history Clinical examination Semen analysis Hormone and genetic tests Magnet resonance imaging
Primary gonadal disorders Anorchia Testicular dysgenesis/cryptrochidism Klinifelter's syndrome Y chromosome microdeletions Androgen insenitivity syndromes 5-alpha-reductase deficiency Myotonic dystrophy Noonan's syndrome Testicular trauma, torsion Tumour, infection Varicocele Drugs, anabolic steroids Cytotoxic therapy, irradiation Systemic diseases (e.g. renal failure, liver cirrhosis, sickle cell disease) Surgery (orchiectomy, herniorrhaphy)	++++	Medical/clinical history Clinical examination Semen analysis Hormone and genetic tests
Disorders of sperm transport Surgery (e.g. vasectomy) Congenital bilateral absence of the vas deferens/cystic fibrosis Infection Young's syndrome	++++	Medical/clinical history Clinical examination Semen analysis Genetic test (CFTR-Gen)

References

1. Zegers-Hochschild F, Adamson GD, de Mouzon J, et al. The International Committee for Monitoring Assisted Reproductive Technology (ICMART) and the World Health Organization (WHO) revised glossary on ART terminology. Hum Reprod. 2009;24(11):2683–7.
2. World Health Organization Department of Reproductive Health and Research. WHO laboratory manual for the examination and processing of human semen. 5th ed. Geneva: WHO; 2010.
3. Cooper TG, Noonan E, von Eckardstein S, et al. World Health Organization reference values for human semen characteristics. Hum Reprod Update. 2010;16(3):231–45.

Proteinuria

4

Bastian Amend and Karl-Dietrich Sievert

4.1 Definition

Proteinuria is defined as the temporary or continuous detection of proteins in the urine, which exceeds an amount of 150–200 mg per 24 h, using a base of urine production of 1,500 ml a day. Regular protein excretion consists of approximately 30 % globulins, 30 % albumin, and 40 % of other proteins, especially Tamm-Horsfall glycoprotein (uromodulin, excreted primarily by the kidney).

In a healthy kidney, limitation of protein loss is regulated by the glomerular filter, with a filtration barrier for proteins larger than 50 kDa and especially negative electrically charged molecules, and the tubular reabsorption of smaller proteins and amino acids which passed the glomerular membrane. Therefore, proteinuria is subdivided into different categories: glomerular (prevalent heavy molecular weight), tubular (prevalent small molecular weight), overflow (increased serum protein concentrations), and also postrenal proteinuria (increased renal excretion or associated infection). Table 4.1 summarizes typical marker proteins.

Microalbuminuria, characterized as a 30–300 mg loss in 24 h or a urine concentration of 20–200 mg albumin per liter, should be considered in patients with diabetes mellitus and/or hypertension as an early marker for nephropathy.

4.2 Medical History

In most cases proteinuria is not a symptom reported by the patient himself/herself. Generally proteinuria is either found during a preventive medical checkup or identified within specific laboratory urine analysis in case of a suspected diagnosis or

B. Amend (✉) • K.-D. Sievert
Department of Urology, Eberhard-Karls-University,
Hoppe-Seyler-Str. 3, Tuebingen 72076, Germany
e-mail: bastian.amend@med.uni-tuebingen.de; karl.sievert@med.uni-tuebingen.de

A.S. Merseburger et al. (eds.), *Urology at a Glance*,
DOI 10.1007/978-3-642-54859-8_4, © Springer-Verlag Berlin Heidelberg 2014

Table 4.1 Marker proteins to categorize the form of proteinuria

Glomerular proteinuria
Selective glomerular proteinuria
Albumin
Transferrin
Unselective glomerular proteinuria
Albumin
Transferrin
Immunoglobulin G
α-2-macrogloculin
Tubular proteinuria
β-2-microglobulin
Alpha-1-acid glycoprotein
Prerenal proteinuria ("overflow")
Myoglobin (muscle trauma)
Hemoglobin (hemolysis, also red urine)
Bence Jones protein (paraneoplastic)
Postrenal
Tubular secret proteins, e.g., Tamm-Horsfall

proved disease. Only in rare cases the patient presents with the specific symptom of foaming urine during micturition.

The initial medical history should focus on the timing of proteinuria. In case of short-term proteinuria, typical signs of infection (fever, exudation, dysuria, malaise) and emotional and physical stress should be explored. Especially in young men, intermittent and light proteinuria is often seen as a so-called orthostatic proteinuria, which can be excluded by repeated morning urine sample analysis. In case of persistent proteinuria, a wide range of diseases with nephrotoxic potential are known. Therefore, a comprehensive anamnesis including acute and chronic diseases, as well as cancer with potential paraneoplastic protein production, should be investigated. Advanced proteinuria can lead to hypoproteinemia with a decreased oncotic pressure resulting in edemas and ascites.

4.3 Diagnostics

Dipstick analysis is the first step to detect proteinuria. The dye for protein analysis changes due to a pH shift. Dipstick tests are most sensitive to albumin; therefore, false-negative results could be obtained, if albumin excretion is not increased (e.g., in case of a Bence Jones proteinuria) or if the urine sample is highly diluted or alkaline. Standard dipstick tests will also not detect microalbuminuria.

If proteinuria is present and reasons for short-term proteinuria (especially urinary tract infection) are excluded, a quantification of the amount of protein loss should be performed over a 24-hour period. Protein electrophoresis of the urine unveils the different molecules of proteinuria based on their molecular weight, which enables the categorization in Table 4.1. If a paraneoplastic "overflow" proteinuria is suspected, immunoelectrophoresis and immunofixation are the methods of choice. Quantification of specific proteins could be achieved either by urine (immuno-) nephelometry or turbidimetry.

In case of continuous proteinuria, urine analysis should be accompanied by the examination of the urine sediment (focus on dysmorphic erythrocytes and urinary casts in case of glomerulonephritis) as well as serum protein analysis.

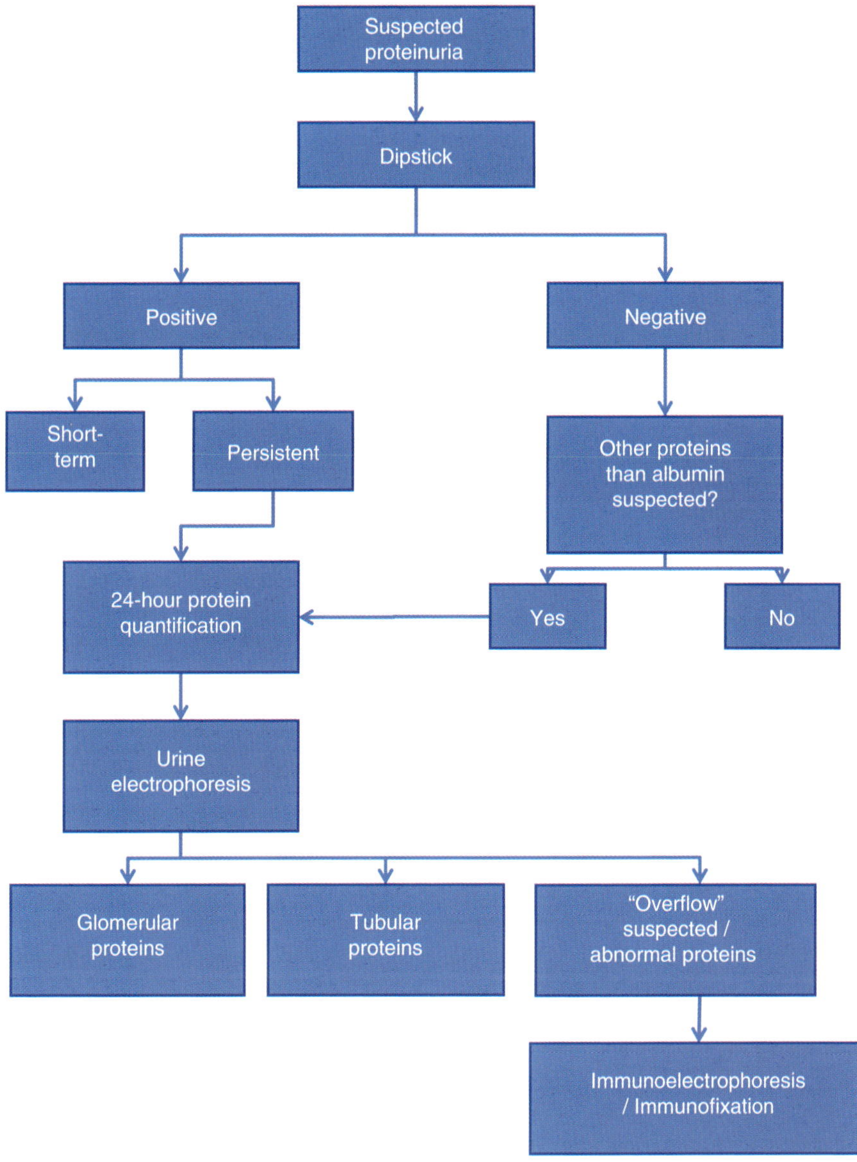

Table 4.2 Examples of different proteinuria-associated diseases

Short-term or intermittent proteinuria
Prerenal ("overflow")
Orthostatic proteinuria
Muscle trauma
Hemolysis
Pre- and/or postrenal
Urinary tract infection
Systemic infections
Physical/emotional stress
Persistent proteinuria
Prerenal ("overflow")
Paraneoplastic proteins: multiple myeloma, Waldenström's macroglobulinemia
Hemolysis
Glomerular
Glomerulonephritis (partially with tubular proteinuria)
Hypertensive nephropathy
Diabetic nephropathy (early stage, late stage: plus tubular proteinuria)
Benign nephrosclerosis
Nephropathy associated with different forms of systemic vasculitis (plus tubular proteinuria)
Renal transplant rejection (plus tubular proteinuria)
Tubular
Interstitial nephritis
Analgesic nephropathy
Fanconi's syndrome
Balkan nephropathy
Tubulotoxic drugs (e.g., aminoglycosides)
HIV nephropathy

4.4 Differential Diagnosis

Differential diagnoses of proteinuria underlying diseases are summarized in Table 4.2 [1–3].

References

1. Herold G. Internal medicine. 1st ed. Gerd Herold: Cologne; 2011.
2. Campbell MF, Wein AJ, Kavoussi LR. Campbell-Walsh urology/editor-in-chief, Alan J. Wein; editors, Kavoussi LR, Novick AC, Partin AW, Peters CA et al. 9th ed. Clinical Decision Making. Evaluation of the Urologic Patient: History, Physical Examination, and Urinanalysis Philadelphia: W.B. Saunders; 2007;1:100–103.
3. Schmidt RF, Lang F, Heckmann M. Physiologie des Menschen: mit Pathophysiologie. 31st ed. Berlin/Heidelberg/New York: Springer; 2010.

Polyuria

5

Hendrik Borgmann

5.1 Definition

Polyuria is defined as an excessive excretion of urine in a 24-h period. Definitions vary but a urine output of more than 3 l in 24 h in adults is usually considered as polyuria. A more accurate method – especially for children – is to calculate the amount of urine in relation to body weight. Polyuria is then defined as a urine output of more than 30 ml/kg body weight/24 h. It must be differentiated from the more common complaints of frequency or nocturia, which are not associated with an increase in the total urine output.

5.2 Medical History

The history of the present illness should cover questions on the amounts of fluid consumed and voided to distinguish between polyuria and urinary frequency. The patient should be asked about the duration of the problem, the rate of onset (abrupt vs gradual), and variations of onset during the day and during the week. Explicit questions should cover recent clinical features potentially causing polyuria like metabolic and endocrinologic disorders, IV fluids, tube feeding, resolution of urinary obstruction, recent surgery, stroke, or head trauma. A review of systems should search for symptoms suggesting causes like dry eye or dry mouth (Sjogren's syndrome) and B symptoms (cancer). Past medical history should focus on conditions associated with polyuria like diabetes mellitus, sarcoidosis, amyloidosis, and hyperparathyroidism. Drug history should look for drugs increasing urine output like

H. Borgmann
Department of Urology, University Hospital Frankfurt,
Theodor-Stern-Kai 7, Frankfurt 60590, Germany
e-mail: hendrik.borgmann@kgu.de

A.S. Merseburger et al. (eds.), *Urology at a Glance*,
DOI 10.1007/978-3-642-54859-8_5, © Springer-Verlag Berlin Heidelberg 2014

diuretics, caffeinated beverages, and alcohol as well as drugs associated with nephrogenic diabetes insipidus like cidofovir, foscarnet, and lithium. Red flags signalizing severe diseases are abrupt onset of polyuria or onset during the first years of life, B symptoms in combination with a smoking history and psychiatric disorders.

5.3 Diagnostics

The diagnostic workup should start with a physical examination noticing signs of obesity as a risk factor for type 2 diabetes mellitus or undernutrition reflecting underlying cancer or eating disorder with diuretic use. Skin examination should focus on hyper- or hypopigmentations, ulcers, or subcutaneous nodules that may suggest sarcoidosis. Urological disorders should be excluded as well by physical examination and ultrasound. The first step of laboratory investigations should rule out uncontrolled diabetes mellitus by serum or fingerstick glucose determination. Further laboratory investigations include serum and urine electrolytes and serum and urine osmolality. A urine osmolality of >300 mOsm/kg is usually associated with solute diuresis and a urine osmolality of <300 mOsm/kg with water diuresis. Further investigations include (enhanced) water deprivation tests and measurement of plasma ADH to distinguish between different conditions causing water diuresis. The flow chart (Fig. 5.1) demonstrates the pathway from symptoms to diagnosis.

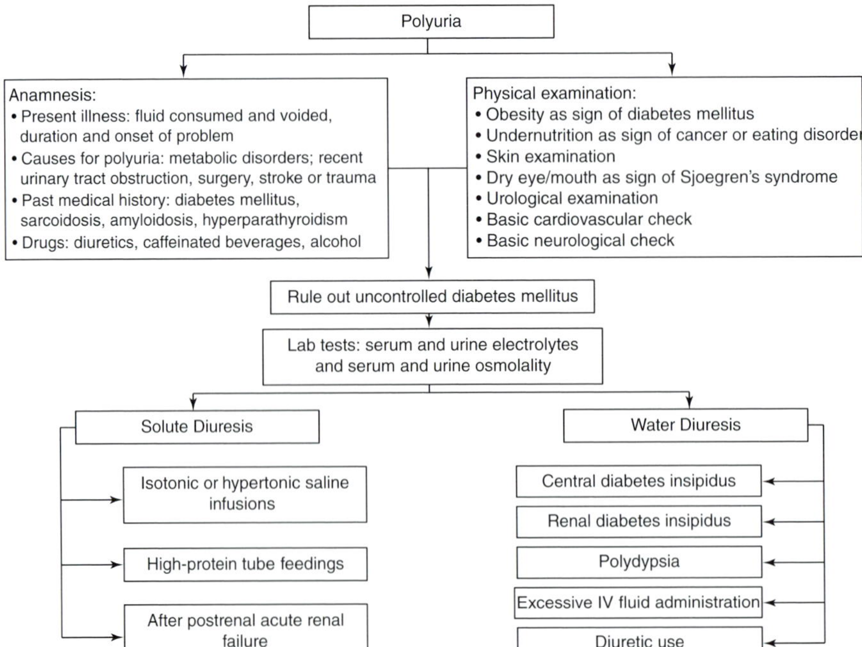

Fig. 5.1 Flow chart demonstrating the pathway from the symptom polyuria to the final diagnosis

5.4 Differential Diagnosis

Reasons for polyuria

Differential diagnosis	Incidence	Diagnostics
Diabetes mellitus	++++	Glucose, oral tolerance test
Isotonic or hypertonic saline infusions	+++	Stopping or slowing rate of administration
High-protein tube feedings	++	Switching to feedings with lower protein content
After acute renal failure	+	Clinical evaluation
Central diabetes insipidus	+	Laboratory and water deprivation test, imaging
Renal diabetes insipidus	+	Laboratory and water deprivation test
Polydipsia	++	Laboratory and water deprivation test
Excessive IV fluid administration	+++	Stopping or slowing rate of administration
Diuretic use	+++	Clinical evaluation

6 Nocturia

Lilia Heit

6.1 Definition

According to the definition of the International Continence Society (ICS), nocturia is a complaint that the individual wakes at night one or more times to void where each micturition is preceded and followed by sleep. The prevalence of nocturia increases with age and occurs almost equally in both men and women. The most common causes for nocturia are benign prostatic hyperplasia (BPH), congestive heart failure, urinary tract infection, and diabetes mellitus. Other causes can be sleep apnea, restless legs syndrome, use of diuretics, polydipsia, or excessive consumption of beverages containing caffeine or alcohol. Nocturnal urinary incontinence or nighttime bed-wetting (enuresis) is distinct from nocturia.

6.2 Medical History

Nocturia is associated with a variety of clinical disorders. Therefore, the diagnosis is challenging. In order to diagnose nocturia properly, the medical history should include both general questions on preexisting illnesses, operations, and medication and specific questions regarding lifestyle factors (e.g., consumption of alcohol, dietary and drinking behavior), insomnia, and if there are any discernible factors to which the patient could trace it back (for instance, change in medication or newly occurred polydipsia). An important consideration is whether the patient is awakened by the need to void or voids after being awakened for another reason (e.g., sleep disorders, restless legs syndrome). The patient should be asked how often he or she arises from sleep to urinate and how much water he or she passes (e.g., a couple of drops or one or more cupfuls) – furthermore, whether he or she has had

L. Heit
Department of Urology and Urological Oncology, Hannover University Medical School, Carl-Neuberg-Str. 1, Hannover 30625, Germany
e-mail: lilia.heit@stud.mh-hannover.de

A.S. Merseburger et al. (eds.), *Urology at a Glance*,
DOI 10.1007/978-3-642-54859-8_6, © Springer-Verlag Berlin Heidelberg 2014

any pain or burning while urinating, difficulty urinating, or experienced any tenderness or upper abdominal pain (possible indication for urinary tract infections). Nocturia is often quoted as the most bothersome of lower urinary tract symptoms. Sleep disturbance caused by nocturnal voiding may result in daytime fatigue, mood changes, increased risk of falling, and decreased cognitive performance, which might negatively affect the quality of life and even cause depression.

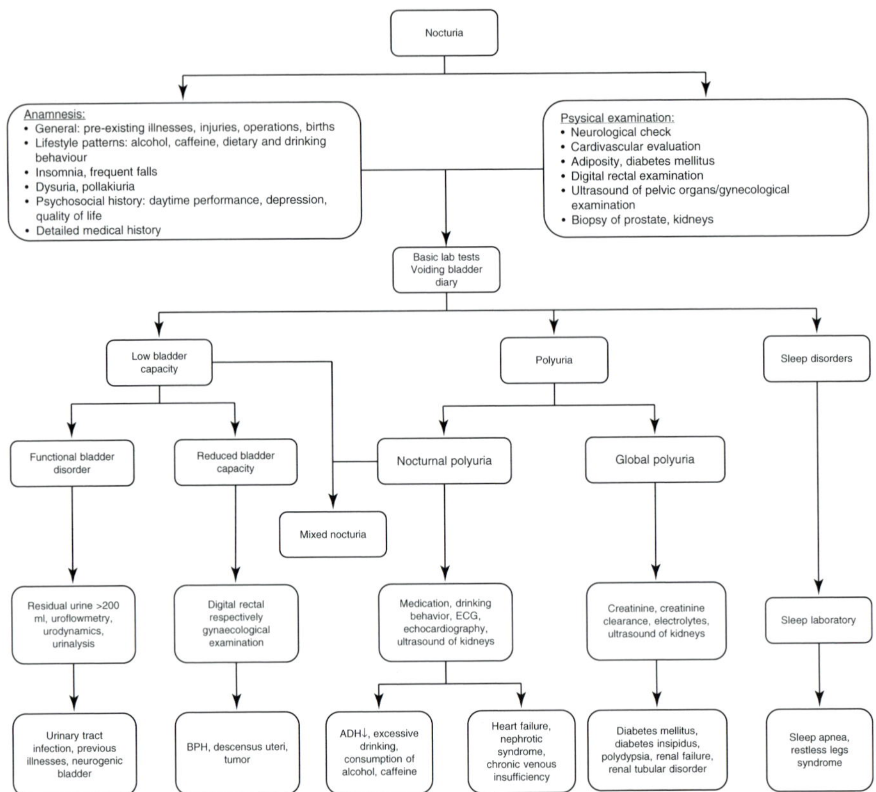

6.3 Diagnostics

The initial workup should consist of a complete physical examination including neurological status and digital rectal examination. To exclude a malignant process, an examination of the pelvis should be done thoroughly, in the case of female patients by a gynecologist. During the physical examination, attention should be paid to overweight, as this can increase the risk for sleep apnea. In cases of suspected sleep apnea, a visit of the sleep laboratory is necessary. Whether the patient is suffering from congestive heart failure can be determined by electrocardiography, echocardiography, and X-ray. Physical examination should be supplemented by blood analysis including glucose tolerance, HbA_{1c}, antidiuretic hormone, serum electrolytes, creatinine, urea, uric acid, BUN, cystatin C, PSA, and urinalysis which should include protein, glucose, white blood cells, red cells, bacteria, casts, and urine culture.

The causes of nocturia can be divided into three categories: low bladder capacity, nocturnal polyuria, and global polyuria. Bladder storage problems and nocturnal polyuria are, however, not mutually exclusive. If they occur simultaneously in one patient, they may even contribute to worsen the symptoms of nocturia. This is known as mixed nocturia. Patients who do not have any kind of polyuria will likely have either a sleep disorder or a reduced nocturnal bladder capacity (NBC). Decreased NBC can be caused by obstructions (e.g., BPH, descensus of the uterus, any kind of tumor or cancer) or it may result out of a functional bladder disorder (e.g., neurogenic bladder, anxiety disorders, learned voiding disorders) which can be excluded by residual urine measurement (≤200 ml), uroflowmetry, and urodynamics. Nocturnal polyuria or nocturnal overproduction of urine is defined by a normal 24-h urine volume, whereas the proportion of nocturnal urine production amounts to more than 35 %. (Formula for nocturnal polyuria index (NPi) is simply nocturnal urine volume (NUV) divided by 24-h urine volume: NPi = NUV/24 h UV). The primary cause is the lack of nocturnal increase in arginine vasopressin level. Secondary causes include diabetes mellitus, congestive heart failure, chronic venous insufficiency, nephrotic syndrome, or lifestyle factors such as excessive drinking before going to sleep. A voiding bladder diary helps differentiate between reduced bladder capacity and nocturnal polyuria. Global polyuria is a continuous increased production of urine which is defined as more than 40 ml/kg and a frequent urination in both day and nighttime. Diabetes mellitus, diabetes insipidus, or primary polydipsia can also result in global polyuria.

6.4 Differential Diagnosis

Reasons for nocturia

Differential diagnosis	Incidence	Diagnostic
Benign prostatic hyperplasia	+++	Ultrasound
Congestive heart failure	+++	Electrocardiography, echocardiography, chest X-ray
Urinary tract infection	+++	Urinalysis, urine culture
Prostate cancer (late stages)	+++	Digital rectal examination, ultrasound, magnetic resonance imaging, biopsy, tumor markers
Diabetes mellitus	+++	Blood glucose, HbA_{1c}
Diabetes insipidus	++	Antidiuretic hormone
Sleep apnea	++	Sleep laboratory
Renal failure	++	Blood analysis (renal retention), ultrasound

Edema

7

Stefan Vallo and Georg Bartsch

7.1 Definition

An edema is an abnormally large fluid volume between interstitial spaces.

7.2 Medical History

It is important to distinguish between a generalized and a local edema. If it is generalized, this is a hint to a dysfunction concerning the whole body. Possible reasons might be heart insufficiency or renal failure. It is important to know if there are other medical conditions like cardiac problems or renal insufficiency. Symptoms like, e.g., shortage of breath or headache have to be asked. Information about regular medication, consumption of drugs, drinking habits, and nutrition is necessary. If the edema is local, the questions should focus on this specific region.

S. Vallo (✉) • G. Bartsch
Department of Urology, University Hospital Frankfurt,
Theodor-Stern-Kai 7, Frankfurt 60590, Germany
e-mail: stefan.vallo@kgu.de; georg.bartsch@kgu.de

A.S. Merseburger et al. (eds.), *Urology at a Glance*,
DOI 10.1007/978-3-642-54859-8_7, © Springer-Verlag Berlin Heidelberg 2014

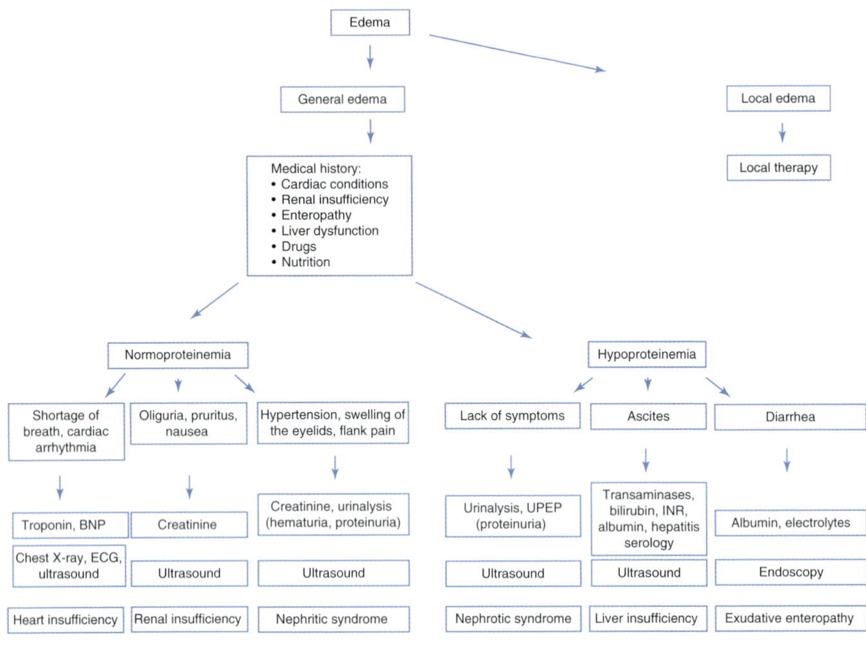

7.3 Diagnostics

During the physical examination, it is important to determine the localization of the edema. One must differentiate if it is generalized and if it is symmetrical. Also, the texture of the swelling indicates the genesis of the edema. This can be verified by pressing the skin. The swelling of an acute edema is mostly soft and easily causes dents, while in chronic edema the texture is firmer [1].

In normoproteinemic patients, heart insufficiency is a common reason for edemas [2]. In this case, the swelling is found mostly in the lower parts of the body, following gravity. In severe cases, genital edemas are also common. ECG, chest X-ray, and echocardiography offer additional information about the cardiac status of the patient.

In addition, drugs can be a reason for normoproteinemic edemas.

In hypoproteinemic edema [3], gravity plays a minor role for the localization of the swelling. Frequently, the face and eyelids are affected. Oliguria might be a symptom of renal insufficiency, which can be uncovered by renal function parameters, urinalysis, and urine protein electrophoresis (UPEP).

If the patient is complaining about diarrhea and abdominal pain, exudative gastropathies like ulcerative colitis might be the reason of an edema.

Another reason can be malnutrition [4]. In western countries this occurs, for example, in alcoholics with a low-protein diet. In addition, a reduced synthesis of proteins in the liver caused by liver insufficiency leads to a hypoproteinemia.

Therefore, one should check transaminases and bilirubin in the serum. In severe cases, the patient has an icteric skin color.

Hypothyroidism might cause myxedemas [5]. There is a pathological deposition of mucopolysaccharides mainly located in the pretibial dermis. Thyroid hormones should be checked if this differential diagnosis is likely.

Differential diagnosis	Incidence	Diagnostics
Heart insufficiency	++++	ECG, chest X-ray, echocardiography, BNP, troponin, cardiac catheter examination
Renal insufficiency	+++	Ultrasound, creatinine, GFR, urinalysis, UPEP, renal biopsy
Liver insufficiency	+++	GOT, GPT, bilirubin, ultrasound, history of alcohol abuse, hepatitis
Thyroid disorders	++	TSH, T3, T4, ultrasound, scintigraphy
Exsudative gastropathies	+	Endoscopy
Drug-induced edema	+	Medical history, drug usage screening
Malnutrition/cachexia	+++	Medical history

References

1. Brunkhorst S. Differentialdiagnostik und Differentialtherapie. Amsterdam: Urban & Fischer Verlag/Elsevier GmbH; 2010.
2. Clark AL, Cleland JG. Causes and treatment of oedema in patients with heart failure. Nat Rev Cardiol. 2013;10(3):156–70.
3. Siddall EC, Radhakrishnan J. The pathophysiology of edema formation in the nephrotic syndrome. Kidney Int. 2012;82(6):635–42.
4. Ahmed T, Rahman S, Cravioto A. Oedematous malnutrition. Indian J Med Res. 2009; 130(5):651–4. Review.
5. Cho S, Atwood JE. Peripheral edema. Am J Med. 2002;113(7):580–6. Review.

Back Pain

8

Kathrin Simonis and Michael Rink

8.1 Definition

Back pain is defined as pain felt in the back that may have various reasons and clinical presentations. The reasons for back pain can be diverse (see also Sect. 8.4): musculoskeletal diseases (e.g., disc herniation, scoliosis), trauma, spinal infections (e.g., discitis, osteomyelitis) or non-spinal infections (e.g., paraspinous muscle abscess, pyelonephritis, pneumonia, pelvic inflammatory disease), tumors or metastasis, urological disorders (e.g., urolithiasis or ureteropelvic junction obstruction), or chronic pain syndromes [1]. Lifting or twisting can release muscle-related pain, while bone-related pain is often aggravated by extension.

The pain may be localized in the neck, the upper or lower back, or across these regions. The pain may radiate into the upper or lower limbs as well as into the ventroinguinal region. Pain character can be acute or chronic, dull or sharp, colicky, intermittent, or permanent.

Back pain may be accompanied by other symptoms such as fever, nausea, vomiting, dysuria, or neurological impairment.

8.2 Medical History

The medical history in patients having back pain should include questions regarding pain onset (> differentiation between acute and chronic pain) and the pain character (e.g., radiating or not, motion-dependent or not, intensity). It is

---

Conflict of Interest
The authors have nothing to disclose

K. Simonis • M. Rink, MD, FEBU (✉)
Department of Urology, University Medical Center Hamburg-Eppendorf,
Martinistrasse 52, Hamburg D-20246, Germany
e-mail: k.simonis@uke.de; m.rink@uke.uni-hamburg.de

A.S. Merseburger et al. (eds.), *Urology at a Glance*,
DOI 10.1007/978-3-642-54859-8_8, © Springer-Verlag Berlin Heidelberg 2014

important to get detailed information about accompanying symptoms such as fatigue, fever and weakness, neurological impairment, weight loss, or dysuria. Besides, current ongoing disorders and preexisting diseases, previous treatments or surgery, current medication, and physical and social activity should be inquired.

In urology, back pain is a common symptom. Pain originating from the kidneys or ureters can be localized in the flanks or lower back. It may radiate into the ipsilateral groin, testis, or labium. Patients with a renal colic usually describe a heavy, colicky pain, often accompanied by parasympathetic symptoms including sweating, nausea, and/or vomiting. Patients with acute renal colic often bent over to the side of pain and hold their flank. In upper urinary tract infections, pain is usually described as more constant and dull combined with fever. Chronic urinary retention, bladder tumors, and upper urinary tract tumors may lead to upper urinary tract dilatation and also may be accompanied by dull flank pain.

8.3 Diagnostics

The flow chart presents an overview of anamnestic and diagnostic steps (Fig. 8.1). A physical examination with inspection and palpation of the back, the flanks, and the genital area is mandatory. The patient should be examined for tenderness on palpation and pain released by percussion, respectively.

If neurological impairment is suspected, a neurological examination should be performed including examination of sensitivity, power, reflexes, and nerve extension pain. For example, spinal disc herniation may compromise the cauda equina resulting in bladder dysfunction, impaired sphincter tonus, and saddle anesthesia. Therefore, voiding and anal sphincter tension should be checked in patients at risk for cauda equina syndrome.

It is of critical importance to recognize serious causes of back pain that need urgent or immediate further diagnostics or treatment (e.g., computed tomography (CT), magnetic resonance imaging (MRI), surgery).

In assumption of an infection, vital signs and body temperature should be taken as well as blood and urine analysis. Blood analysis should be checked for systemic signs of an infection or signs of sepsis; blood cultures should be taken. Urine analysis should comprise dipstick test and urine culture.

In patients presenting with flank pain accompanied by dysuria, fever, or hematuria, ultrasound of the abdomen (kidneys, urinary bladder, retroperitoneum, and testis) should be performed. In addition, the liver, gallbladder, and pancreas should be examined to rule out concomitant disorders.

Patients with a renal colic due to urinary tract stones might have a consecutive dilation of the renal pelvis in ultrasound. Elevated creatinine level and microscopic hematuria help confirm the diagnosis. Nowadays, a native CT scan is the diagnostic tool of choice in renal and ureter stones (Fig. 8.2a, b).

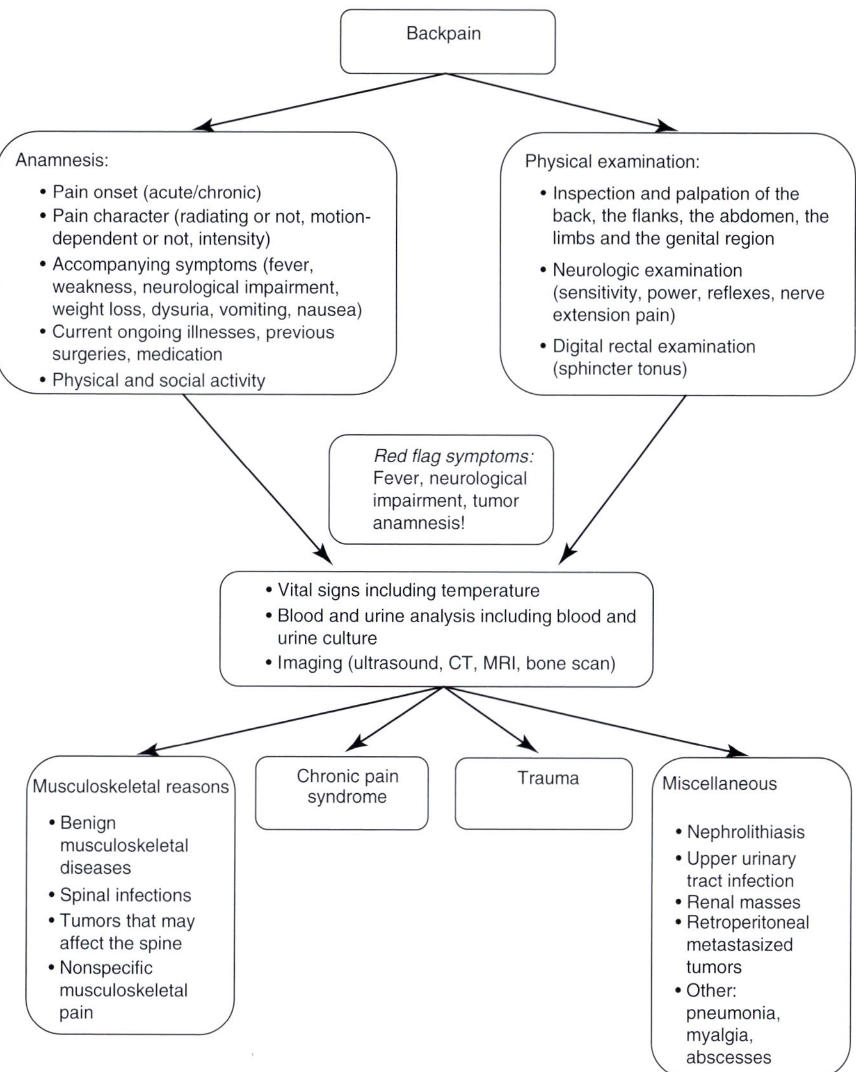

Fig. 8.1 Flow chart demonstrating the pathway from symptoms to diagnosis in patients presenting with back pain

Other urological reasons for flank and lower back pain might be renal masses (renal cell carcinoma, upper tract urothelial carcinoma), retroperitoneal lymph node metastasis in almost any urological carcinoma (i.e., prostate, bladder, renal cell, upper urinary tract, or testicular cancer), or an abscess-forming pyelonephritis (Fig. 8.3a, b). In case of malignancies, additional diagnostic tests should be performed to complete the staging.

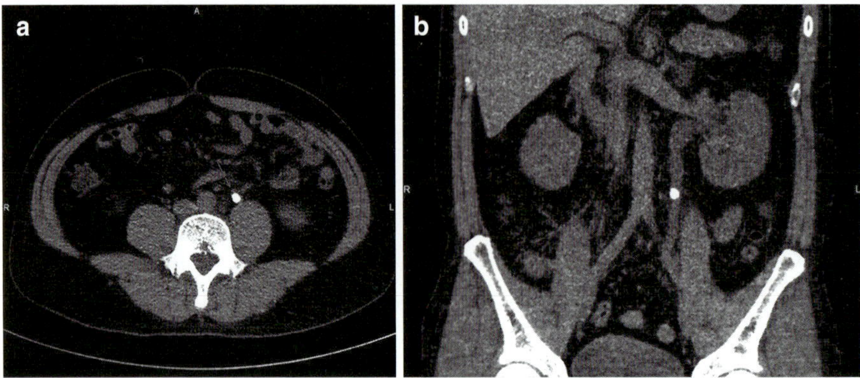

Fig. 8.2 Native CT scan of a 43-year-old male patient showing an impacted 7 mm stone in the ureter on the left-hand side. (**a**) Transverse plane; (**b**) Coronal plane

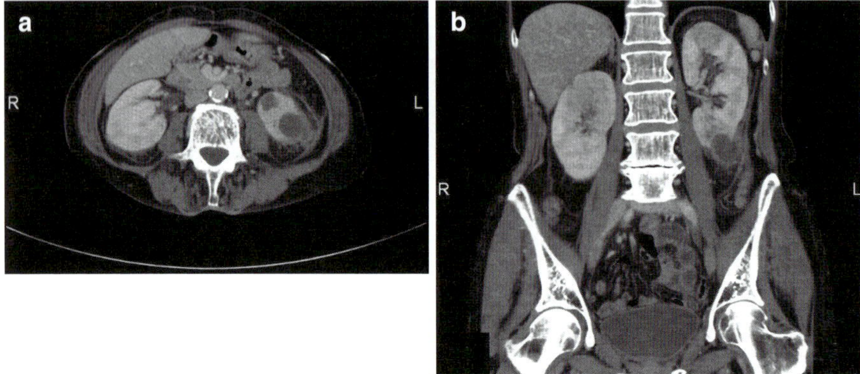

Fig. 8.3 Contrast enhanced CT scan of a 56-year-old female patient showing an abscess-forming pyelonephritis on the left-hand side. (**a**) Transverse plane; (**b**) Coronal plane

8.4 Differential Diagnosis

There are several differential diagnoses that may be the reasons for back pain. An interdisciplinary assessment is recommended when diagnosis remains inconclusive at first sight. Physicians from general, trauma, and/or spine surgery, internal medicine (including rheumatology), urology, gynecology, and/or neurology may be involved in the initial workup procedure.

Table 8.1 presents an overview of differential diagnosis and related diagnostic procedures to confirm diagnosis.

Table 8.1 Differential diagnosis and diagnostic procedures for back pain workup

Differential diagnosis	Diagnostics
Benign musculoskeletal diseases	
Spondylolysis	Physical examination
Scoliosis	Imaging (X-ray, MRI)
Spinal disc herniation	
Degenerative spinal disc changes	
Spinal infections	
Discitis	Physical examination
Vertebral osteomyelitis	Laboratory features (CRP, leukocytes)
Epidural abscess	Imaging (CT, MRI)
Tumors that may affect the spine	
Leukemia	Laboratory features (complete blood count)
Lymphoma	Imaging (CT, MRI, bone scan)
Sarcoma	
Neurofibroma	
Trauma	Anamnesis
	Physical examination
	Imaging (depending on anamnesis)
Nonspecific musculoskeletal pain	Anamnesis
	Physical examination
Nephrolithiasis	Anamnesis
	Laboratory features (creatinine, microscopic hematuria)
	Ultrasound, CT
Pyelonephritis	Anamnesis
	Physical examination
	Laboratory features (CRP, leukocytes, leukocyturia)
	Urine culture
	Imaging (Ultrasound, CT)
Renal masses	Anamnesis
	Ultrasound, CT
Retroperitoneal metastasized tumors	Anamnesis
	Physical examination
	Ultrasound, CT
Chronic pain syndrome	Anamnesis
Others	
Pneumonia	Anamnesis
Myalgia	Physical examination
Paraspinous muscle abscess	Laboratory features (CRP, leukocytes)
	Imaging (dependent on suspected diagnosis)

Reference

1. Nigrovic P. Back pain in children and adolescents: overview of causes [Internet]. UpToDate; 2013. Available from: www.uptodate.com/store.

9 Shock

Thenappan Chandrasekar and Derya Tilki

9.1 Definition

Shock is a clinical diagnosis of multi-organ hypoperfusion. As defined by the Oxford English Dictionary, shock is "an acute medical condition associated with a fall in blood pressure, caused by such events as loss of blood, severe burns, bacterial infection, allergic reaction, or sudden emotional stress, and marked by cold, pallid skin, irregular breathing, rapid pulse, and dilated pupils" [12]. According to the American College of Surgeons, shock is defined more succinctly as "tissue hypoperfusion due to an imbalance between oxygen supply and demand in the tissues of the body" [5]. Ultimately, however, it should be noted that shock is a clinical diagnosis.

Shock is a life-threatening medical emergency that requires early recognition, diagnostics, and intervention. Despite the emphasis placed on this, however, mortality rates still exceed 20–50 % [7].

Shock has been further subdivided into five basic categories, first described by Blalock: cardiogenic, neurogenic, hypovolemic, anaphylactic, and septic shock [10, 3]. Additional subdivisions have been described in the recent literature. While all of these types of shock are medical emergencies, within the realm of urology however, hypovolemic and septic shock predominate. In particular, septic shock from urosepsis is an important etiology of shock in the urologic patient.

Hypovolemic or hemorrhagic shock is characterized by a rapid reduction in blood volume. It is further divided by degree into Class I–IV, based on percentage of blood volume lost: Class I (0–15 %), Class II (15–30 %), Class III (30–40 %), and Class IV (>40 %).

T. Chandrasekar, MD • D. Tilki, MD (✉)
Department of Urology, University of California, Davis, Medical Center,
4860 Y Street, Suite 3500, Sacramento, CA 95817, USA
e-mail: thenappan.chandrasekar@ucdmc.ucdavis.edu;
derya.tilki@ucdmc.ucdavis.edu, dtilki@me.com

A.S. Merseburger et al. (eds.), *Urology at a Glance*,
DOI 10.1007/978-3-642-54859-8_9, © Springer-Verlag Berlin Heidelberg 2014

Table 9.1 Definitions of the sepsis spectrum

Bacteremia	Presence of viable bacteria in the blood
SIRS (systemic inflammatory response syndrome)	Presence of more than one of the following clinical findings
	1. Body temperature >38 or <36 °C
	2. Heart rate >90 beats/min
	3. Hyperventilation (resp. rate >20/min OR $PaCO_2$ <32 mmHg)
	4. WBC >12,000 cells/μL or <4,000 cells/μL
Sepsis	SIRS criteria plus evidence of infection
Severe sepsis	Sepsis and presence of organ dysfunction
Septic shock	Sepsis and evidence of acute circulatory failure/evidence of shock

Levy et al. [8]
Dellinger et al. [4]

On the SIRS (systemic inflammatory response syndrome) spectrum, sepsis and septic shock represent the most severe manifestations. The full spectrum with definitions can be found in Table 9.1. Sepsis and septic shock in the urology patient are the most common presentations of shock, typically due to infection from the genitourinary (GU) tract. Mortality rates due to septic shock range from 30 to 60 % [1, 2, 9], and a urinary source accounts for 9–31 % of all septic shock [9].

9.2 Medical History

A high index of suspicion is necessary for early diagnosis and management of patients in shock. As such, a thorough history and physical exam are critical in early workup. However, the resuscitative efforts should NOT be delayed for medical history taking, physical exam, or diagnostics.

The history is an important portion of any evaluation of a critically ill patient. However, in a patient in shock, a full history may not be directly available. It may be necessary to question support staff, family members, and other individuals to obtain the necessary history. History should be focused on identifying key points that will help narrow the etiology of shock.

The physical exam is a critical portion of the evaluation as shock is often a clinical diagnosis. The exam should also be focused, with an emphasis on vital signs, neurologic status, cardiorespiratory function, and end-organ perfusion. From a urologic perspective, a Foley catheter or urine output monitoring is an important component of evaluation and should be placed early in the evaluation of the patient.

Some of the key physical exam findings include [11] hypotension (brachial artery systolic blood pressure <90 mmHg), tachycardia (HR >90 beats/min) or bradycardia (HR <60 beats/min) as a sign of decompensation, tachypnea (respiratory rate >20 breaths/min), altered mental status, oliguria, and hypoxemia. Certain findings may be more specific to certain categories of shock, including temperature extremes in septic or inflammatory shock and cutaneous hypoperfusion in all other forms of shock.

9.3 Diagnostics

Diagnostic testing for patients in shock occurs simultaneously to the clinical assessment of the patient, as time is of the essence.

Laboratory tests to obtain include but are not limited to the following: (1) basic metabolic panel to assess renal function, evidence of electrolyte disturbances, bicarbonate deficit, and blood sugar disturbances; (2) complete blood count with differential to assess for leukocytosis or leukopenia, evidence of bleeding, or thrombocytopenia or thrombocytosis; (3) coagulation factors to assess for bleeding diathesis; (4) arterial blood gas to assess for acid/base status, need for ventilation or oxygenation, and correctable metabolic disturbances; (5) lactic acid to assess for hypoperfusion and ischemia; and (6) urinalysis. Other lab tests that may be indicated based on clinical picture include blood cultures, urine or sputum culture, type and cross, amylase/lipase, D-dimer and fibrin assays, toxicology screen, and cardiac enzymes.

Initial radiographic and functional assessment of the patient includes a standard upright chest x-ray and 12-lead electrocardiogram. Additional testing can be ordered based on the suspected etiology of the shock and the patient's clinical and social history. These studies include abdominal plain films, CT abdomen/pelvis, CT chest, CT head, or echocardiogram.

Invasive monitoring may also need to be placed in a patient in acute shock. Typical monitoring includes (1) arterial line for more accurate blood pressure monitoring and (2) central venous catheter for central pressure assessment, fluid status assessment, additional venous access for interventions, and possible pulmonary artery catheterization. As mentioned before, Foley catheter placement or equivalent method of draining the bladder is strongly recommended.

9.4 Differential Diagnosis

The differential diagnosis of shock is very broad. Classification of shock into different categories based on initial presentation, as described earlier, helps direct initial interventions and management. However, in conjunction with early management, efforts should be made to identify and treat the underlying pathology. Refer to Fig. 9.1 for a review of the etiologies and initial workup of a patient in shock.

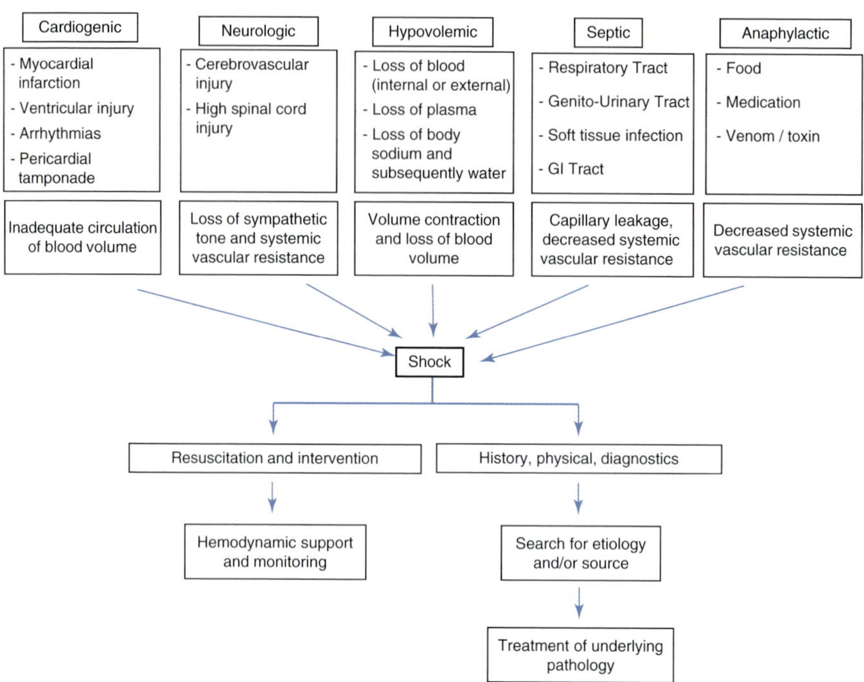

Fig. 9.1 Flowchart: differential diagnosis and initial management of a patient in shock

References

1. Angus DC, Linde-Zwirble WT, Lidicker J, Clermont G, Carcillo J, Pinsky MR. Epidemiology of severe sepsis in the United States: analysis of incidence, outcome, and associated costs of care. Crit Care Med. 2001;29(7):1303–10.
2. Annane D, Aegerter P, Jars-Guincestre MC, Guidet B. Current epidemiology of septic shock: the CUB-Rea network. Am J Respir Crit Care Med. 2003;168(2):165–72.
3. Blalock A. Acute circulatory failure as exemplified by shock and haemorrhage. Surg Gynecol Obstet. 1934;58:551.
4. Dellinger RP, Levy MM, Rhodes A, Annane D, Gerlach H, Opal MO, et al. Surviving sepsis campaign: international guidelines for the management of severe sepsis and septic shock: 2012. Crit Care Med. 2013;41:580.
5. Holcroft JT, Anderson JT, Sena MJ. Section 8, Chapter 3: Shock. ACS surgery: principles and practice. New York: Web MD Publishing; 2007.
6. Holmes CL, Walley KR. The evaluation and management of shock. Clin Chest Med. 2003;24:775–89.
7. Jones AE, Kline JA. Chapter 4: Shock. In: Marx JA, Hockberger RS, Walls RM, Adams JG, Barsan WG, Biros MH, Danzl DF, Gausche-Hill M, Ling LJ, Newton EJ, editors. Rosen's emergency medicine. 7th ed. Philadelphia: WB Saunders; 2010.
8. Levy MM, Fink MP, Marshall JC, Abraham E, Angus DC, Cook D, Cohen J, Opal SM, Vincent JL, Ramsay G. 2001 SCCM/ESICM/ACCP/ATS/SIS international sepsis definitions conference. Crit Care Med. 2001;31(4):1250–6.

9. Levy MM, Artigas A, Phillips GS, Rhodes A, Beale R, Osborn T, Vincent JL, Townsend S, Lemeshow S, Dillinger RP. Outcomes of the surviving sepsis campaign in intensive care units in the USA and Europe: a prospective cohort study. Lancet Infect Dis. 2012;12:919–24.
10. Millham FH. A brief history of shock. Surgery. 2010;148:1026–37.
11. Moore LJ, Moore FA. Section 8, Chapter 4: Early management of sepsis, severe sepsis and septic shock in the surgical patient. ACS surgery: principles and practice. New York: Web MD Publishing; 2007.
12. Oxford English Dictionary [Internet]. Oxford University Press. Shock. Available from: http://oxforddictionaries.com/us/definition/american_english/shock. Cited 8 Aug 2013.
13. Schaeffer AJ, Schaeffer EM. Chapter 10: Infections of the urinary tract. In: Wein AJ, Kavoussi LR, Partin AW, Peters CA, editors. Campbell–Walsh urology. 10th ed. Philadelphia: WB Saunders; 2011.
14. Wagenlehner FMA, Lichtenstern C, Rolfes C, Mayer K, Ulfe F, Weidman W, Weigand MA. Diagnosis and management for urosepsis. Int J Urol. 2013;20:963–70. Epub May 2013.
15. Wagenlehner FMA, Weidman W, Naber KG. Optimal management of urosepsis from the urologic perspective. Int J Microb Agents. 2007;30:390–7.

Urosepsis

10

Axel Heidenreich and Andrea Thissen

10.1 Definition

Urosepsis is defined as sepsis caused by urinary tract infection (UTI) and accounts for 25 % of all sepsis cases [1]. Patients with anatomical and/or functional abnormalities of the urinary tract and patients with comorbidities such as poor-regulated diabetes mellitus or immunosuppressive therapy are predisposed to sepsis syndrome [2]. Severe sepsis is a potentially life-threatening condition related to a mortality rate ranging between 30 and 50 % [3]. Hence, early goal-directed therapy and empirical antibiotic treatment are crucial aspects of patient care in urosepsis.

10.2 Medical History

Patients should be questioned regarding symptoms of urinary tract infection, such as dysuria, flank pain, or fever and chills (see Fig. 10.1). Pain and its duration, localization, and quality must be carefully gathered and patient's medication reviewed. Furthermore, information about age and underlying illnesses such as diabetes mellitus, cancer, or other forms of compromising disorders contributes to acquiring a realistic assessment of the patient's condition.

10.3 Diagnostics

Physical examination with assessment of vital signs (body temperature, heart and respiratory rate, blood pressure, urine output, vigilance) and results of laboratory data (white blood cell count, c-reactive protein, procalcitonin, AT III, liver enzymes, blood gas analysis) are essential parameters for the evaluation of the disease

A. Heidenreich • A. Thissen (✉)
Department of Urology, RWTH University Aachen, Pauwelsstr. 30, Aachen 52074, Germany
e-mail: aheidenreich@ukaachen.de; anthissen@ukaachen.de

A.S. Merseburger et al. (eds.), *Urology at a Glance*,
DOI 10.1007/978-3-642-54859-8_10, © Springer-Verlag Berlin Heidelberg 2014

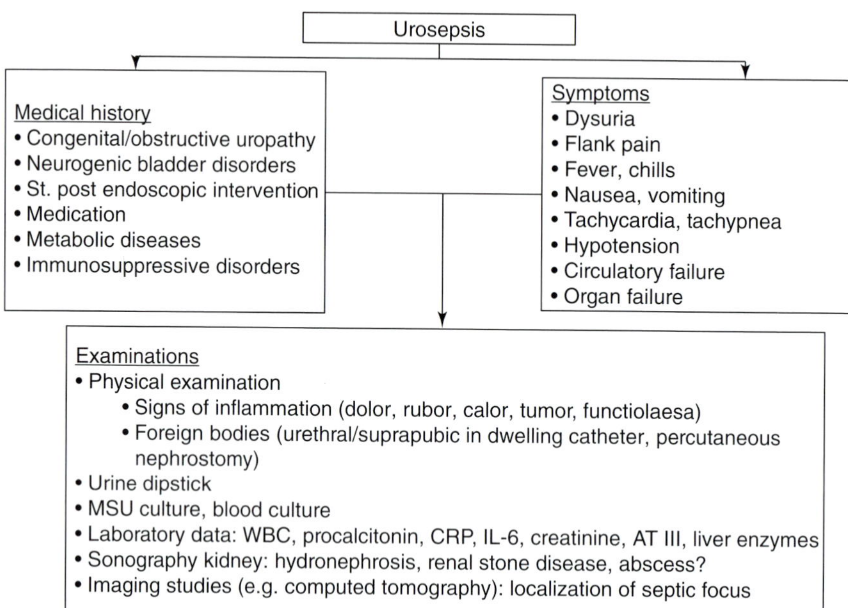

Fig. 10.1 Flow chart demonstrating the pathway from symptoms to diagnosis

severity in sepsis. Procalcitonin has emerged as an early reliable marker suggestive of severe bacterial infection and may help decide if an immediate urological intervention is required or not [4]. Blood and urine cultures as well as local swabs (e.g., of abscesses) ought to be taken before beginning with antibiotic treatment. Evaluation of the upper urinary tract should be performed by sonography to rule out obstructive uropathy. Additional imaging studies such as computed tomography may be helpful to confirm a potential source of infection and localize the septic focus, such as perinephric or intrarenal abscess formation.

10.4 Differential Diagnosis

Nosocomial infection	Indwelling foreign body infections, HAP (hospital-acquired pneumonia), wound infection
Respiratory system	Pneumonia, pyothorax, lung abscess
Cardiac system	Endocarditis
Gastrointestinal tract	Cholecystitis, pancreatitis, perforated sigma diverticulitis, peritonitis
Central nervous system	Meningococcal disease

10.5 General Facts

Predominant pathogens identified on urine culture in uroseptic patients are enterobacteria, with *Escherichia coli* being the most common microorganism. *Pseudomonas aeruginosa* and *Serratia* sp. are likely to be multiresistant and difficult to treat [2]. Risk factors for bacteremia are complicated UTIs, such as pyelonephritis or obstructive uropathy. Elderly and immunocompromised patients (diabetes mellitus, cancer diseases, or immunosuppressive therapy) are at higher risk to experience severe complications of genitourinary infections, for instance, perinephric (emphysematous) or renal abscesses or xanthogranulomatous pyelonephritis [5–7]. Depending on the severity of the condition, sepsis can be classified into four groups: SIRS (systemic inflammatory response syndrome), sepsis, severe sepsis, and septic shock, first defined in 1991 by the American College of Chest Physicians (ACCP) and Society of Critical Care Medicine (SCCM) [8]. SIRS is a clinical syndrome resulting from a noninfectious insult and can be diagnosed when two or more of the criteria below are present (Table 10.1).

Severe sepsis, defined by the presence of symptoms of organ dysfunction, is related to UTI in 5 % [2], causing mortality in 30–50 % [3]. Main cause of mortality is a hemodynamic collapse due to the release of pro-inflammatory cytokines, such as interleukin-1 and interleukin-6 (IL-1, IL-6), and tumor necrosis factor-alpha (TNF-α), which is activated by bacterial components. The excessive production of pro-inflammatory cytokines increases the permeability of endothelial cells leading to blood shift into the interstitial space and triggers proanticoagulant mechanisms with occurrence of multiple intravascular thrombi [3]. Endothelial damage prevents the activation of protein C, which is important for the downregulation of proanticoagulant mechanisms. As a consequence of the homeostatic imbalance toward coagulation, impaired blood flow to vital organs may lead to circulatory and organ failure. Hence, interdisciplinary management, including early transfer to intensive care unit, is essential to prevent fatal outcome.

Table 10.1 Clinical diagnostic criteria of SIRS, sepsis, and septic shock [2]

Disorder	Definition
Systemic inflammatory response syndrome (SIRS)	Temperature >38° or <36° Heart rate >90 bpm Respiratory rate >20 breaths/min or $PaCO_2$ <32 mmHg WBC >12,000 cells/mm^3 or <4,000 cells/mm^3
Sepsis	Activation of the inflammatory process due to infection
Severe sepsis	Organ dysfunction, hypoperfusion, or hypotension
Septic shock	Sepsis with hypoperfusion despite adequate fluid resuscitation

10.6 Symptoms, Classification, and Grading

Symptoms of urosepsis can range from fever and chills, flank pain, abdominal tenderness, tachypnea, and tachycardia to more severe symptoms such as hypothermia and confusion. Further complications are drop of blood pressure, circulatory failure, and oliguria/anuria. SIRS can evolve into sepsis and septic shock, with endothelial injury being one of the hallmarks. As a result of capillary leakage, venous pooling and peripheral vasodilatation may occur, leading to intravascular volume depletion, tissue hypoxia, and consecutive organ failure. Refractory septic shock presents the most severe complication in patients with urosepsis, with non-response to fluid and pharmacological interventions causing a significant increase of morbidity and mortality.

10.7 Therapy

The optimal approach to uroseptic patients involves three goals: early recognition, causal treatment with relief of urinary tract obstruction, and timely administration of antimicrobial agents [2]. Any delay in the initiation of adequate therapy is potentially lethal. Causal treatment requires urological interventions, such as performance of percutaneous or surgical drainage of renal abscesses, placement of percutaneous nephrostomy for infected hydronephrosis, or insertion of suprapubic catheter in bacterial prostatitis. Prostate abscesses need to be drained immediately either by perineal placement of a drain or by TURP depending on the patient's general condition. Empirical antibiotic treatment should be promptly initiated with reassessment of microbiological and clinical data to narrow antimicrobial coverage in the course of the therapy. Critically ill patients have to be provided with life-sustaining circulatory and respiratory support at the intensive care unit, where maintenance of balance between oxygen delivery and oxygen demand is crucial in the prevention of metabolic acidosis and consecutive organ failure. It should be constantly monitored by the assessment of central venous oxygenation saturation, lactate concentration, serum pH, and base excess.

Supportive and adjunctive therapy, including volume resuscitation with crystalloids and catecholamines, remain the mainstay in the strategy of septic shock and contribute to a significant reduction of mortality [2]. The administration of human recombinant activated protein C with its anticoagulant properties aims at improving sepsis-induced coagulopathy and outcome [9]. Interdisciplinary management, early goal-directed therapy, source control, continuous monitoring, management of fluid and electrolyte balance, and correction of coagulation abnormalities present the crucial therapeutic challenges of urosepsis (Fig. 10.2).

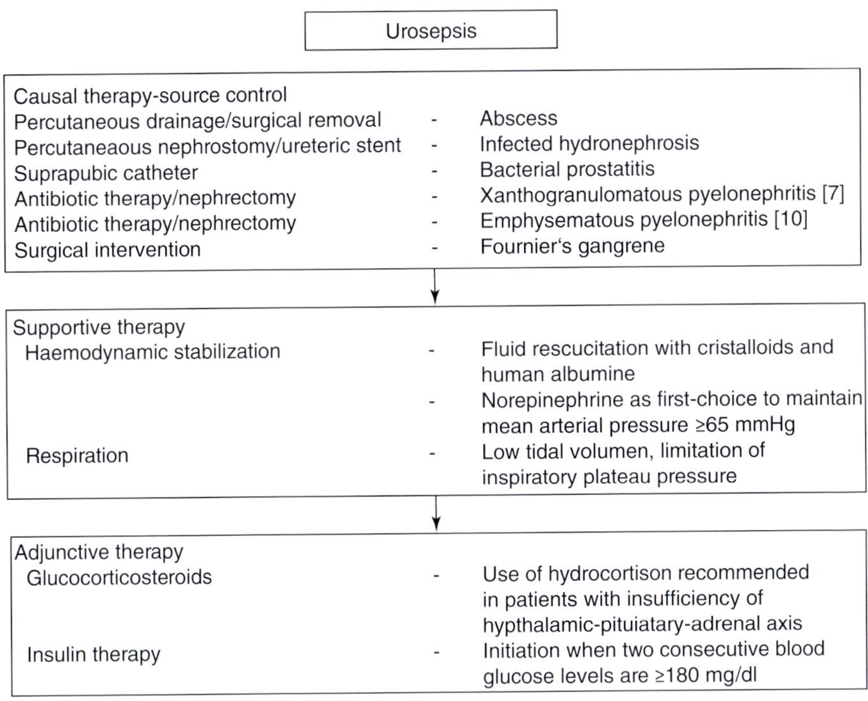

Fig. 10.2 Flow chart demonstrating the pathway from diagnosis to therapy [2, 7, 10, 11]

10.8 Complications

Fournier's gangrene, a necrotizing fasciitis of the perineal, perianal, and genital region, presents a rare but life-threatening complication of urogenital infections [2]. Since it is a rapidly progressing disorder of the fascia and subcutaneous soft tissue, mortality and morbidity rate is high [12]. Hence, urgent surgical debridement with wide excision of the necrotic tissue and the immediate administration of broad-spectrum antibiotic therapy present the only way of improving the chances for patient's survival [12].

In general, mortality rate of severe sepsis has decreased in recent years, although it is still a very serious condition. The degree of organ dysfunction and coagulopathy, microbiological etiology, and comorbidities are essential prognostic factors for an adverse outcome. As sepsis develops rapidly, with symptoms frequently imitating those of other conditions, early and accurate diagnosis and prompt therapy remain significant clinical challenges and key elements in the care of septic patients.

References

1. Wagenlehner FME, Pilatz A, Weidner W. Urosepsis–from the view of the urologist. Int J Antimicrob Agents. 2011;38(Suppl):51–7.
2. Grabe M (chair), Bartoletti R, Bjerklund-Johansen TE, Çek HM, Pickard RS, Tenke P, Wagenlehner F, Wullt B. European Association of Urology 2014. Guidelines on urological infections. Sepsis syndrome in urology (Urosepsis). 2014;(5):34–8.
3. Satran R, Almog Y. The coagulopathy of sepsis: pathophysiology and management. Isr Med Assoc J. 2003;5(7):516–20.
4. Assicot M, Gendrel D, Carsin H, Raymond J, Guilbaud J, Bohuon C. High serum procalcitonin concentrations in patients with sepsis and infection. Lancet. 1993;341(8844):515–8.
5. Wagenlehner FM, Lichtenstern C, Rolfes C, Mayer K, Uhle F, Weidner W, Weigand MA. Diagnosis and management for urosepsis. Int J Urol. 2013;20(10):963–70.
6. Nicolle LE. Urinary tract infection. Crit Care Clin. 2013;29(3):699–715.
7. Li L, Parwani AV. Xanthogranulomatous pyelonephritis. Arch Pathol Lab Med. 2011; 135(5):671–4.
8. American College of Chest Physicians/Society of Critical Care Medicine Consensus Conference. Definition for sepsis and organ failure and guidelines for the use of innovative therapies in sepsis. Crit Care Med. 1992;20(6):86.
9. Glück T, Opal SM. Advances in sepsis therapy. Drugs. 2004;64(8):837–59.
10. Archana S, Vijaya C, Geethamani V, Savitha AK. Emphysematous pyelonephritis in a diabetic leading to renal destruction: pathological aspects of a rare case. Malays J Pathol. 2013; 35(1):103–6.
11. Dellinger RP, Levy MM, Rhodes A, Annane D, Gerlach H, Opal SM, Sevransky JE, Sprung CL, Douglas IS, Jaeschke R, Osborn TM, Nunnally ME, Townsend SR, Reinhart K, Kleinpell RM, Angus DC, Deutschman CS, Machado FR, Rubenfeld GD, Webb S, Beale RJ, Vincent JL, Moreno R, Surviving Sepsis Campaign Guidelines Committee Including the Pediatric Subgroup. Surviving sepsis campaign: international guidelines for management of severe sepsis and septic shock, 2012. Intensive Care Med. 2013;39(2):165–228.
12. Yanar H, Taviloglu K, Ertekin C, Guloglu R, Zorba U, Cabioglu N, Baspinar I. Fournier's gangrene: risk factors and strategies for management. World J Surg. 2006;30(9):1750–4.

Erectile Dysfunction

11

Axel S. Merseburger

11.1 Definition

Erectile dysfunction (ED) is defined as a sexual dysfunction characterized by the inability to develop or maintain an erection of the penis during sexual performance. Psychic or organic reasons can be the reason and also a combination of both. Older men tend to have an organic reason, whereas younger men are more often affected by psychogenic reasons. The most common organic causes are cardiovascular disease and diabetes, neurological problems (e.g., nerve damage from pelvic surgery), drug side effects, and hormonal insufficiencies (hypogonadism).

A.S. Merseburger
Department of Urology and Urological Oncology, Hannover University Medical School, Hannover, Germany
e-mail: merseburger.axel@mh-hannover.de

A.S. Merseburger et al. (eds.), *Urology at a Glance*,
DOI 10.1007/978-3-642-54859-8_11, © Springer-Verlag Berlin Heidelberg 2014

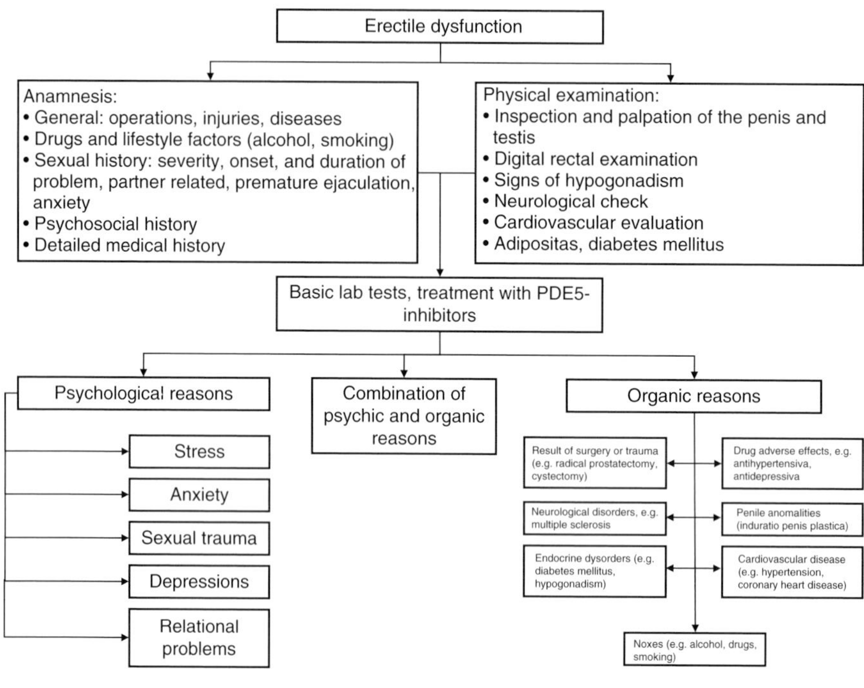

11.2 Medical History

The medical history consists of a general part covering questions on previous illness, operations, injuries, and interviewing for any symptoms from other diseases. Additionally lifestyle factors, smoking, alcohol, and prescribed medicine should be asked for. The sexual history should be covered in detail best using standardized questioners. Are there full erections at some times, e.g., in the morning or at night? Psychological questions on performance anxiety, mental disorders, stress, and depression should be asked. In general, if the patient never has an erection, the problem is likely to be physiological; if in some occasions an erection is possible, both can be the reason.

11.3 Diagnostics

The diagnostic workup should always begin with a physical examination, including an inspection and palpation of the penis and testis and digital rectal examination. Blood tests are performed to exclude underlying diseases, such as diabetes, hypogonadism, or prolactinoma. In details, tests should include glucose tolerance, triglycerides, cholesterin, TSH, creatinine, transaminases, and morning testosterone.

Following initial workup initial treatment will be performed with phosphodiesterase-5-inhibitors. Further semi-invasive diagnostic includes penile injections with prostaglandin E1 (SKAT) with integrated duplex ultrasound to test penile cavernous-arterial perfusion. The bulbocavernosus reflex (squeeze of the glans causes anus to contract) gives the physician answers if there is sufficient nerve sensation in the penis. Noctural penile tumescence and penile biothesiometry using electromagnetic vibration to evaluate sensitivity are additional rare diagnostic tests. In case of suspected altered blood supply, a cavernosography can be performed. Here a contrast medium is injected in the corpus cavernosum with a butterfly needle to visualize the blood flow and irregularities. Nowadays often magnetic resonance angiography (MRA) is performed which results in an enhanced resolution.

11.4 Differential Diagnosis

Reasons of erectile dysfunction

Differential diagnosis	Incidence	Diagnostics
Hypogonadism	–	Morning testosterone and sexual hormone-binding globulin, FSH, LH
Thyroid disorders	+	TSH
Penile anomalies	+	
Surgery, trauma	+	Medical history
Diabetes mellitus	++++	Glucose, oral tolerance test
Cardiovascular disease	++++	Cholesterin, triglycerides
Neurological disorders	++	Specific neurological diagnostic
Drug side effects	+++	Medical history
Noxes	++	Anamnesis
Psychogenic reasons	+++	Psychological/psychiatric workup

Uremia

12

Reinhard Brunkhorst

12.1 Definition

Uremia is defined as a number of clinical symptoms observed in stages 4 and 5 (GFR 15–29 and <15 ml/min resp.) of chronic kidney disease (CKD). These symptoms may vary in order and severity. Without improvement of renal function or initiation of dialysis treatment, uremia leads to death. In stage 4, CKD symptoms of anemia as fatigue and dyspnea may be the first signs of uremia, often followed by itching, uremic fetor, nausea in the morning, and vomiting. Uremic serositis may cause pericarditis or pleuritis. Without dialysis in CKD 5, diarrhea, dyspnea caused by hyperhydration, and neurologic complications as seizures, somnolence, and coma are observed.

12.2 Medical History

Specific questions for uremic symptoms have to be asked in all CKD 4 and 5 patients in regular intervals in order to notice severe uremic organ involvement as, e.g., gastroenteritis or pulmonary edema. For clarifying the cause of CKD questioning for hereditary disease (Alport syndrome, polycystic kidney disease), diabetes mellitus, arterial hypertension, acute disease in the last weeks (fever, diarrhea, severe vomiting), and nephrotoxic medication (NSAR, antibiotics, chemotherapeutics etc.) have to be performed thoroughly. Medical history should further consist of questions for systemic autoimmune or tumor disease, prostatic disease, and urolithiasis (Fig. 12.1).

R. Brunkhorst
Klinik für Nieren-, Hochdruck- und Gefässerkrankungen, Klinikum Oststadt-Heidehaus, Klinikum Region Hannover GmbH, Podbielskistr. 380, Hannover 30659, Germany
e-mail: sekretariat.brunkhorst.oststadt@klinikum-hannover.de

A.S. Merseburger et al. (eds.), *Urology at a Glance*,
DOI 10.1007/978-3-642-54859-8_12,

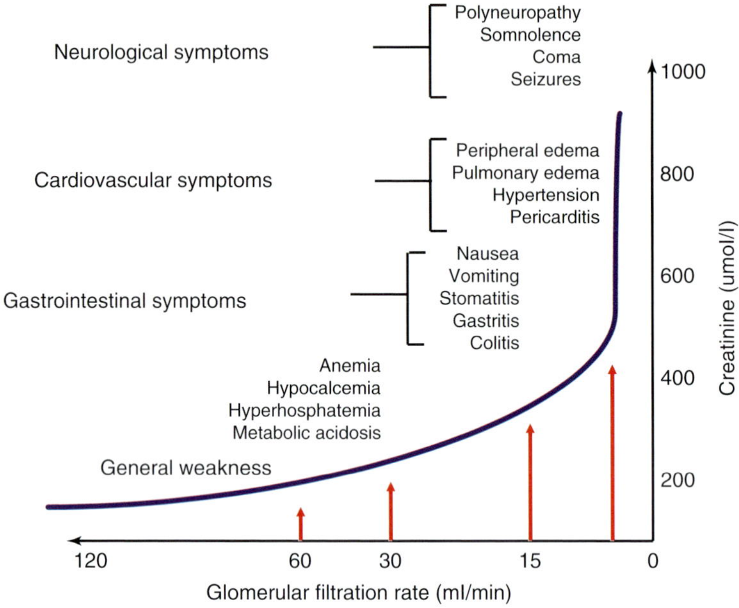

Fig. 12.1 Frequent uremic symptoms in correlation to the decline of renal glomerular filtration rate

12.3 Diagnostics

12.3.1 Physical Examination

In most cases of uremia, blood pressure is elevated. Auscultation of heart and lung is considerably important to exclude pericarditis and pulmonary edema. Furthermore, presence of peripheral edema, anasarca, and alterations of the retina (diabetic or hypertensive retinopathy) has to be excluded. Neurologic examination has to pay attention to peripheral neuropathy, urologic to enlargement of the prostate, and the palpation of the abdomen may detect large cysts in polycystic disease. The gynecologist may find tumors as a cause of postrenal obstruction.

12.3.2 Laboratory Analysis

S-creatinine and urea are elevated; glomerular filtration rate (creatinine clearance) is reduced to <30, in most cases below 15 ml/min. In CKD renal anemia, hyperphosphatemia, and metabolic acidosis are common findings. Serum parathyroid hormone levels may be elevated and S-calcium reduced. High alkaline phosphatase levels may be found in renal bone disease but also in multiple myeloma and metastatic bone disease. Hyperkalemia leads to characteristic alterations in the ECG (sharp inversion of the T-waves, in leads III and aVF, arrhythmias).

In search for the cause of uremia inflammation markers (CRP, BSR, procalcitonine), immune markers (ANA's, ANCA's, etc.), and indicators for multiple myeloma (S-light chains, S-electrophoresis) have to be investigated.

Urine analysis for quantitative proteinuria and hematuria, and as appropriate to exclude nephritic syndrome phase contrast microscopy for dysmorphic erythrocytes and erythrocyte cylinders, should be performed.

As one of the first diagnostic steps (see algorithm), ultrasound of the kidneys is indicated to exclude urinary obstruction and to assess kidney size and parenchymal damage. Chest X-ray disclaims pulmonary edema and effusion. In case of unknown cause of renal failure, kidney biopsy should be performed in order to evaluate prognosis and therapeutic options.

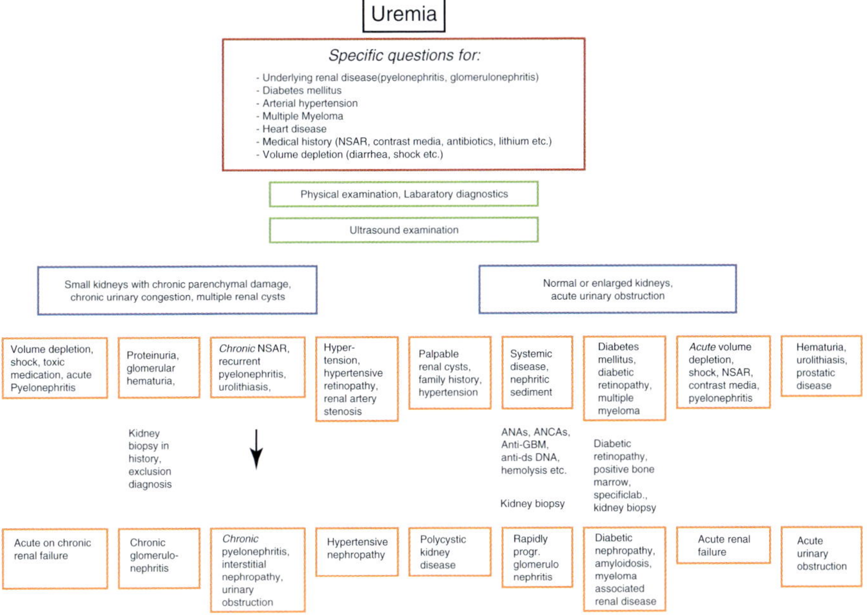

12.4 Differential Diagnosis

Causes of uremia		
Diagnosis	Frequency	Diagnostic measures
Diabetic nephropathy	++++	Normal size in ultrasound, diabetic retinopathy, renal biopsy
Hypertensive nephropathy	+++	Hypertensive retinopathy, echocardiography
Glomerulonephritis	++	Hematuria, proteinuria, renal biopsy
Chronic pyelonephritis, chronic urinary obstruction	++	Urinary sediment, ultrasound
Polycystic kidney disease	+	Ultrasound, family history
Renal involvement in systemic disease	+	Nephritic urinary sediment, renal biopsy, immunologic testing
Toxic nephropathy	+	Medication history, ultrasound
Alport syndrome	(+)	Family history, hearing deficit

Acute Kidney Injury (AKI) 13

Marcus Hiß and Jan T. Kielstein

13.1 Definition

Acute kidney injury (formerly known as acute renal failure) is a complex disorder with many underling conditions. It is seen in SIRS/sepsis and associated with a mortality of 60 % [1]. In 2007, a uniform definition was proposed which now replaces the more than 30 definitions that existed previously [2]. The diagnostic criteria for AKI were proposed based on acute alterations in serum creatinine or urine output. The Acute Kidney Injury Network (AKIN) criteria (Table 13.1) are based on epidemiological studies. Those studies indicated that modest changes in serum creatinine were significantly associated with mortality, hospital length of stay, and costs [3]. The old classification of prerenal, renal, and postrenal AKI is becoming less important as more than 90 % of the AKI patients suffer from a combination of prerenal and renal AKI.

The incidence of AKI is increasing worldwide. From 2000 to 2009, the incidence of dialysis-requiring AKI in the USA increased about 10 % per year [4]. This increase in incidence was evident in all age, sex, and race subgroups examined. The total number of deaths associated with dialysis-requiring AKI rose from 18,000 in 2000 to nearly 39,000 in 2009 [4]. Old age, higher degree of baseline renal impairment, and advanced diagnostic and therapeutic procedures epitomized by high-dose chemotherapy or implantation of cardiac assist devices are factors associated with this increase.

There is no specific treatment for AKI! Dozens of compounds that were tested to be effective in preclinical studies failed in the clinical setting; hence preventive measures are of importance. Prevention starts by identifying patients at risk. Table 13.2 summarizes risk factors.

M. Hiß (✉) • J.T. Kielstein
Department of Nephrology and Hypertension, Hannover Medical School, Carl-Neuberg-Str. 1, Hannover 30625, Germany
e-mail: hiss.marcus@mh-hannover.de; kielstein@yahoo.com

A.S. Merseburger et al. (eds.), *Urology at a Glance*,
DOI 10.1007/978-3-642-54859-8_13, © Springer-Verlag Berlin Heidelberg 2014

Table 13.1 AKIN criteria for the diagnosis of AKI

Stage	Serum creatinine	Urine output
1	1.5–1.9 times baseline OR >0.3 mg/dl (>26.5 μmol/l) increase	<0.5 ml/kg/h for 6–12 h
2	2.0–2.9 times baseline	<0.5 ml/kg/h for ≥12 h
3	3.0 times baseline OR Increase in serum creatinine to >4.0 mg/dl (>353.6 μmol/l) OR Initiation of renal replacement therapy OR in patients <18 years, decrease in eGFR to <35 ml/min/1.73 m^2	<0.3 ml/kg/h for >24 h OR Anuria for >12 h

Table 13.2 Causes of AKI: exposures and susceptibilities for nonspecific AKI

Exposures	Susceptibilities
Sepsis	Dehydration or volume depletion
Critical illness	Advanced age
Circulatory shock	Female gender
Cardiac surgery (especially with CPB)	Chronic diseases (heart, lung, liver)
Trauma	Diabetes mellitus
Major noncardiac surgery	Anemia
Nephrotoxic drugs	Cancer
Radiocontrast agents	CKD

Adapted from Kellum and Lameire [5]

There are currently no studies supporting the use of specific drugs for the prevention of AKI. This holds true for the infamous "renal dose dopa" [6] as well as for the use of diuretics which have been shown to have a detrimental effect on renal function and mortality [7, 8]. However, the early consultation of a nephrologist is associated with a better outcome of AKI patients [9]. In contrast to the disappointing results of pharmacological interventions, volume expansion with either isotonic sodium chloride or sodium bicarbonate solutions has repeatedly shown to ameliorate or prevent AKI, especially in the setting of radio contrast exposure. Care must be taken that volume replacement does not lead to prolonged fluid accumulation, which has been shown to be associated with adverse outcome [10].

Although there is consensus that renal replacement therapy (RRT) needs to be emergently initiated if life-threatening changes in fluid, electrolyte, and acid-base balance exist or the patients are intoxicated with a dialyzable toxin, the timing of RRT initiation in general is more complex. There is no specific urea/BUN that should trigger the start of RRT, but rather the broader clinical context and the presence of conditions that can be modified with RRT have to be integrated into the decision making.

In contrast to previous assumptions that AKI, once survived, will not have long-term sequela, we now know that this is not true. In a large, community-based cohort

Table 13.3 The AKI ABC

A	Address drugs	Look for/discontinue NSAIDs, inhibitors of renin–angiotensin–aldosterone system, nephrotoxic antibiotics
B	Boost blood pressure	Required perfusion pressure for the kidney might be higher in severe atherosclerosis, abdominal compartment syndrome use Doppler sonography Consider functional hemodynamic monitoring and use of pressors
C	Calculate fluid balance	Persistent (>3 days) hypervolemia in AKI is associated with adverse outcome; hence, persistent hypervolemia should be avoided
D	Dip urine	Urinary sediment analysis to diagnose acute glomerulonephritis, vasculitis, interstitial nephritis, thrombotic Microangiopathy
E	Exclude obstruction	Obstruction has to be excluded in every patient with AKI by sonography

of patients with CKD, an episode of superimposed dialysis-requiring AKI was associated with very high risk for non-recovery of renal function. Dialysis-requiring AKI also seemed to be an independent risk factor for long-term risk for death or chronic dialysis dependency [11] (Table 13.3).

References

1. Uchino S, Kellum JA, Bellomo R, Doig GS, Morimatsu H, Morgera S, Schetz M, Tan I, Bouman C, Macedo E, Gibney N, Tolwani A, Ronco C. Acute renal failure in critically ill patients: a multinational, multicenter study. JAMA. 2005;294:813–8.
2. Mehta RL, Kellum JA, Shah SV, Molitoris BA, Ronco C, Warnock DG, Levin A. Acute Kidney Injury Network (AKIN): report of an initiative to improve outcomes in acute kidney injury. Crit Care. 2007;11:R31.
3. Chertow GM, Burdick E, Honour M, Bonventre JV, Bates DW. Acute kidney injury, mortality, length of stay, and costs in hospitalized patients. J Am Soc Nephrol. 2005;16:3365–70.
4. Hsu RK, McCulloch CE, Dudley RA, Lo LJ, Hsu CY. Temporal changes in incidence of dialysis-requiring AKI. J Am Soc Nephrol. 2013;24:37–42.
5. Kellum JA, Lameire N. Diagnosis, evaluation, and management of acute kidney injury: a KDIGO summary (part 1). Crit Care. 2013;17:204.
6. Friedrich JO, Adhikari N, Herridge MS, Beyene J. Meta-analysis: low-dose dopamine increases urine output but does not prevent renal dysfunction or death. Ann Intern Med. 2005;142:510–24.
7. Lassnigg A, Donner E, Grubhofer G, Presterl E, Druml W, Hiesmayr M. Lack of renoprotective effects of dopamine and furosemide during cardiac surgery. J Am Soc Nephrol. 2000;11: 97–104.
8. Mehta RL, Pascual MT, Soroko S, Chertow GM. Diuretics, mortality, and nonrecovery of renal function in acute renal failure. JAMA. 2002;288:2547–53.
9. Mehta RL, McDonald B, Gabbai F, Pahl M, Farkas A, Pascual MT, Zhuang S, Kaplan RM, Chertow GM. Nephrology consultation in acute renal failure: does timing matter? Am J Med. 2002;113:456–61.
10. Bouchard J, Soroko SB, Chertow GM, Himmelfarb J, Ikizler TA, Paganini EP, Mehta RL. Fluid accumulation, survival and recovery of kidney function in critically ill patients with acute kidney injury. Kidney Int. 2009;76:422–7.
11. Hsu CY, Chertow GM, McCulloch CE, Fan D, Ordonez JD, Go AS. Nonrecovery of kidney function and death after acute on chronic renal failure. Clin J Am Soc Nephrol. 2009;4:891–8.

Ileus

14

Armin Pycha and Salvatore Palermo

14.1 Definition

Ileus is a mechanical or functional obstruction of the intestines, preventing the normal propulsive ability of the gastrointestinal tract. Mechanical obstruction can occur at any level of the intestine distally from the duodenum and can be caused by three types of abnormalities [1]:

1. Obturation of the intestinal lumen [1, 2] by polypoid tumors of the bowel, intussusception, foreign bodies, bezoars, fecal impaction, fecaloma, and endometriosis.
2. Intrinsic bowel lesions [1, 2] which are often congenital as atresia, Hirschsprung's disease, or congenital stenosis. These are seen most frequently in infants and are a domain of pediatric surgery. In adults the common causes are strictures, which may follow neoplasms or inflammatory bowel disease as in Crohn's disease or iatrogenic maneuvers as after radiation therapy or a surgical anastomotic stricture.
3. Lesions extrinsic to the bowel [1, 2] are mostly caused by adhesions from previous surgical procedures which lead to kinking or angulation or by creating bands of tissue that strangulate the bowel. Strangulation can also happen by external and internal hernias as well as by a volvulus.

A paralysis or an atony of any degree of intestinal muscles is called paralytic ileus [1, 3, 4]. It is a common side effect of intestinal surgery, which leads to intestinal distension. But also distension of a ureter or a retroperitoneal hematoma or a renal or a spinal trauma can lead to a paralytic ileus [5]. Also peritonitis; severe hypothyroidism; electrolyte imbalance, particularly hypopotassemia; diabetic

A. Pycha, MD, FEBU (✉) • S. Palermo, MD, FEBU
Department of Urology, Central Hospital of Bozen/Bolzano,
Lorenz Böhler Street 5, Bozen/Bolzano 39100, Italy
e-mail: armin.pycha@libero.it

A.S. Merseburger et al. (eds.), *Urology at a Glance*,
DOI 10.1007/978-3-642-54859-8_14, © Springer-Verlag Berlin Heidelberg 2014

ketoacidosis; and drugs like opiates or antimuscarinics contribute to paralytic ileus by interfering with the normal ionic movements during smooth muscle contraction [6]. Finally, ischemia of the intestine rapidly inhibits motility [6].

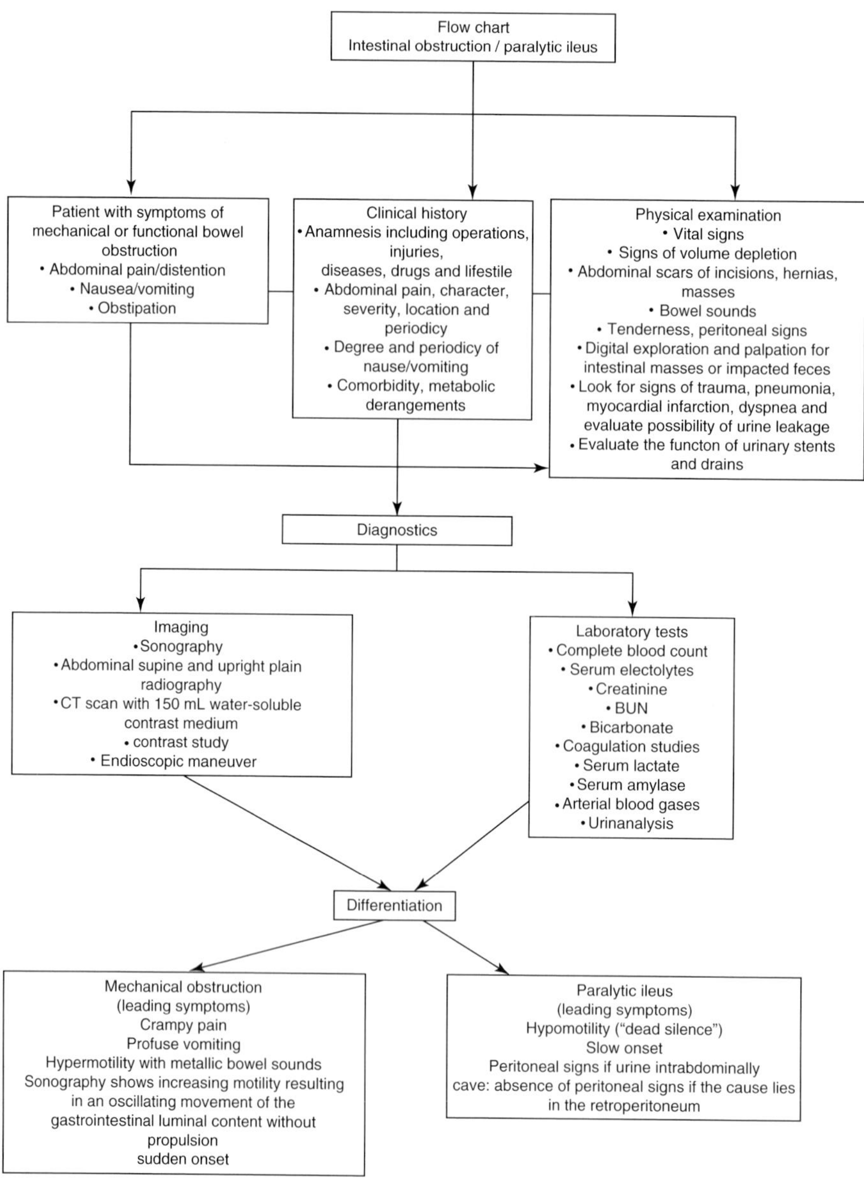

14.2 Medical History

The medical history consists of a general part, covering questions of previous surgery, especially abdominal operations, known hernias or previous illness, recent traumas, neurologic disorders, medication, and smoking history. Detail should be paid to previous severe inflammatory illness like Crohn's disease [7], diverticulitis or previous peritonitis, last flatulence, and defecation [1–3].

The dynamics of moderate abdominal discomfort at the beginning to abdominal pain later on, nausea, vomiting, obstipation, abdominal distension, and lack of flatulence should be covered in detail. Crampy pain at a 4–5-min interval in the proximal ileus is often associated with profuse vomiting (small bowel obstruction) [3, 8]. The more distal obstruction is the less frequent, accompanied by vomiting, and the symptoms have a delayed onset (large bowel obstruction) [5, 8, 9]. In case of a mechanical obstruction, hypermotility with metallic sounds can be observed in the beginning, which decrease with time and become later completely paralytic [1]. Paradox stool can happen until the bowel distally from the obstruction is emptied. Obstipation and failure to pass gas are signs of complete obstruction/paralysis [1, 2, 8].

In the urological field different causes can lead to an obstruction/ileus. Previous surgeries such as a cystectomy with neobladder or a conduit are risk factors for intestinal obstruction by band adhesion as well as for a paralytic ileus. After lymphadenectomies in the pelvis, one must always think about possible mechanical obstructions by adhesion of small bowel loops in the right fossa obturatoria. Urine with its high concentration of nitrogen causes a strong tissue reaction in the peritoneum leading to uremic peritonitis and paralytic ileus. Therefore, urine leakage has to be considered at all times. But also urine in the retroperitoneum can cause a reflectory paralytic ileus as well as hematomas after surgery, traumas, or overlooked rupture of the fornix in an occluding stone [3].

14.3 Diagnostics

The diagnostic workup should always begin with a complete physical examination including the search of surgical scars for etiological reasons, listening to the abdomen with a stethoscope, and classification of abdominal sounds as absent or increasing high pitch, metallic, or tinkling [1].The palpation of the abdomen is mandatory to define abdominal distension, localized or rebound tenderness, and guarding, which would suggest peritonitis. Hydration status should be estimated by evaluation of skin turgor and moisture of the tongue [1].

Heart frequency and blood pressure recording are mandatory, because tachycardia and hypotension may indicate severe dehydration, peritonitis, or both. Rectal examinations have to be done to exclude rectal endoluminal masses [1, 2, 4, 5, 8].

The presence or absence of feces should be noted and if present examination for occult blood has to be performed. Blood indicates the presence of cancer, intussusception, or intestinal infarction [1, 6].

Supine and upright abdominal radiographic examination may show abnormally large quantities of gas in the bowel, indicating an organ distension and multiple gas fluid levels and inverted U-shaped loops and the absence of gas distally of the obstruction [1, 10].

Ultrasonography may be showing extended loops of small or large intestine with loss of motility in a paralytic ileus, whereas a mechanic obstruction shows an increasing motility resulting in an oscillating movement of the gastrointestinal luminal content without propulsion.

CT scan or magnetic resonance imaging [11] can be useful to determine the level of obstruction, whether the obstruction is partial or complete. It is also helpful to define the cause of obstruction [1, 5, 12].

Endoscopic procedures are requested if a pseudo-obstruction is to be excluded [13]. In this case the diagnostic approach is also the therapy.

Any patient which is suspected to have an intestinal obstruction should have blood tests including a complete blood count (CBC), electrolytes, and prothrombin time (PT). Serum chemistries, blood urea nitrogen (BUN), bicarbonate, creatinine, lactate, amylase, urinalysis, and arterial blood gases also may be done (Figs. 14.1 and 14.2).

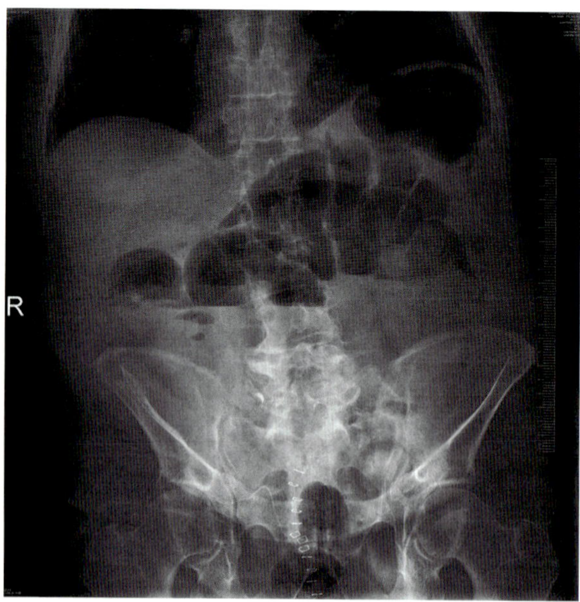

Fig. 14.1 The upright abdominal radiographic examination shows distended small bowel loops and abnormally large quantities of gas in the bowel indicating an organ distension and inverted U-shaped loops in a paralytic ileus

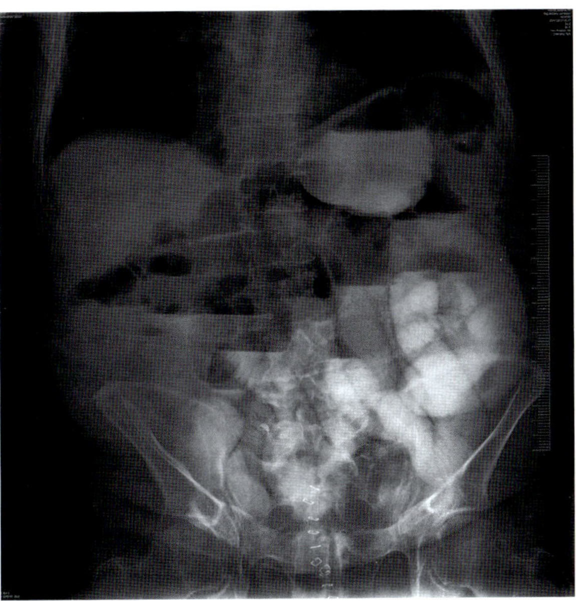

Fig. 14.2 Radiographic examination 4 h after a contrast medium meal. Gaseous distension is somewhat uniformly present in the stomach, small bowel, and left colonic flexure. The small bowel pattern occupies the more central portion of the abdomen showing multiple gas fluid levels in distended bowel with inverted U-loops. Colonic haustral markings occupy a part of the transverse colon; no gas in the colon descendens and rectum (large bowel obstruction)

14.4 Differential Diagnosis

Differential diagnosis	Incidence	Diagnostics
Pseudo-obstruction (Ogilvie's syndrome)	+	Plain X-ray
Peritonitis	++	Physical examination, blood count, sonography
Kidney stones	+	Sonography, CT scan
Spinal cord lesions	++	Neurologic evaluation
Megarectum	+	Medical history, plain X-ray, CT scan, colonoscopy
Alcoholic ketoacidosis	++	
Cholecystitis	++	Ultrasonography, blood count
Biliary colic	++	Ultrasonography
Cholelithiasis	++	Ultrasonography, blood count
Diverticular disease	++	History, ultrasonography, physical examination, laboratory tests
Endometriosis	+	MRI
Inflammatory bowel disease	+++	History, ultrasonography, physical examination, laboratory tests, MRI
Mesenteric ischemia	++	History, physical examination, CT scan
Abdominal hernias	++	Physical examination, CT scan
Appendicitis	+	History, physical examination, rebound tenderness
Renal trauma	++	History, ultrasonography, CT scan
Retroperitoneal urinoma	++	Urography, CT scan

(continued)

Differential diagnosis	Incidence	Diagnostics
Pseudomembranous colitis	+	Colonoscopy with biopsy
Toxic megacolon	+++	Plain X-ray
Paralytic ileus	+++	Abdominal radiography, "death silence"
Anastomotic leakage	++	Physical examination, CT scan, laboratory tests
Anastomotic stricture	+++	Ultrasonography
Intestinal stricture	+++	Ultrasonography
Acute gastroenteritis	++	History, physical examination, laboratory tests
Acute pancreatitis	+	Amylase, CT scan
Cancer of the gastrointestinal tract	+++	CT scan, colonoscopy
Crohn's disease	+++	MRI, ultrasonography
Ovarian cancer	+	CT scan
Adhesions	++	Physical examination, sonography, CT scan

References

1. Sabiston Jr DC, editor. Textbook of surgery: the biological basis of modern surgical practice. 14th ed. Philadelphia: W.B. Saunders Company; 2012.
2. Maung AA, Johnson DC, Piper GL, Barbosa RR, Rowell SE, Bokhari F, Collins JN, Gordon JR, Ra JH, Kerwin AJ, Eastern Association for the Surgery of Trauma. Evaluation and management of small-bowel obstruction: an Eastern Association for the Surgery of Trauma practice management guideline. J Trauma Acute Care Surg. 2012;73(5 Suppl 4):362–9.
3. Dayton MT, Dempsey DT, Larson GM, Posner AR. New paradigms in the treatment of small bowel obstruction. Curr Probl Surg. 2012;49(11):642–717.
4. Kim M, Isbert C. Anorectal functional diagnostics. Therapy algorithm for obstruction and incontinence. Chirurg. 2013;84(1):7–14.
5. Doorly MG, Senagore AJ. Pathogenesis and clinical and economic consequences of postoperative ileus. Surg Clin North Am. 2012;92(2):259–72.
6. Scali ST, Waterman A, Feezor RJ, Martin TD, Hess Jr PJ, Huber TS, Beck AW. Treatment of acute visceral aortic pathology with fenestrated/branched endovascular repair in high-surgical-risk patients. J Vasc Surg. 2013;58(1):56–65.
7. Lu KC, Hunt SR. Surgical management of Crohn's disease. Surg Clin North Am. 2013;93(1):167–85.
8. Ahn BK, Lee KH. Characteristics and prognoses of small obstructing colorectal cancers: the combination of gross findings has value in predicting recurrence after curative therapy. Am Surg. 2013;79(5):544–7.
9. Winner M, Mooney SJ, Hershman DL, Feingold DL, Allendorf JD, Wright JD, Neugut AI. Management and outcomes of bowel obstruction on patients with stage IV colon cancer: a population-based cohort study. Dis Colon Rectum. 2013;56(7):834–43.
10. Hayakawa K, Tanikake M, Yoshida S, Urata Y, Yamamoto E, Morimoto T. Radiological diagnosis of large bowel obstruction: neoplastic etiology. Emerg Radiol. 2013;20(1):69–76.
11. Masselli G, Gualdi G. MR imaging of the small bowel. Radiology. 2012;264(2):333–48.
12. Hope JM, Pothuri B. The role of palliative surgery in gynecologic cancer cases. Oncologist. 2013;18(1):73–9.
13. Ertberg P, Vilandt J, Bodker B. Diagnosis and treatment of acute colonic pseudo-obstruction. Ugeskr Laeger. 2013;175(17):1176–80.

Incontinence

15

Omar M. Aboumarzouk, Jan Adamowicz, Piotr L. Chłosta, and Tomasz Drewa

15.1 Definitions

Urinary incontinence (UI) is defined as an involuntary loss of urine. It is subdivided into (a) stress incontinence whereby involuntary loss of urine is on physical exertion or effort or on sneezing or coughing, (b) urgency incontinence is involuntary loss of urine when associated with or preceded by urgency, and (c) mixed incontinence is a mixture of the two types whereby involuntary loss of urine is associated with both urgency and on physical exertion or effort or on sneezing or coughing. Urgency is defined as 'the complaint of a sudden compelling desire to pass urine' [1].

Two main pathophysiological entities that cause UI are bladder abnormalities and sphincter abnormalities. Bladder abnormalities include detrusor overactivity (DO) and low bladder compliance (LBC). DO is characterized by spontaneous or provoked

O.M. Aboumarzouk, MBChB, MSc, PhD, MRCS (Glasg) (✉)
College of Medicine, Islamic University of Gaza, Gaza, Occupied Palestine
e-mail: aboumarzouk@gmail.com

J. Adamowicz
Department of Tissue Engenering and Urology, Collegium Medicum, University of Nicolaus Copernicus, Toruń, Poland

Katedra i Klinika Urologii Collegium, Medicum Uniwersytetu Jagiellońskiego, ul. Grzegórzecka 18, Kraków, Poland

P.L. Chłosta, MD, PhD, DSci, FEBU
Department of Urology, Jagiellonian University in Krakow, ul. Grzegorzecka 18, Krakow 31-531, Poland
e-mail: piotr.chlosta@gmail.com

T. Drewa
Department of Urology, Nicolaus Copernicus Hospital, Batory 17-19 str., Toruń 87-100, Poland

Katedra i Klinika Urologii Collegium, Medicum Uniwersytetu Jagiellońskiego, ul. Grzegórzecka 18, Kraków, Poland
e-mail: tomaszdrewa@wp.pl, sekurol@med.torun.pl

A.S. Merseburger et al. (eds.), *Urology at a Glance*,
DOI 10.1007/978-3-642-54859-8_15, © Springer-Verlag Berlin Heidelberg 2014

involuntary detrusor contraction during the filling phase of the micturition cycle and shows various patterns such as phasic, terminal, or in combination DO [1]. Phasic DO is characteristically wave form contractions +/– UI and may or may not have any sensation to void. Terminal DO is a single involuntary contraction which cannot be suppressed and leads to UI. DO incontinence is involuntary detrusor contraction in patients with normal sensation, whereby urgency is experienced just before incontinence episodes. DO are of two main types, neurogenic, which is caused by a neurological condition (supraspinal lesions: stroke, Parkinson disease, hydrocephalus, brain tumour, brain traumatic injury, multiple sclerosis; suprasacral spinal lesions: spinal cord injury or tumour, multiple sclerosis, myelodysplasia, transverse myelitis), and idiopathic DO with no specific cause found but can be associated with bladder infection, stones, tumors, and foreign body or bladder outlet obstruction.

LBC is characterized by having an abnormal decreased volume to pressure relationship, whereby there is an increase in the intravesicular pressure as the bladder fills with urine. It is mainly caused by changes in the elastic properties of the bladder wall, changes in the bladder muscle tone, or a combination. Causes of LBC are either neurogenic (myelodysplasia, Shy-Drager syndrome, suprasacral spinal cord injury or lesions), operations (hysterectomy or abdominoperineal resection of the rectum), or non-neurogenic (more collagen/elastic property changes related) (tuberculous cystitis, radiation cystitis, long-term catheterisation, bladder outlet obstruction).

Sphincter abnormalities vary between men and women. In men, it is more commonly due to damage to the sphincter mechanism after prostate surgery or in rare instances caused by trauma, radiation therapy, or neurological abnormalities. While in women, the sphincter weakness can be caused by urethral hypermobility (anatomical support defect, i.e. prolapse) or intrinsic sphincter insufficiency. Urethral hypermobility is more commonly due to pregnancy, vaginal delivery, or pelvic/gynecological operations. Intrinsic sphincter insufficiency can be seen in patients who had previous urethral surgery (urethral diverticulum or anti-incontinence surgery), pelvic radiation therapy, or neurological damage or insults (herniated disks, diabetic neuropathy, multiple sclerosis, spinal cord tumors, after extensive pelvic surgery).

15.2 Medical History

A complete history is always vital to establish a direction of management, dividing the history into specific questions of the presenting complaint of incontinence, followed by general questions.

Specific question of incontinence should be tailored around identifying precipitating or aggravating factors and establishing a predominant type of incontinence and association with other urinary symptoms. The main risk factors associated with UI are listed in Table 15.1 and should be asked on or about during the history taking.

The patient should be questioned about the duration of incontinence, the onset and frequency of leakage, diurnal variation, and fluid consumption and type. Questioning whether or not the leakage occurs with physical activity, coughing, sneezing, and straining or if it is associated with a sense of urgency or without any sensation at all should be asked. If a mixture of the symptoms is present, which one is predominant? Determining if the patients' symptoms are bothersome and affect

Table 15.1 Main risk factors for incontinence

Risk factor in women	Risk factor in men
Increasing age [3]	Increasing age [4]
Obesity [5, 6]	Lower urinary tract symptoms [7]
Parity [5, 8, 9]	Urinary tract infections [10]
Pregnancy [11, 12]	Neurological disease [13, 14]
Vaginal delivery [15]	Diabetes [14]
Race [16]:	Prostatectomy [17]
Stress incontinence: white race	
Urge incontinence: black race	
Menopausal replacement therapy [18, 19]	Sedentary lifestyle/lack of exercise/impaired physical activity [10, 17]
Hysterectomy [20]	
Caffeine [21]	
Sedentary lifestyle/lack of exercise/impaired physical activity [22]	

their daily activities should also be asked to establish if risks of treatment complications of side effects outweigh the benefits of treatment. Alarming symptoms such as pain, dysuria, recurrent urinary tract infections, haematuria, or recent unexpected weight loss should be elicited; as may lead to more urgent investigations.

General questions to be asked include past medical and surgical history, in women the history should include questions regarding menstrual, gynacological and obstetric, and sexual histories. Drug and medication history, social, psychological, smoking, alcoholic, and work histories should also be asked about.

15.3 Diagnostics

Physical examination is the initial and vital step in establishing the diagnosis of incontinence. Physical examination of the body as a whole is vital and should ideally have started when the patient walks into the room looking for any neurological gaits or frailty. Look for a palpable bladder or previous surgery scars during the abdominal examination. In women, a pelvic examination should include the external genitalia, urethra, vagina, cervix, uterus, and adnexa. A digital rectal examination should be done to assess the prostate gland in men and the rectovaginal septum in women, identifying a rectocele or masses in the rectum, in addition for assessment of the anal sphincter tone (S2–4 function). A full neurologic examination is important as well.

Specific tests conducted during an exam include the Q-tip test and assessment of pelvic organ prolapse (POP) and the stress test. Q-tip test is done to evaluate urethra mobility. A Q-tip is inserted into the bladder through the urethra, and the angle that the Q-tip sits in while in its final position when the patient strains is measured. Hypermobility is considered when the Q-tip angle is more than 30° from the horizontal plane. Assessment for POP is performed in both lithotomy and standing positions with the aid of a speculum. Also stress test can be performed while using the speculum, involving the observation of urine loss during coughing or Valsalva manoeuvre.

Aiding both the history and examination are a series of investigations (questionnaires and tests) required to establish a functional diagnosis:

- Patient questionnaires such as symptom scores, symptom questionnaires, patient reported outcome measures (PROMS), or health-related quality of life (HRQoL) measures. These can not only assess severity of symptoms but also monitor the effects of treatment.
- Voiding diaries: the patient records the frequency and volume of urine voided, incontinence episodes, pad usage, fluid intake, and degree of urgency.
- Pad test: carried out by asking the patient to wear continence pads for a set period of time. The pad test was designed to quantify the volume of urine loss by weighing it before and after leakage. A measure loss of more than 1.3 g of urine in a 24-h period is considered positive.
- Urine dip stick and urinalysis: to detect the presence of haematuria, pyuria, glycosuria, or proteinuria. Nitrites and leucocyte esterase may indicate an infection, protein may indicate an infection or renal disease, blood may indicate in infection or malignancy, and glucose may indicate diabetes mellitus.
- Post-voiding residual (PVR) volume: defined as the amount of urine in the bladder after voiding. Can be measured either by an ultrasound scan or by the use of an in-out catheter. Used to detect impaired bladder emptying.
- Cystoscopy: looking for pathology either in the urethra (strictures, diverticulum, foreign bodies, fistulas) or bladder (tumors, stones, inflammation, foreign bodies, previous pelvic floor reconstructive surgical material eroding into the bladder).
- Urodynamics: used in patients with mix incontinence to distinguish urgency or obstructive symptoms and in patients with high PVRs or neurologic disease.
  - Simple urodynamics: determine bladder sensation, compliance, stability, and capacity, as well as outlet competence and PVR.
  - Multichannel urodynamics: more extensive evaluation of the filling/storage phase by filling cystometrogram and the voiding/emptying phase by uroflowmetry. Used in patients when conservative treatment fails, when the diagnosis is unclear, or diagnostic procedures are inconclusive; in patients who had radiation therapy, neurologic disease, or prior failed pelvic floor reconstruction or anti-incontinence surgery; or when patients describe symptoms which are not clinically elicited.
  - Videourodynamics (electromyogram (EMG) and fluoroscopic imaging): can demonstrate the anatomy in the upright position and can confirm incontinence in patients in whom the diagnosis is difficult and can provide an accurate measure of leak point pressure, used in assessing suspicion of detrusor-sphincter dyssynergia or primary bladder neck obstruction and evaluating for vesicoureteral reflux.
- Imaging:
  - Voiding cystourethrogram: can be used in patients with recurrent urinary tract infections looking for urethral diverticulum or vesicoureteric reflux. It can also provide visualisation of subtle leakage with coughing or straining and give information regarding the position of the bladder base and neck during voiding.
  - Ultrasound: looking for signs of high pressure disease such as hydroureteronephrosis, upper tract pathology (stones, tumours), and can also be used to assess the bladder neck for urine leakage and descent during stress [2].
  - Magnetic resonance imaging (MRI): to evaluate the anatomy of the bladder neck and urethra, pelvic floor relaxation, and POP and to identify urethral

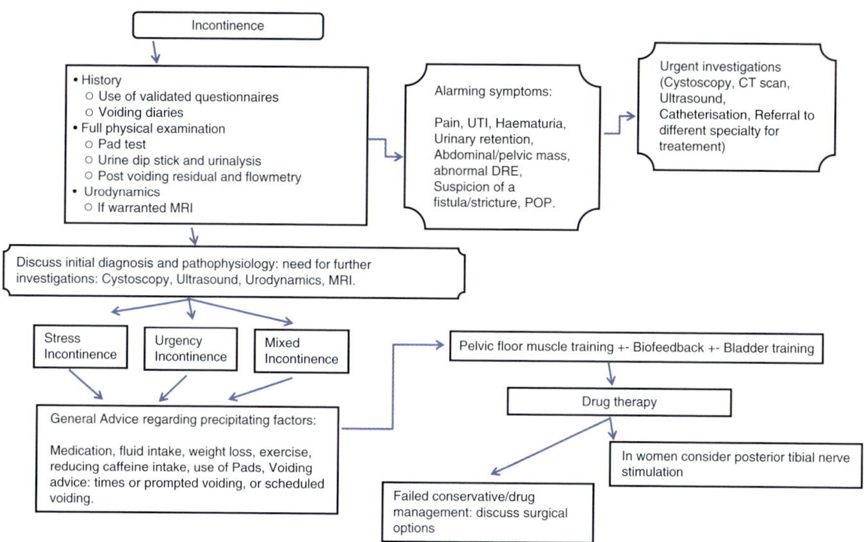

Fig. 15.1 Flow diagram of assessment and treatment of incontinence

diverticulum. MRI can be used to plan out surgical procedures (urethral diverticulum or pelvic floor reconstructions).

15.4 Differential Diagnosis

Differentiating between the different types of UI (stress, urgency, or mixed) can aid in the treatment. Also a distinction needs to be made from other types of incontinences:

- Overflow incontinence, which is the leakage of urine associated with urinary retention
- Nocturnal enuresis which is the loss of urine during sleep
- Post micturition dribbling which is dribbling loss of urine occurring after voiding due to pooling of urine in the bulbous urethra after voiding
- Extra-urethral incontinence which is urine leakage through passages other than the urethra, such as through fistulas or ectopic ureter, immediately after passing urine (See Fig. 15.1)

References

1. Abrams P, Cardozo L, Fall M, Griffiths D, Rosier P, Ulmsten U, et al. The standardisation of terminology of lower urinary tract function: report from the Standardisation Sub-committee of the International Continence Society. NeurourolUrodyn. 2002;21(2):167–78. Epub 2002/02/22.
2. Martin JL, Williams KS, Sutton AJ, Abrams KR, Assassa RP. Systematic review and meta-analysis of methods of diagnostic assessment for urinary incontinence. NeurourolUrodyn. 2006;25(7):674–83; discussion 84. Epub 2006/10/04.
3. Hannestad YS, Rortveit G, Sandvik H, Hunskaar S. A community-based epidemiological survey of female urinary incontinence: the Norwegian EPINCONT study. Epidemiology of

incontinence in the county of Nord-Trondelag. J Clin Epidemiol. 2000;53(11):1150–7. Epub 2000/12/07.
4. Markland AD, Goode PS, Redden DT, Borrud LG, Burgio KL. Prevalence of urinary incontinence in men: results from the national health and nutrition examination survey. J Urol. 2010; 184(3):1022–7. Epub 2010/07/21.
5. Danforth KN, Townsend MK, Lifford K, Curhan GC, Resnick NM, Grodstein F. Risk factors for urinary incontinence among middle-aged women. Am J Obstet Gynecol. 2006;194(2): 339–45. Epub 2006/02/07.
6. Hunskaar S. A systematic review of overweight and obesity as risk factors and targets for clinical intervention for urinary incontinence in women. NeurourolUrodyn. 2008;27(8):749–57. Epub 2008/10/28.
7. Diokno AC, Brock BM, Brown MB, Herzog AR. Prevalence of urinary incontinence and other urological symptoms in the noninstitutionalized elderly. J Urol. 1986;136(5):1022–5. Epub 1986/11/01.
8. Grodstein F, Fretts R, Lifford K, Resnick N, Curhan G. Association of age, race, and obstetric history with urinary symptoms among women in the Nurses' Health Study. Am J Obstet Gynecol. 2003;189(2):428–34. Epub 2003/10/02.
9. Rortveit G, Hannestad YS, Daltveit AK, Hunskaar S. Age- and type-dependent effects of parity on urinary incontinence: the Norwegian EPINCONT study. Obstet Gynecol. 2001;98(6):1004–10. Epub 2002/01/05.
10. Ueda T, Tamaki M, Kageyama S, Yoshimura N, Yoshida O. Urinary incontinence among community-dwelling people aged 40 years or older in Japan: prevalence, risk factors, knowledge and self-perception. Int J Urol. 2000;7(3):95–103. Epub 2000/04/06.
11. Morkved S, Bo K. Prevalence of urinary incontinence during pregnancy and postpartum. Int Urogynecol J Pelvic Floor Dysfunct. 1999;10(6):394–8. Epub 1999/12/30.
12. Marshall K, Thompson KA, Walsh DM, Baxter GD. Incidence of urinary incontinence and constipation during pregnancy and postpartum: survey of current findings at the Rotunda Lying-In Hospital. Br J Obstet Gynaecol. 1998;105(4):400–2. Epub 1998/06/03.
13. Resnick NM, Yalla SV. Detrusor hyperactivity with impaired contractile function. An unrecognized but common cause of incontinence in elderly patients. JAMA. 1987;257(22):3076–81. Epub 1987/06/12.
14. Shamliyan TA, Wyman JF, Ping R, Wilt TJ, Kane RL. Male urinary incontinence: prevalence, risk factors, and preventive interventions. Rev Urol. 2009;11(3):145–65. Epub 2009/11/18.
15. Press JZ, Klein MC, Kaczorowski J, Liston RM, von Dadelszen P. Does cesarean section reduce postpartum urinary incontinence? A systematic review. Birth. 2007;34(3):228–37. Epub 2007/08/28.
16. Waetjen LE, Liao S, Johnson WO, Sampselle CM, Sternfield B, Harlow SD, et al. Factors associated with prevalent and incident urinary incontinence in a cohort of midlife women: a longitudinal analysis of data: study of women's health across the nation. Am J Epidemiol. 2007;165(3):309–18. Epub 2006/11/30.
17. Hunskaar S. One hundred and fifty men with urinary incontinence. I. Demography and medical history. Scand J Prim Health Care. 1992;10(1):21–5. Epub 1992/03/01.
18. Grady D, Brown JS, Vittinghoff E, Applegate W, Varner E, Snyder T. Postmenopausal hormones and incontinence: the heart and estrogen/progestin replacement study. Obstet Gynecol. 2001;97(1):116–20. Epub 2001/01/12.
19. Grodstein F, Lifford K, Resnick NM, Curhan GC. Postmenopausal hormone therapy and risk of developing urinary incontinence. Obstet Gynecol. 2004;103(2):254–60. Epub 2004/02/03.
20. Forsgren C, Lundholm C, Johansson AL, Cnattingius S, Zetterstrom J, Altman D. Vaginal hysterectomy and risk of pelvic organ prolapse and stress urinary incontinence surgery. Int Urogynecol J. 2012;23(1):43–8. Epub 2011/08/19.
21. Hannestad YS, Rortveit G, Daltveit AK, Hunskaar S. Are smoking and other lifestyle factors associated with female urinary incontinence? The Norwegian EPINCONT Study. BJOG. 2003;110(3):247–54. Epub 2003/03/12.
22. Danforth KN, Shah AD, Townsend MK, Lifford KL, Curhan GC, Resnick NM, et al. Physical activity and urinary incontinence among healthy, older women. Obstet Gynecol. 2007;109(3): 721–7. Epub 2007/03/03.

Metabolic Alkalosis

16

Michael Gierth, Bernhard Banas, and Maximilian Burger

16.1 Definition

Metabolic alkalosis is a metabolic condition with an elevated pH beyond the normal range (7.35–7.45). This is the result of primarily increased bicarbonate plasma concentrations or decreased hydrogen ion concentration leading to a relative excess of plasma bicarbonate. Secondary or compensatory processes that cause an elevation in plasma bicarbonate should be separated from primary processes [1, 2].

16.2 Pathophysiology

Three main mechanisms lead to the development of a metabolic alkalosis:

1. Net loss of hydrogen ions from the extracellular fluid (ECF), either gastrointestinal or renal
2. Net addition of bicarbonate or bicarbonate precursors to the ECF
3. External loss of fluids containing high chloride but low bicarbonate concentrations (leading to the so-called contraction alkalosis)

The initiating processes for metabolic alkalosis may be a gain of alkali in the ECF (extracellular fluid) from an exogenous or an endogenous source or the loss of

Conflict of Interest
The authors declare that there is no conflict of interest in relation to this article.

M. Gierth • M. Burger, MD (✉)
Department of Urology, Caritas St. Josef Medical Centre, University of Regensburg,
Landshuter Strasse 65, Regensburg 93053, Germany
e-mail: michael.gierth@ukr.de; maximilian.burger@ukr.de

B. Banas
Department of Nephrology, University of Regensburg,
Landshuter Strasse 65, Regensburg 93053, Germany
e-mail: bernhard.banas@ukr.de

A.S. Merseburger et al. (eds.), *Urology at a Glance*,
DOI 10.1007/978-3-642-54859-8_16, © Springer-Verlag Berlin Heidelberg 2014

protons from ECF via kidneys or via the stomach. Beside hepatic metabolism of citrate, lactate or acetate to bicarbonate can cause a brief metabolic alkalosis. Chloride depletion reduced glomerular filtration rate (GFR), potassium depletion and ECF volume depletion can lead to persisting metabolic alkalosis [3, 4].

In some disorders (e.g. vomiting), volume depletion and potassium depletion may coexist. Severe potassium depletion alone can cause a metabolic alkalosis but typically of a mild to moderate degree. The mechanism is related to an intracellular shift of H+ in exchange for K+. While alkalosis is generated predominantly due to non-renal mechanisms, renal mechanisms are frequently involved in potassium depletion [5].

Volume depletion is implicated in maintenance of alkalosis since hypovolaemia is associated with increased fluid and sodium reabsorption in the proximal renal tubule. Bicarbonate is reabsorbed in preference to chloride, leading to maintenance of alkalosis [6]. Nevertheless, the coexisting chloride depletion is the most important factor for the persistence of alkalosis.

Diuretics can cause excess renal loss of nonvolatile (= fixed) acid anions and result in alkalosis. Their use can lead to depletion of chloride, water, and potassium. These factors together maintain the alkalosis.

Renal compensation for metabolic alkalosis consists of increased excretion of bicarbonate, as the filtered load of bicarbonate exceeds the ability of the renal tubule to reabsorb it, which is only efficiently excreted if concentration exceeds 24 mmol/l. Impairment of renal bicarbonate excretion can in turn cause persistence of the metabolic alkalosis. Since renal compensation for metabolic alkalosis is much more effective than respiratory, metabolic alkalosis rarely occurs in healthy renal status. However, in pathological renal status, compensatory mechanisms for metabolic alkalosis are mainly respiratory. Hypoventilation leads to the retention of carbon dioxide (CO_2), which is then transformed to carbonic acid, thus decreasing pH. In turn, PCO_2 is increased inhibiting hypoventilation by stimulating central chemoreceptors sensitive to the partial pressure of CO_2 increasing respiration again [7–9].

In urological care metabolic alkalosis may also be caused by excess intake of bicarbonate applied for correction of metabolic acidosis related to continent urinary diversion.

16.3 Diagnostic and Differential Diagnosis

While dehydration is the most prominent clinical symptom of metabolic alkalosis, symptoms often may not be noticeable [10]. Laboratory tests show blood pH >7.45. Levels of potassium, sodium, and chloride fall below normal ranges. Bicarbonate levels in the blood will usually exceed 29 mEq/l. Urine pH may rise to 7.0.

Assessment of urinary chloride can be useful and define two subgroups: Firstly, urinary chloride levels lower than 10 mmol/l usually originate from previous thiazide diuretic therapy, from vomiting, or in fewer cases from volume depletion with

Table 16.1 Differential diagnoses of metabolic alkalosis

Addition of base to ECF
Milk-alkali syndrome
Excessive $NaHCO_3$ intake
Recovery phase from organic acidosis (excess regeneration of HCO_3)
Massive blood transfusion (due metabolism of citrate)
Chloride depletion
Loss of acidic gastric juice
Diuretics
Post-hypercapnia
Excess faecal loss (e.g. villous adenoma)
Potassium depletion
Primary hyperaldosteronism
Cushing's syndrome
Secondary hyperaldosteronism
Some drugs (e.g. carbenoxolone)
Kaliuretic diuretics
Excessive liquorice intake (glycyrrhizic acid)
Bartter's syndrome
Severe potassium depletion
Other disorders
Laxative abuse
Severe hypoalbuminaemia

increased proximal tubular reabsorption of bicarbonate or from saline infusion. Secondly, urinary chloride levels higher than 20 mmol/l originate from severe hypokalaemia, current diuretic therapy, or Bartter's syndrome and are often associated with volume expansion and resistance to therapy with saline infusion. The urinary chloride/creatinine ratio may be elevated in extra-renal alkalosis [6]. Table 16.1 shows differential diagnoses for metabolic alkalosis.

16.4 Treatment

While the underlying cause of metabolic alkalosis must be corrected, symptomatic treatment focuses on correcting the aforementioned imbalances. Intravenous correction of hypovolaemia, chloride, or potassium is indicated in more severe cases. Drugs to regulate blood pressure or heart rate or to control nausea and vomiting might be given. Vital signs like pulse, respiration, blood pressure, and body temperature will be monitored [10]. Figure 16.1 demonstrates the typical pathway of metabolic alkalosis.

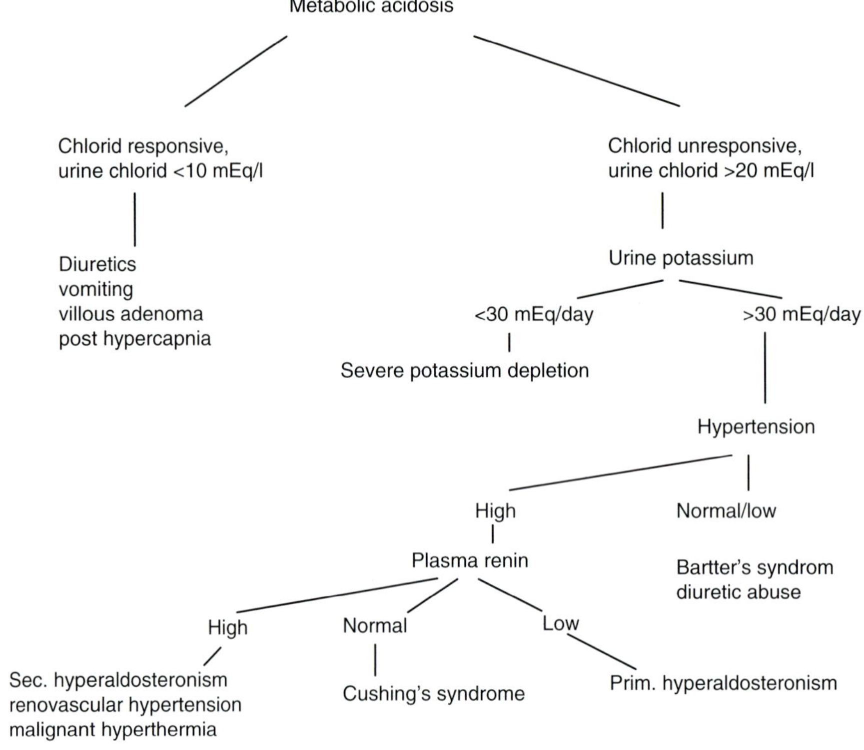

Fig. 16.1 Clinical pathway of metabolic alkalosis [6, 7, 11]

References

1. Khanna A, Kurtzman NA. Metabolic alkalosis. Respir Care. 2001;46:354–65.
2. Pahari DK, Kazmi W, Raman G, et al. Diagnosis and management of metabolic alkalosis. J Indian Med Assoc. 2006;104:630–4, 636.
3. Driscoll DF, Bistrian BR, et al. Development of metabolic alkalosis after massive transfusion during orthotopic liver transplantation. Crit Care Med. 1987;15:905–8.
4. Berger BE, Cogan MG, Sebastian A. Reduced glomerular filtration and enhanced bicarbonate reabsorption maintain metabolic alkalosis in humans. Kidney Int. 1984;26:205–8.
5. Hernandez RE, Schambelan M, Cogan MG, et al. Dietary NaCl determines severity of potassium depletion-induced metabolic alkalosis. Kidney Int. 1987;31:1356–67.
6. Palmer BF, Alpern RJ. Metabolic alkalosis. J Am Soc Nephrol. 1997;8:1462–9.
7. Gluck SL. Acid-base. Lancet. 1998;352:474–9.
8. Gennari FJ. Pathophysiology of metabolic alkalosis: a new classification based on the centrality of stimulated collecting duct ion transport. Am J Kidney Dis. 2011;58:626–36.
9. Jacobson HR. Medullary collecting duct acidification. Effects of potassium, HCO3 concentration, and pCO2. J Clin Invest. 1984;74:2107–14.
10. Webster NR, Kulkarni V. Metabolic alkalosis in the critically ill. Crit Rev Clin Lab Sci. 1999;36:497–510.
11. Adrogue HJ, Madias NE. Management of life-threatening acid-base disorders. Second of two parts. N Engl J Med. 1998;338:107–11.

Metabolic Acidosis

17

Christian Niedworok and Christian Rehme

17.1 Definition

A reduction of serum bicarbonate (HCO_3^-) and decrease of blood pH combined with a decrease of the arterial partial pressure of carbon dioxide (pCO_2) represent the measurable changes in the metabolism of a metabolic acidosis. The metabolic acidosis can occur as an acute (hours to days) or chronic (weeks to years) disease, presenting itself in different clinical symptoms. The acute form of the metabolic acidosis usually occurs when an oversupply of acidotic metabolic waste products overwhelms the physiologic extinction mechanisms for acid compounds. Loss of bicarbonate and renal insufficiency most frequently are the reasons for a chronic metabolic acidosis [1].

There is a wide range of clinical symptoms characterizing a metabolic acidosis. Mild forms are clinically inapparent, and moderate and severe forms lead to cardiovascular disorders like hypo- or hypertension, cardiac arrhythmias, venoconstriction, impairment of cardiac contractility, and development of edema. Apart from cardiovascular disorders numerous metabolic effects can be affected and appear as loss of weight by wasting of muscle tissue, increasing risk of skeletal events (e.g., bone fractures), prediabetic metabolic state by cellular insulin resistance, reduced answer to infectious diseases by changes in leukocyte function and interleukin production, and changes in mental status and behavior [2–4]. Chronic metabolic acidosis also can result in osteoporosis and pathological fractures when undetected.

C. Niedworok, FEBU (✉) • C. Rehme
Department of Urology, Essen Medical School, University Duisburg-Essen,
Hufelandstrasse 55, Essen 45122, Germany
e-mail: christian.niedworok@uk-essen.de; christian.rehme@uk-essen.de

A.S. Merseburger et al. (eds.), *Urology at a Glance*,
DOI 10.1007/978-3-642-54859-8_17, © Springer-Verlag Berlin Heidelberg 2014

17.2 Medical History

The patient should be questioned about his general physical condition and whether the symptoms began slowly or acute. The medical history of a patient should also include detailed questions about operations the patient has had. In urologic patients a metabolic acidosis can occur when an operative bladder removal was performed due to a bladder disease. An acquired lacking of the bladder requires the construction of a urinary diversion. The urine is diverted either by performing a ureterocutaneostomy or by using intestine tissue for constructing an intracorporal reservoir as continent or an ileum conduit or colon conduit as incontinent urinary diversion [5]. Commonly used intestinal tissue for urinary diversions is either small or large intestine; in selected cases a ureterosigmoideostomy can be performed. Rarely the stomach is used to create a urinary diversion [6]. All urinary diversions using intestinal tissue tend to develop a metabolic acidosis except from the stomach that tends to develop an alkalosis. Reason for this finding is the fact that the intestinal tissue keeps its absorption abilities. Thereby one of the crucial factors for developing a metabolic acidosis is the time the urine comes in contact with the intestinal tissue. For this reason, incontinent diversions like the ileum conduit have lower tendency to develop metabolic status [7]. The probability for metabolic status increases when continent diversions are performed. Patients with urine transportation disorders after urologic operations or obstructions in the efferent urinary tract tend to develop metabolic acidosis due to a reduction in the renal capability of elimination of acid compounds.

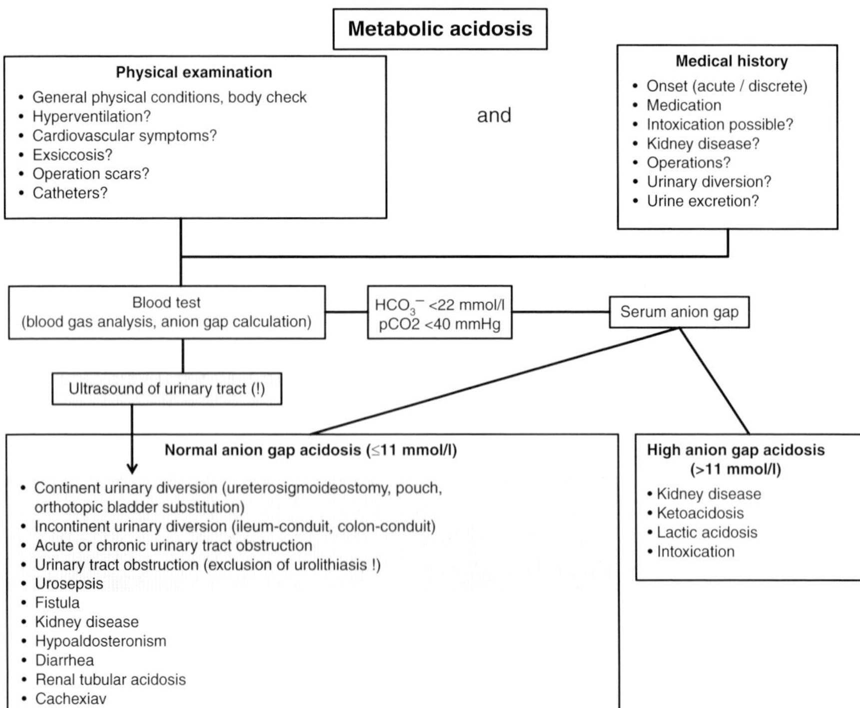

17.3 Diagnostics

Pathophysiologic mechanism of metabolic acidosis due to urinary diversion is a reabsorption of ammonium (NH_4^+) and chloride (Cl^-) from the urine. To secrete ammonium (NH_4^+), bicarbonate (HCO_3^-) is secreted and a proton (H^+) and chloride (Cl^-) are absorbed, resulting in a hyperchloremic acidosis with a lack of bicarbonate [8]. An immediate reaction of the respiratory tract, characterized by hyperventilation, is an acute consequence of metabolic acidosis. This reaction of the organism is easy to notice and the first step in diagnostic approach that should always include a thoroughly physical examination. In severe cases a Kussmaul breathing, presented as deep and labored breathing, is a pathognomonic sign of acidotic metabolic status [9]. Initially, a mild hypocapnia caused by hyperventilation compensates a decrease of serum pH. Further diagnostic bases upon a blood gas analysis and further blood diagnostics. Loss of bicarbonate results in decreased serum bicarbonate levels and a reduction of the base excess (reference level 0 ±2 mmol/l). The blood pH (reference 7, 35–7, 42) also can be reduced, although in mild chronic acidosis, blood pH may be within the normal range. To evaluate additional effects of metabolic status, checking of serum electrolyte levels is mandatory. A further helpful diagnostic means in the management of metabolic acidosis is the calculation of the anion gap. The serum anion gap is defined as the difference between the cation sodium and the anions chloride and bicarbonate ($Na^+ - [Cl^- + HCO_3^-]$, reference 3–11 mmol/l). Usually the loss of bicarbonate is compensated by elevation of chloride. But the anion gap also can be compensated by further anionic acids like ketone bodies, lactate, phosphate, or sulfate which are not analyzed in anion gap calculation. The analysis of the anion gap then gives evidence about the origin of the metabolic disorder [10]. Typically, in patients with urinary diversions and metabolic acidosis, a normal anion gap is found because the loss of bicarbonate triggers a hyperchloremic acidosis, and the stoichiometric difference between chloride and bicarbonate is balanced.

Frequently an acidotic metabolic status implicates a variety of different symptoms. An often seen concomitant symptom is an exsiccosis which should moderately be compensated to prevent further electrolyte disturbances. In urologic patients with a history of urinary diversion, an ultrasound examination of the intracorporal urine reservoir (if existing) and the kidneys should always be performed. If a urinary transportation disorder is seen and suspect as reason for the metabolic situation, the ectasia should be released by catheterization or a draining puncture in the acute situation. An obstruction of the urinary tract can occur in combination with an infection in the section proximal of the obstruction. This circumstance can result in a urosepsis with a possible consecutive need to intensive care treatment in severe cases. Every patient who is known or estimated for chronic metabolic status should be questioned about bone pain or muscle cramps to perform special examinations (conventional X-ray investigation, CT scan, bone densitometry, or skeletal scintigraphy) if necessary. As chronic acidosis can cause calculosis, every patient known for long-lasting acidotic metabolism should be questioned and examined particularly with regard to urolithiasis [11].

17.4 Differential Diagnosis

See Fig. 17.1.

Chronic or acute pre-, intra- or postrenal kidney disease
Intoxikation by digestion- or inhalation (e.g. ethanol, methanol, glycol, carbon monoxid or dioxid, organic and anorganic solvents)
Drug intoxication (NSAR, spironolactone, amiloride, pentamidine, paracetamol, triamterene, ciclosporin)
Ketoacidosis (diabetic, alcoholic, fasting)
Lactic acidosis
Urinary diversions (ileum conduit, ureterosigmoideostomy, orthotopic bladder substitute, pouch)
Urinary tract obstruction
Fistula (vesicointestinal, biliodigestive, pancreaticodigestive, intestinal)
Chronic or acute infection, sepsis, urosepsis
Adrenal insufficiency
Renal tubular acidosis
Diarrhea
Tumor related cachexia
Hypoaldosteronism

Fig. 17.1 Differential diagnosis of metabolic acidosis

References

1. Kraut JA, Kurtz I. Metabolic acidosis of CKD: diagnosis, clinical characteristics, and treatment. Am J Kidney Dis. 2005;45(6):978–93.
2. Kraut JA, Madias NE. Metabolic acidosis: pathophysiology, diagnosis and management. Nat Rev Nephrol. 2010;6(5):274–85.
3. World Health Organization (WHO) Consensus Conference on Bladder Cancer, Hautmann RE, Abol-Enein H, Hafez K, Haro I, Mansson W, Mills RD, Montie JD, Sagalowsky AI, Stein JP, Stenzl A, Studer UE, Volkmer BG. Urinary diversion. Urology. 2007;69(1 Suppl):17–49.
4. Mills RD, Studer UE. Metabolic consequences of continent urinary diversion. J Urol. 1999;161(4):1057–66.
5. Oosterlinck W, Lobel B, Jakse G, Malmström PU, Stöckle M, Sternberg C, European Association of Urology (EAU) Working Group on Oncological Urology. Guidelines on bladder cancer. Eur Urol. 2002;41(2):105–12.
6. Zugor V, Schreiber M, Klein P, Schott GE. Urinary bladder augmentation using the stomach in patients with compensated renal insufficiency [article in German]. Urologe A. 2007;46(6):667–70.
7. Davidsson T, Lindergård B, Månsson W. Long-term metabolic and nutritional effects of urinary diversion. Urology. 1995;46(6):804–9.
8. Weiner ID, Hamm LL. Molecular mechanisms of renal ammonia transport. Annu Rev Physiol. 2007;69:317–40.
9. Kussmaul A. Zur Lehre vom Diabetes mellitus. Über eine eigenthümliche Todesart bei Diabetischen, über Acetonämie, Glycerin-Behandlung des Diabetes und Einspritzungen von Diastase in's Blut bei dieser Krankheit. Deutsches Archiv klinische Medicin, Leipzig. 1874;14:1–46. [Thomas CC. English translation in Ralph Hermon Major (1884–1970), classic descriptions of disease. Springfield; 1932. 2nd ed, 1939. 3rd ed, 1945].
10. Emmett M. Anion-gap interpretation: the old and the new. Nat Clin Pract Nephrol. 2006;2(1):4–5.
11. Wagner CA, Mohebbi N. Urinary pH and stone formation. J Nephrol. 2010;23 Suppl 16:S165–9.

Hypo-/Hypercalcemia 18

Mehmet Özsoy and Christian Seitz

18.1 Definition

Calcium (Ca) is a vital element of human physiology. It acts as an important regulator in numerous intracellular and extracellular processes within the human body including hormone release, transmitting nerve signals, muscle contraction, plasma coagulation, and enzyme regulation.

Almost all of body Ca is stored in bones. Plasma calcium levels are strictly regulated. Approximately 1 % of bone Ca is freely exchangeable with extracellular fluid and can be used to regulate plasma Ca balance.

Total plasma Ca levels in healthy individuals range from 2.20 to 2.60 mmol/l (8.8–10.4 mg/dl). Approximately 40 % of total plasma Ca is bound to plasma proteins mainly albumin. The remaining consists of ionized Ca and Ca complexed with phosphate and citrate. Ideally the ionized Ca should be determined as this is the physiologically active form.

A balanced dietary Ca intake, Ca absorption from GI tract in jejunum and proximal ileum, and renal Ca excretion help maintain the necessary calcium storage and plasma calcium concentration.

Kidneys filter approximately 270 mmol of calcium and must reabsorb more than 98 % of it to keep body's Ca levels in balance. The main renal reabsorption site is the proximal tubule.

Calcium and phosphate balance is dependent on parathyroid hormone (PTH), vitamin D, and calcitonin.

M. Özsoy (✉) • C. Seitz
Department of Urology, Medical University of Vienna,
Waehringer Guertel 18-20, Vienna A-1090, Austria
e-mail: mehmet.oezsoy@meduniwien.ac.at; drseitz@gmx.at

A.S. Merseburger et al. (eds.), *Urology at a Glance*,
DOI 10.1007/978-3-642-54859-8_18, © Springer-Verlag Berlin Heidelberg 2014

Hypocalcemia is a decrease in total plasma calcium concentration below 2.20 mmol/l (8.8 mg/dl) in the presence of normal plasma protein concentration. The most common causes are hypoparathyroidism, idiopathic hypoparathyroidism, pseudoparathyroidism, vitamin D deficiency, renal tubular disease, hypoproteinemia, and hypomagnesemia.

Hypercalcemia is an increase in total plasma calcium concentration above 2.60 mmol/l (10.4 mg/dl). Excessive bone resorption resulting from increased PTH levels or malignancies with bone metastasis, excessive GI calcium absorption, Addison's disease, and prolonged treatment with thiazide diuretics are some of the most common causes.

18.2 Medical History

Medical history taking should start with a thorough questioning of previous illnesses that could cause hypo-/hypercalcemia. In addition patient's nutritional habits should be questioned in order to evaluate excessive or insufficient Ca intake. Regular daily medication should also be investigated as prolonged intake of certain medicines such as phenytoin, phenobarbital, rifampin, and furosemide or thiazide diuretics could alter Ca hemostasis. Irregularities in defecation such as diarrhea or obstipation are not just symptoms but can also manifest as causes for Ca balance disturbances.

18.3 Diagnostics

Diagnosis is established through measurement of blood calcium levels. Both hypo- and hypercalcemia especially in their mild state are mostly asymptomatic and often diagnosed accidentally during routine laboratory screening.

Clinical manifestations of hypocalcemia arise from neuromuscular irritability due to altered cellular membrane potential. Muscle cramps and mild/diffuse encephalopathy resulting in depression or dementia are some of the common symptoms. Prolonged hypocalcemia can lead to papilledema or cataracts. Severe hypocalcemia with Ca levels <1.75 mmol/l (<7 mg/dl) can manifest with tetany, laryngospasm, or generalized convulsions. Hyperventilation-induced tetany due to anxiety disorders should be taken into consideration as a possible differential diagnosis. Furthermore, arrhythmias can occasionally develop among severe cases. In ECG prolongation of QTc and ST intervals, T peaking, or T inversion can be observed. In chronic hypocalcemia, dry skin, coarse hair, and brittle nails can be seen. Candida infections occasionally occur especially in patients with idiopathic hypoparathyroidism.

PTH deficiency or absence causes hypoparathyroidism. This is almost always accompanied with hypocalcemia and hyperphosphatemia and is often associated with tetany. Hypoparathyroidism could be a result of accidental removal of parathyroid glands during thyroidectomy or operation on the parathyroid gland itself. If PTH levels are undetectable, idiopathic parathyroidism should be taken into consideration as the cause. This is a rare condition that can occur sporadically or be inherited and is characterized with atrophy or absence of parathyroid glands. It manifests as an early onset during childhood and may be associated with Addison's disease.

Pseudoparathyroidism is a group of disorders resulting not from a PTH deficiency but target organ resistance to it. Type 1 pseudoparathyroidism manifests itself with hypocalcemia and normal or even elevated levels of PTH. These patients fail to present normal renal response to PTH and lack phosphaturia. The diagnosis of Type 2 pseudoparathyroidism requires the exclusion of vitamin D deficiency.

In patients with osteomalacia, plasma phosphate levels are mildly reduced and alkaline phosphatase is elevated. In order to distinguish between vitamin D deficiency from vitamin D-dependent states, hydroxycholecalciferol and calcitriol levels should be measured.

Clinical manifestations of hypercalcemia are constipation, nausea, vomiting, abdominal pain, ileus, polyuria, nocturia, and polydipsia. In severe cases confusion, delirium, psychosis, and coma can occur. Neuromuscular involvement may result in skeletal muscle weakness. Hypercalciuria (urinary calcium excretion greater than 4 mg/kg/day) is the most common abnormality identified in calcium stone formers. Hypercalcemia may also cause reversible acute renal failure or irreversible renal damage due to precipitation of Ca salts in kidney parenchyma (nephrocalcinosis). In severe hypercalcemia, a shortened QT interval is observed on ECG; cardiac arrhythmias may also occur. Hypercalcemia with Ca levels greater than 4.50 mmol/l (18 mg/dl) can result in renal failure, shock, and death.

Primary hyperparathyroidism is a common cause of hypercalciuria and is often associated with nephrolithiasis. It manifests with hypercalcemia, hypophosphatemia, and excessive bone resorption. In hospitalized patients, on the other hand, immobilization with prolonged bed rests such as after orthopedic or spinal surgeries can cause hypercalcemia due to accelerated bone resorption. Malignancy-associated hypercalcemia is another common cause of hypercalciuria in hospitalized patients. Tumors produce PTH-related protein (PTHrP) which over humoral pathways activates osteoclasts and results in bone lysis and hence hypercalcemia.

Many granulomatous diseases are known to cause hypercalcemia including tuberculosis, sarcoidosis, histoplasmosis, etc. Sarcoidosis is commonly associated with urolithiasis.

Besides medical history and clinical findings, radiographic evidence of bone disease may also help diagnose underlying cause of hypercalcemia.

Familial hypocalciuric hypercalcemia is a syndrome defined by the presence of hypermagnesemia and hypercalcemia without excessive renal calcium excretion. These patients normally do not develop nephrolithiasis.

18.4 Differential Diagnosis

Hypocalcemia	Hypercalcemia
Hypoparathyroidism	Hyperparathyroidism
Pseudohypoparathyroidism	Malignant tumors
Vitamin D deficiency	Vitamin D toxicity
Renal tubular disease	Hyperthyroidism
Renal failure	Sarcoidosis
Magnesium depletion	Addison's disease
Acute pancreatitis	Pheochromocytoma
Hungry bone syndrome	Immobilization
Septic shock	Lithium intoxication
Hyperphosphatemia	Primary increase in 1, 25(OH)2D
Furosemide intake	Thiazide intake
	Paget disease

18.5 Diagnostic Work Flow

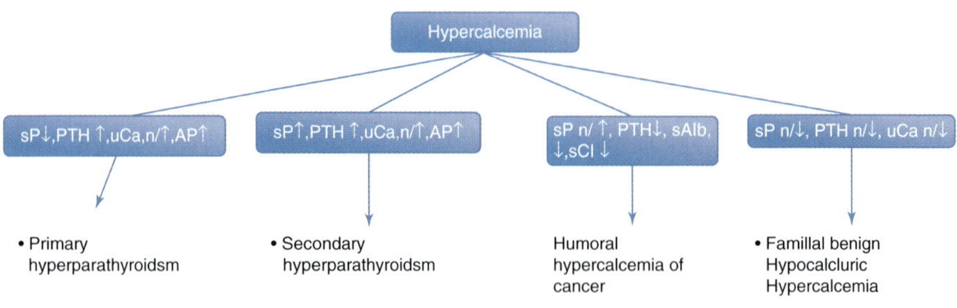

P Phosphate, PTH Parathyroid hormone, Ca Calcium, AP Alkaline Phosphatase,Alb Albumin, Cl Chloride, s Serum levels, n normal

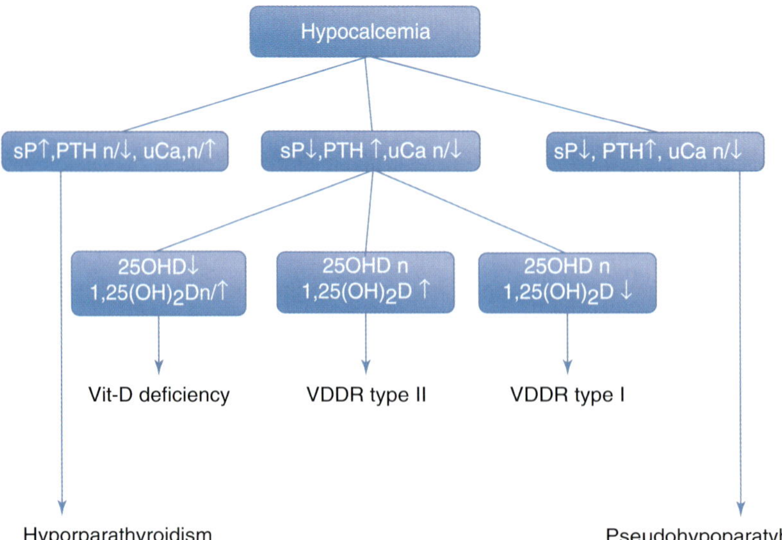

P Phosphate, PTH Parathyroid hormone, Ca Calcium, 25OHD hydroxycholecalciferol, 1.25(OH)2D Calcitriol, s Serum levels, n normal, VDDR Vitamin D Dependent Rickets

Hypokalemia

19

Reinhard Brunkhorst

19.1 Definition

Hypokalemia is defined as a serum potassium of <3.5 mmol/l. It is graded in mild (potassium 3–3.5 mmol/l, whole body deficit 130–300 mmol/l), moderate (potassium 2.5–3.0 mmol/l, whole body deficit 300–500 mmol/l), and severe (potassium <2.5 mmol/l, whole body deficit >500 mmol/l).

19.2 Medical History

Most of the causes of hypokalemia such as severe vomiting, diarrhea, eating disorder, and medication (diuretics, laxative abuse, steroids, cisplatin, etc.) become evident by history. Mild hypokalemia may cause a small elevation of blood pressure and cardiac arrhythmias. Moderate hypokalemia may cause muscular weakness, myalgia, muscle cramps, and constipation. With more severe hypokalemia, flaccid paralysis and hyporeflexia may result. There are reports of rhabdomyolysis and respiratory depression.

R. Brunkhorst
Klinik für Nieren-, Hochdruck- und Gefässerkrankungen, Klinikum Oststadt-Heidehaus, Klinikum Region Hannover GmbH, Podbielskistr. 380, Hannover 30659, Germany
e-mail: sekretariat.brunkhorst.oststadt@klinikum-hannover.de

A.S. Merseburger et al. (eds.), *Urology at a Glance*,
DOI 10.1007/978-3-642-54859-8_19, © Springer-Verlag Berlin Heidelberg 2014

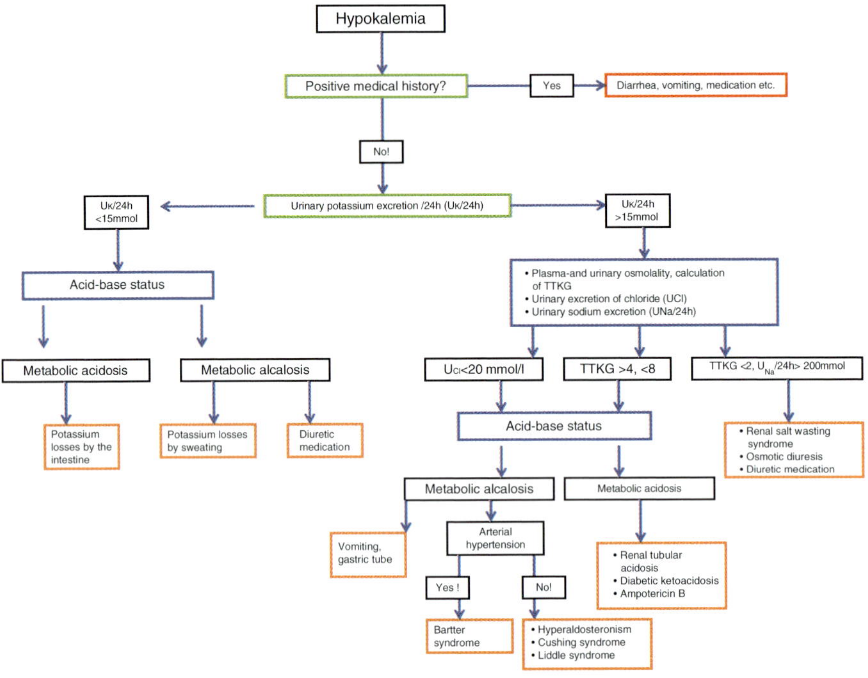

19.3 Diagnostics

Electrocardiographic (ECG) findings associated with hypokalemia include *flattened or inverted T waves*, a U wave, ST depression, and a wide PR interval. Laboratory tests include urinary sodium excretion per day, plasma and urinary osmolality, acid-base status, chloride excretion, and serum sodium.

19.4 Differential Diagnosis

The *trans-tubular potassium gradient* (*TTKG*) is helpful when urinary potassium losses (>15 mmol/24 h) are present; it estimates the ratio of potassium in the lumen of the cortical collecting ducts of the kidney to that in the peritubular capillaries. The following is the formula for calculating the TTKG:

$$\mathrm{TTKG} = \frac{\mathrm{urine}_{\mathrm{K}}}{\mathrm{plasma}_{\mathrm{K}}} \div \frac{\mathrm{urine}_{\mathrm{osm}}}{\mathrm{plasma}_{\mathrm{osm}}}$$

During high potassium intake, more potassium than normal (TTKG 8–9) should be excreted in the urine and the TTKG should be above ten. Low levels (<7) during hyperkalemia may indicate mineralocorticoid deficiency, especially if accompanied by hyponatremia and high urine Na. During potassium depletion or hypokalemia, the TTKG should fall to less than three, indicating appropriately reduced urinary excretion of potassium (Fig. 19.1).

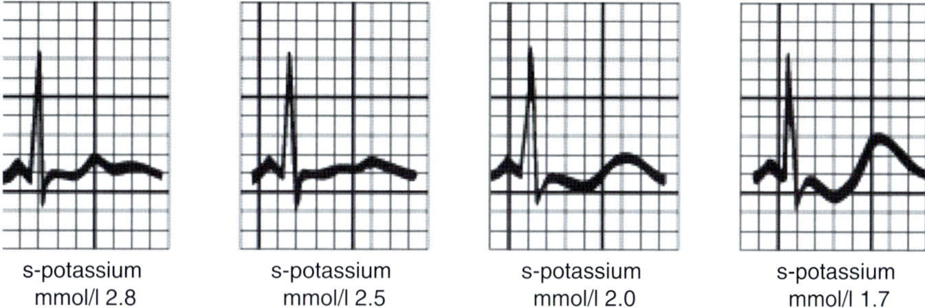

Fig. 19.1 Typical ECG during hypokalemia: *flattened or inverted T waves*, a U wave, and a wide PR interval

Causes of hypokalemia		
Diagnosis	Frequency	Diagnostic measures
Renal losses		
Medication: diuretics, corticosteroids	+++	Medical history, U_K, acid-base status, TTKG
Primary and secondary hyperaldosteronism	+	U_K, TTKG, acid-base status
Osmotic diuresis	+	U_K, TTKG, acid-base status
Enteral losses		
Severe vomiting	+	Medical history, U_K, TTKG, acid-base status, U_{CL}
Chronic diarrhea, laxative abuse	+++	U_K, TTKG, acid-base status
Intracellular shift		
Ileus	++	Medical history, X-ray, and ultrasound of the intestine
Insulin treatment in diabetic ketoacidosis	+	Medical history, U_K, acid-base status, TTKG
Medication: β_2-agonists, theophylline	+	Medical history
Nutritional deficit		
Anorexia nervosa	+	Medical history
Alcoholism	++	Medical history
Rare diseases		
Bartter syndrome	(+)	U_K, TTKG, acid-base status
Liddle syndrome	(+)	U_K, TTKG, acid-base status
Renal tubular acidosis	(+)	U_K, TTKG, acid-base status

Hyperkalemia

20

Reinhard Brunkhorst

20.1 General Facts

Normal serum potassium levels are between 3.5 and 5.0 mmol/l; hyperkalemia refers to serum potassium >5.5 mmol/l. About 98 % of the body's potassium is found inside cells, with the remainder in the extracellular fluid including the blood. Extreme hyperkalemia is a medical emergency due to the risk of potentially fatal arrhythmias.

20.2 Medical History

Medical history should focus on kidney disease and medication use (as, e.g., ACE inhibitors, sartans, aldosterone antagonists), as these are the main causes. The combination of abdominal pain, hypoglycemia, and hyperpigmentation may be signs of Addison's disease. Symptoms are nonspecific and generally include malaise, palpitations, and muscle weakness; mild hyperventilation may indicate a compensatory response to metabolic acidosis, which is one of the possible causes of hyperkalemia. Often, however, hyperkalemia is found during screening or after complications have developed, such as cardiac arrhythmia or sudden death.

R. Brunkhorst
Klinik für Nieren-, Hochdruck- und Gefässerkrankungen, Klinikum Oststadt-Heidehaus, Klinikum Region Hannover GmbH, Podbielskistr. 380, Hannover 30659, Germany
e-mail: sekretariat.brunkhorst.oststadt@klinikum-hannover.de

A.S. Merseburger et al. (eds.), *Urology at a Glance*,
DOI 10.1007/978-3-642-54859-8_20, © Springer-Verlag Berlin Heidelberg 2014

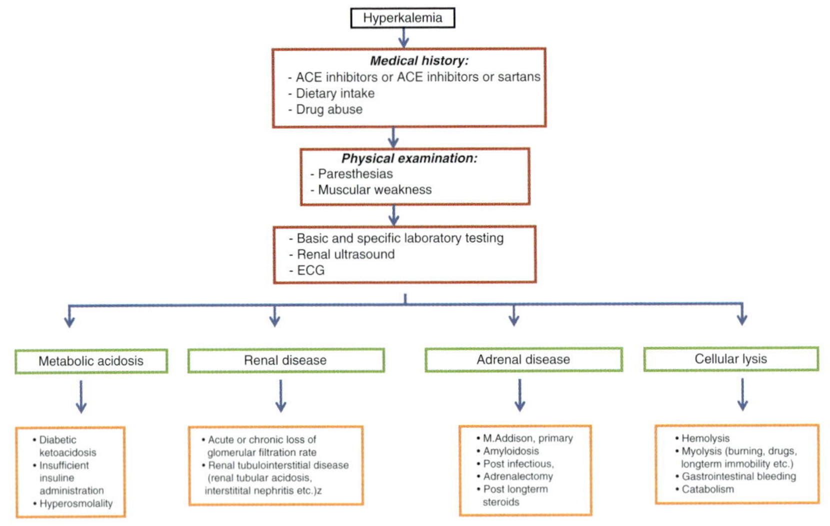

20.3 Diagnostics

Measurement of potassium needs to be repeated, as the elevation can be due to hemolysis in the first sample. Generally, blood tests for renal function (creatinine, blood urea nitrogen), acid–base status, creatine kinase, lactate dehydrogenase, glucose, and occasionally cortisol and aldosterone will be performed. Measuring plasma and urinary osmolality and calculating the trans-tubular potassium gradient can sometimes help in differential diagnosis.

In many cases, renal ultrasound will be performed, since hyperkalemia often is caused by chronic kidney disease and eventually by an adrenal tumor.

ECG: With mild to moderate hyperkalemia, there is reduction of the size of the P wave and development of peaked T waves. Severe hyperkalemia results in a widening of the QRS complex, and the ECG complex can evolve to a sinusoidal shape. Bradycardia, extra systoles, complex ventricular arrhythmias, and bundle branch blocking are frequently observed. Without rapid intervention (i.v. glucose/insulin, sodium bicarbonate, calcium carbonate, hemodialysis), arrhythmias may be fatal (Fig. 20.1).

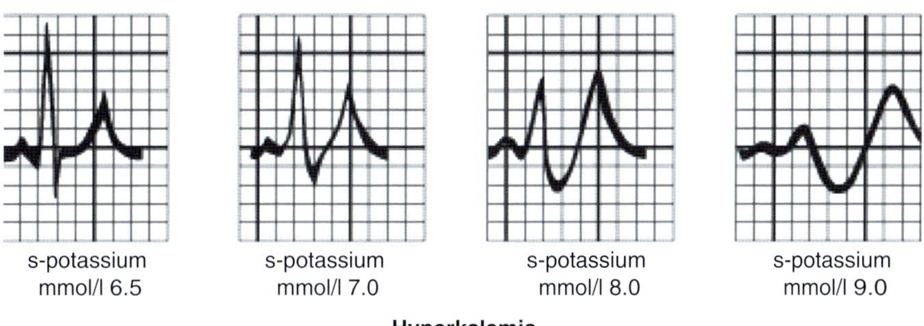

Fig. 20.1 Peaked T waves, widening of the QRS complex, and a ECG complex evolving to a sinusoidal shape with increasing hyperkalemia

20.4 Differential Diagnosis

Diagnosis	Frequency	Diagnostic measures
Acute or chronic kidney disease	++++	Serum creatinine, glomerular filtration rate, renal ultrasound (urinary stasis, kidney size), acid–base status
Diabetes mellitus with insufficient insulin administration	+++	Blood glucose, acid–base status
Myolysis with "crush kidney"	+	Drug abuse, creatine kinase, lactate dehydrogenase
Renal tubular acidosis	+	Acid–base status, urinary electrolytes, serum creatinine, TTKG
M. Addison, M. Cushing	+	Serum–urinary aldosterone and cortisol, ACTH test

Hypogonadism

21

Chris Protzel, Oliver W. Hakenberg, and Kay G. Ballauf

21.1 Definition

The male hypogonadism is an endocrinological disorder with a testosterone deficiency. In the axis hypothalamus, pituitary and testes, the primary hypogonadism and the secondary hypogonadism can be defined by the origin of disturbance.

The primary (hypergonadotropic) hypogonadism is an impaired (either congenital or acquired) testicular function leading to decreased levels of testosterone and elevated levels of gonadotropins. A disorder in the hypothalamic and pituitary area with an abnormal releasing hormone secretion mainly leads to decreased gonadotropins and testosterone levels and is called secondary (hypogonadotropic) hypogonadism (Fig. 21.1).

The lack of testosterone as a result of mixed conditions – as described in primary and secondary hypogonadism – is named late-onset hypogonadism. The recently described term is often accompanied by symptoms of a metabolic syndrome and predominately affects the older men [6].

Other causes of male hypogonadism can be the resistance of androgens in target organs caused by mutations of the androgen receptor or the enzyme deficiency of 5-alpha-reductase with a lack of the active metabolite dihydrotestosterone.

21.2 Medical History

The medical history should include secondary illnesses, chronic diseases, previous operations and injuries. The beginning of puberty and the change of voice should be registered. Questions regarding a decreased performance, hot flushes, less beard growth, psychological changes (lack of interests, weakness and depressions),

C. Protzel (✉) • O.W. Hakenberg • K.G. Ballauf
Department of Urology, University of Rostock,
Ernst-Heydemann-Straße 6, Rostock 18055, Germany
e-mail: chris.protzel@med.uni-rostock.de

A.S. Merseburger et al. (eds.), *Urology at a Glance*,
DOI 10.1007/978-3-642-54859-8_21, © Springer-Verlag Berlin Heidelberg 2014

Symptoms of hypogonadism		
Before puberty	**Feature**	**After puberty**
Unclosed epiphyses Eunuchoid habitus	**Skeletal**	Osteoporosis
Gynaecomastia Lipomastia	**Breast tissue**	Gynaecomastia Lipomastia
Minimal body hair	**Hair**	Loss of body hair
Sarcopenia	**Musculature**	Sarcopenia
Small testes Infertility	**Gonads**	Arrest of spermatogenesis
	Central nervous system	Fatigue depression Hot flushes
Lack of libido	**Sexuality**	Decreased libido Erectile dysfunction

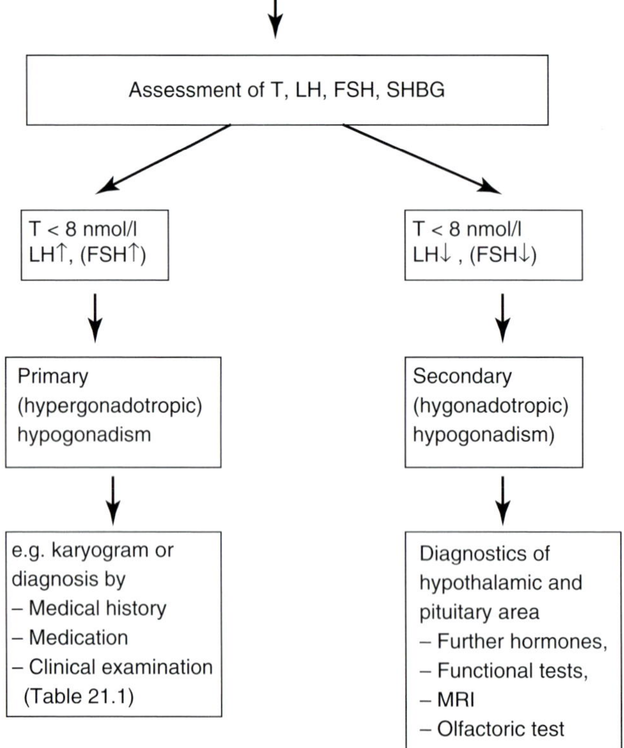

Fig. 21.1 Hypogonadism – from symptoms to diagnosis. *T* testosterone

decreased libido, erectile dysfunction or unvoluntary childlessness are necessary. A detailed history of prescribed medicines and the abuse of anabolics, alcohol, nicotine and drugs are relevant [3].

The versatile symptoms of hypogonadism show a wide range of severity, depending on the first onset and the duration and the degree of the androgen deficiency. In addition genetic factors like the androgen resistance influence the clinical picture [7]. The early onset of male hypogonadism is often related to a delayed, a partial or a lack of puberty. Symptoms of a late-onset hypogonadism are often less impressive [4].

21.3 Diagnostics

The physical examination should include measuring the body mass index (BMI), sagittal abdominal diameter and the observation of body hair or gynaecomastia. A mandatory inspection and palpation of the testes and the penis is completed by an ultrasound of the testes. The transrectal ultrasound can be added to the digital rectal examination. If diagnostics of the hypothalamic-pituitary region are indicated, a magnet resonance imaging (MRI) is needed. Olfactoric test for diagnosing a Kallmann syndrome is necessary.

Basic blood tests are the assessment of testosterone, the gonadotropins (LH, FSH) and sexual hormone binding globulin (SHBG).

For further diagnostics, the assessment of free testosterone, prolactin, TSH, blood lipids, oestradiol, the bone density and a spermiogram can be needed.

The measurement of testosterone should be done in the morning. A value <8 nmol/l is pathologic and its measurement (also LH) must be repeated [1].

For testosterone values between 8 until 12 nmol/l, the calculation of free testosterone is useful [5]. If a secondary hypogonadism is suspected, a GnRH stimulation test is recommended. In cases of a primary hypogonadism, a karyogram is often needed.

21.4 Differential Diagnostics (Table 21.1)

Table 21.1 Reasons for hypogonadism (summary of EAU-guidelines) [2]

Primary hypogonadism	Secondary hypogonadism
Klinefelter syndrome 47 XXY	Hyperprolactinaemia or other pituitary adenomas
46 XX male syndrome	Kallmann syndrome
Anorchia, maldescended or ectopic testis	Idiopathic hypogonadotropic hypogonadism (IHH)
Radiation, trauma operation of the testes	Radiation, trauma, ischemia, operation of the pituitary
Chemotherapy	Haemochromatosis
Orchitis	Secondary GnRH disorders
Testicular tumours	Prader-Willi syndrome
Drugs, medication, toxins, systemic diseases (liver cirrhosis, renal insufficiency)	Drugs, medication
Late-onset hypogonadism	

References

1. Bhasin S, Cunningham GR, Hayes FJ, et al. Testosterone therapy in men with androgen deficiency syndromes: an Endocrine Society clinical practice guideline. J Clin Endocrinol Metab. 2010;95(6):2536–59.
2. Dohle GR, Arver S, Bettocchi C, Kliesch S, Punab M, De Ronde W. J Reproduc Med Endokrime 2013;10(5–6):279–92.
3. Hall SA, Esche GR, Araujo AB, Travison TG, Clark RV, Williams RE, McKinlay JB. Correlates of low testosterone and symptomatic androgen deficiency in a population-based sample. J Clin Endocrinol Metab. 2008;93(10):3870–7.
4. Nieschlag E, Behre HM, editors. Andrology: male reproductive health and dysfunction. 3rd ed. Berlin: Springer; 2010.
5. Vermeulen A, Verdock L, Kaufman JM. A critical evaluation of simple methods for the estimation of free testosterone in serum. J Clion Endocrinol Metab. 1999;74:939–42.
6. Wu FC, Tajar A, Beynon JM, Pye SR, Silman AJ, Finn JD, O'Neill TW, Bartfai G, Cassanueva FF, Fort G, Giwercman A, Han TS, Kula K, Lean ME, Pendleton N, Punab M, Boonen S, Vanderschueren D, Labrie F, Huhtaniemi IT, EMAS Group. Identification of late-onset hypogonadism in middle-aged and elderly men. N Engl J Med. 2010;362(2):123–35.
7. Zitzmann M. Pharmacogenetics of testosterone replacement therapy. Pharmogenomics. 2009;10(8):1341–9.

Hypo- und Hyperglycaemia

22

Robert Wagner and Katarzyna Linder

22.1 Definition

Hyperglycaemia is defined as an inappropriately high plasma glucose which is generally considered at glucose levels higher than 200 mg/dl (11 mmol/l). For the fasting state, glucose values exceeding 126 mg/dl (7 mmol/l) are consistent with hyperglycaemia and diabetes. However, symptoms of hyperglycaemia may often be noticeable only with much higher plasma glucose levels. The cause of hyperglycaemia is a relative or an absolute insulin deficiency which is most often a consequence of diabetes.

The plasma glucose threshold typically used to define *hypoglycaemia* is 70 mg/dl (3.9 mmol/l). The single most prevalent cause of hypoglycaemia is iatrogenic (the use of antidiabetic drugs that cause hypoglycaemia, such as insulin and sulfonylureas). Rare causes include critical illness (sepsis, liver failure and heart failure), adrenal insufficiency, insulin-producing tumours and nonislet cell tumours.

22.2 Medical History

A thorough medical history has to be obtained from patients with hyper- or hypoglycaemia. A key part of the medical history is listing the known conditions, major previous illnesses and former surgical interventions. For patients who are not aware of their chronic diseases, medication history can provide important

R. Wagner, MD (✉) • K. Linder, MD
Division of Endocrinology, Diabetology, Angiology, Nephrology and Clinical Chemistry, Department of Internal Medicine, Eberhard Karls University, University Hospital Tübingen, Otfried-Müller-Str. 10, Tübingen 72076, Germany
e-mail: robert.wagner@med.uni-tuebingen.de; katarzyna.linder@med.uni-tuebingen.de

A.S. Merseburger et al. (eds.), *Urology at a Glance*,
DOI 10.1007/978-3-642-54859-8_22, © Springer-Verlag Berlin Heidelberg 2014

hints for the diagnoses they are being treated for. It cannot be stressed enough how important it is to acquire an exact list of the currently used medications. Often, patients have to be explicitly asked about regular injections (e.g. insulin). Previously known diabetes or the use of antidiabetic drugs can explain both hyperglycaemia and hypoglycaemia. Insulin, sulfonylureas (usually glibenclamide/glyburide, glimepiride, glipizide) and glinides (nateglinide, repaglinide) can lead to sometimes protracted hypoglycaemia. On the other hand, even well-controlled diabetes can cause hyperglycaemia at times of severe stress, infections and sepsis. Infections, often urinary tract infections, can be a potential cause of hyperglycaemia and ketoacidosis. Glucocorticoid (e.g. prednisolone, dexamethasone) use is another important cause of hyperglycaemia in patients with or without previously known diabetes.

The classic symptoms of hyperglycaemia and diabetes are polyuria, polydipsia and weight loss. Patients can also experience erectile dysfunction, blurred vision, dry skin, recurrent infections (often fungal infection of the genitals), poor wound healing and fatigue. High glucose levels can associate with diabetic ketoacidosis, which is a life-threatening condition manifesting with nausea/vomiting, altered consciousness (somnolence, stupor, coma) and sometimes abdominal pain (pseudoperitonitis diabetica). Another serious complication of severe hyperglycaemia is the hyperglycaemic hyperosmolar state, which usually manifests in the elderly and may lead to neurologic abnormalities and coma. Chronic hyperglycaemia can damage a series of organs and leads to the typical diabetes-related complications (most notably kidneys, retina and peripheral nerves).

Hypoglycaemia first causes autonomic-neurogenic symptoms such as nervousness, tremor, sweating, palpitations and hunger, which can progress to neuroglycopenia marked by behavioural changes, weakness, reduced attention, aggressiveness, disorientation, seizures, loss of consciousness and, if untreated, coma. It is important to know that patients with long diabetes duration and frequent episodes of hypoglycaemia can miss autonomic symptoms and develop hypoglycaemia with neurologic deficits much faster. The term severe hypoglycaemia is used when a patient is dependent on external help to counteract hypoglycaemia. Hypoglycaemia, or suspected hypoglycaemia in unconscious patients, has to be treated without delay to avoid the deterioration of the neurologic status of the patient and prevent potentially serious consequences of a loss of consciousness (e.g. aspiration).

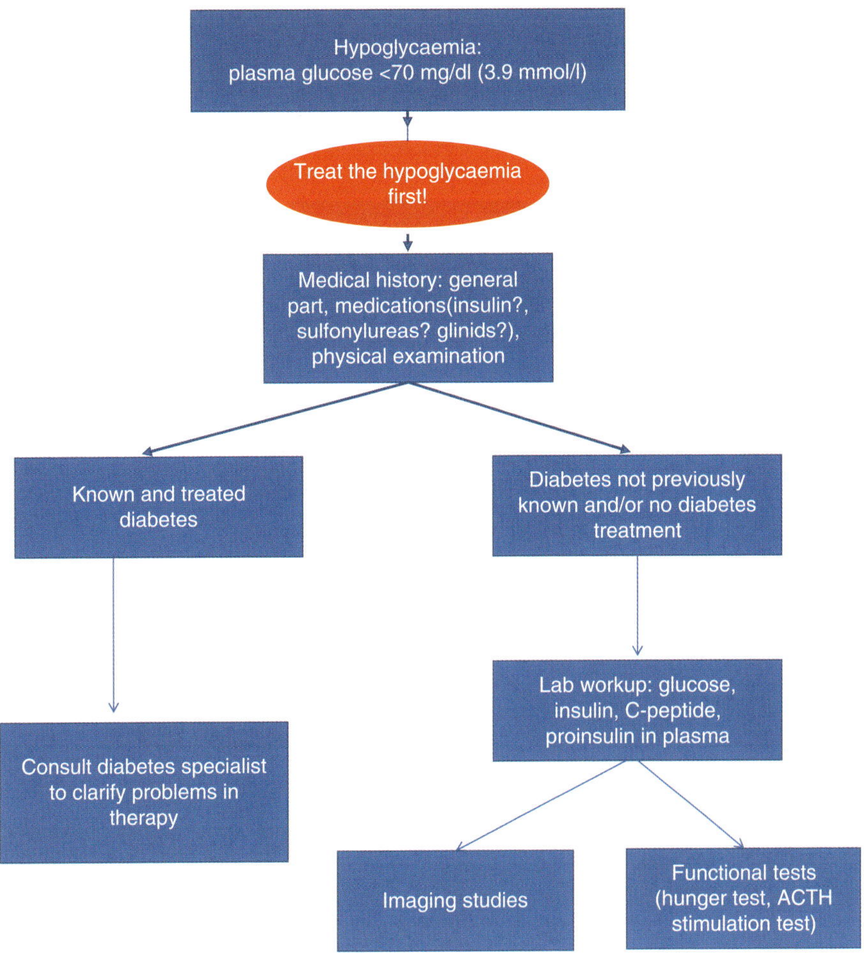
Hypoglycaemia:
plasma glucose <70 mg/dl (3.9 mmol/l)
Treat the hypoglycaemia first!
Medical history: general part, medications(insulin?, sulfonylureas? glinids?), physical examination
Known and treated diabetes
Diabetes not previously known and/or no diabetes treatment
Consult diabetes specialist to clarify problems in therapy
Lab workup: glucose, insulin, C-peptide, proinsulin in plasma
Imaging studies
Functional tests (hunger test, ACTH stimulation test)

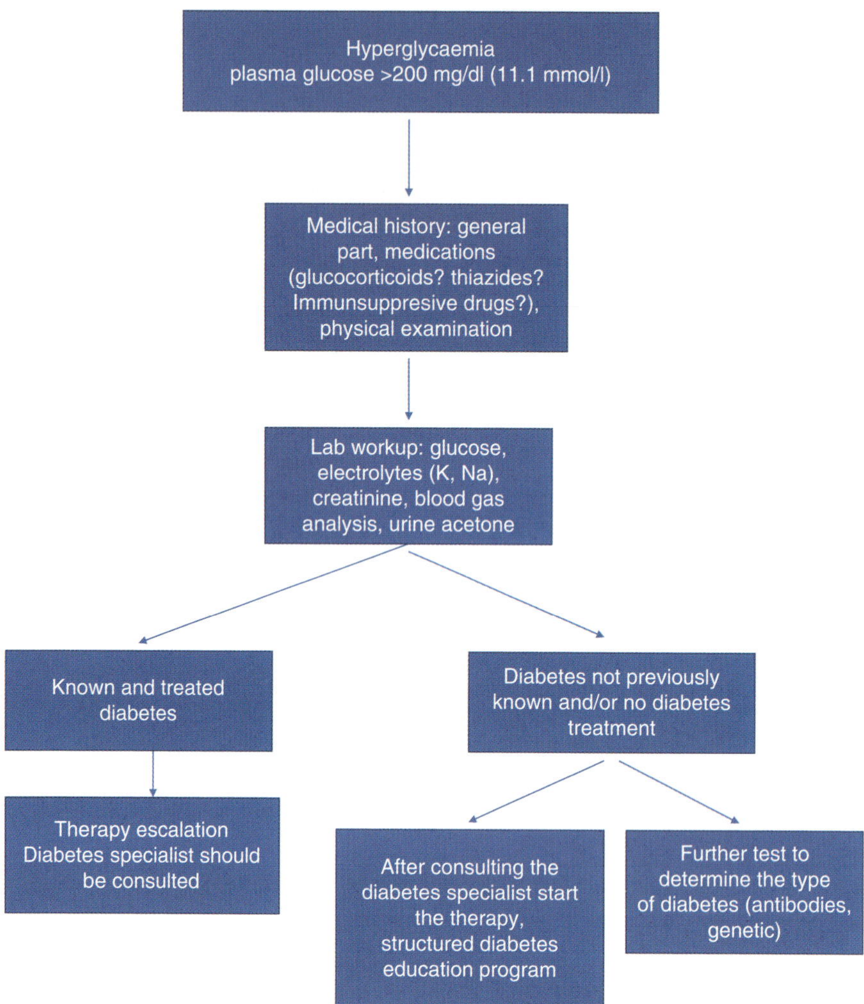

22.3 Diagnostics

Physical examination has to begin with the assessment of vital signs (blood pressure, heart rate, respiratory rate, temperature). A quick neurologic examination should be performed. In addition to an altered mental status and a high-frequency, laboured breathing pattern (Kussmaul breathing) diabetic ketoacidosis can be suspected from a fruity, ketotic odour. Basic anthropometric data (height, weight) have to be at least estimated. The skin, especially the feet, has to be thoroughly examined for diabetic ulcers.

Plasma glucose can be measured with commercially available, bedside blood glucose metres, but such devices are often unable to measure very high or low values. Accurate measurements have to be performed from venous blood with well-calibrated laboratory methods. Most point-of-care blood gas analysers are suitable to quickly determine both the plasma glucose and pH, which are crucial measurements in the acute care of patients with hyperglycaemia. Further important laboratory parameters are blood cell count and C-reactive protein to assess the possibility of an infection. Hyperglycaemia is nearly always associated with volume depletion, and plasma electrolytes (Na, K) should be checked together with plasma creatinine. In the case of unexplained hypoglycaemia, the early determination of both insulin and C-peptide levels can be helpful. High insulin and low C-peptide levels, in conjunction with hypoglycaemia, are consistent with exogenous insulin administration as a cause. *If patients with known diabetes require medical attention because of hypoglycaemia or hyperglycaemia, a diabetes specialist has to be consulted as soon as possible to elucidate causes and adjust therapy.*

When laboratory parameters suggest an infection, additional workup should be performed in a timely manner to uncover the site of infection (chest x-ray, urine routine and microscopy, abdominal ultrasound).

If iatrogenic causes of a symptomatic hypoglycaemia have been ruled out, the patient has to be seen by an endocrinologist for further diagnostics. The classic test is a 72-h supervised fast (hunger test) aiming to reproduce the hypoglycaemia with the concomitant measurement of plasma insulin levels.

22.4 Differential Diagnosis

Reasons for hypoglycaemia

Differential diagnosis	Incidence	Diagnostics
Exogenous insulin injections	+++	Plasma insulin, C-peptide in conjunction with plasma glucose
Antidiabetic drugs (sulfonylureas, glinides)	++	Medication history, drug levels in plasma (sulfonylureas)
Insulin-producing tumours	--	Plasma insulin, C-peptide and proinsulin levels in conjunction with plasma glucose, imaging studies
Nonislet cell tumours	---	Plasma insulin, C-peptide and proinsulin levels, IGF-1 (insulin like growth factor), imaging studies
Adrenal insufficiency	–	Cortisol and ACTH, stimulation tests
Critical illness	–	Underlying critical illness (cardiac failure, liver failure, sepsis) usually apparent at presentation, further workup in the intensive care unit

Hyperuricemia 23

Annika Simon

23.1 Definition

Hyperuricemia is present when the uric acid level in serum exceeds the standard value of 3.5–7.0 mg/dl for male and of 2.5–5.7 mg/dl for women. Since the serum is generally saturated at a concentration of about 7.0 mg/dl, higher values may lead to deposition of the so-called urate crystals [1, 3].

These crystals can deposit in the joints and trigger gout seizures. The causes of hyperuricemia can be classified into two different types: an increased purine synthesis and a decreased renal excretion. Finally, primary and secondary hyperuricemia can be distinguished [1, 3].

23.2 Medical History

If there is an elevated uric acid level in serum, especially two points – which are comorbidities and medication – have to be clarified in the context of medical history. Other important questions refer to lifestyle, e.g., dietary habits and alcohol abuse. Women are generally less affected by high levels of uric acid value and gout seizures; the peak age is mainly after the menopause.

A. Simon, Dipl.-Psych.
Department of Urology and Urological Oncology,
Hannover University Medical School, Carl-Neuberg-Str. 1,
Hannover 30625, Germany
e-mail: psychosomatik.simon@googlemail.com

A.S. Merseburger et al. (eds.), *Urology at a Glance*,
DOI 10.1007/978-3-642-54859-8_23, © Springer-Verlag Berlin Heidelberg 2014

23.3 Diagnostics

The main points of the physical examination are the inspection and palpation of the joints to discover changes and gout tophi and a check of the patients' weight (obesity). In addition, secondary causes of hyperuricemia should be ruled out on physical examination [1].

In case of primary hyperuricemia, further diagnostic tests like imaging (ultrasound to exclude kidney stones) and urine/blood analysis come to use. The most common diseases are gout, nephrolithiasis, and urate nephropathy. However, only a few patients with abnormally high uric acid levels in serum become symptomatic [2, 3].

23.4 Differential Diagnosis [1]

Differential diagnosis	Incidence	Diagnostics
Drug side effects	++++	Medical history
Renal failure	+++	Medical history, anamnesis, laboratory investigation (e.g., serum creatinine/urea, GFR)
Proliferative diseases	+++	Medical history, anamnesis, specific diagnostic tests
Nutrition	+++	Anamnesis
Ketoacidosis, lactic acidosis	++	Anamnesis, laboratory investigations
Endocrinological disease (e.g., hypothyroidism, hyperparathyroidism)	++	Anamnesis, laboratory investigation (phosphate, parathyroid hormone, TSH, ft3, ft4)
Psoriasis	+	Anamnesis, specific dermatological tests
Enzyme defects (e.g., hypoxanthine-guanine phosphoribosyltransferase deficiency)	–	Molecular genetic investigations, DNA analysis
Glycogen storage disease (glycogenosis types I, II, IV, VII)	–	Molecular genetic investigations, DNA analysis

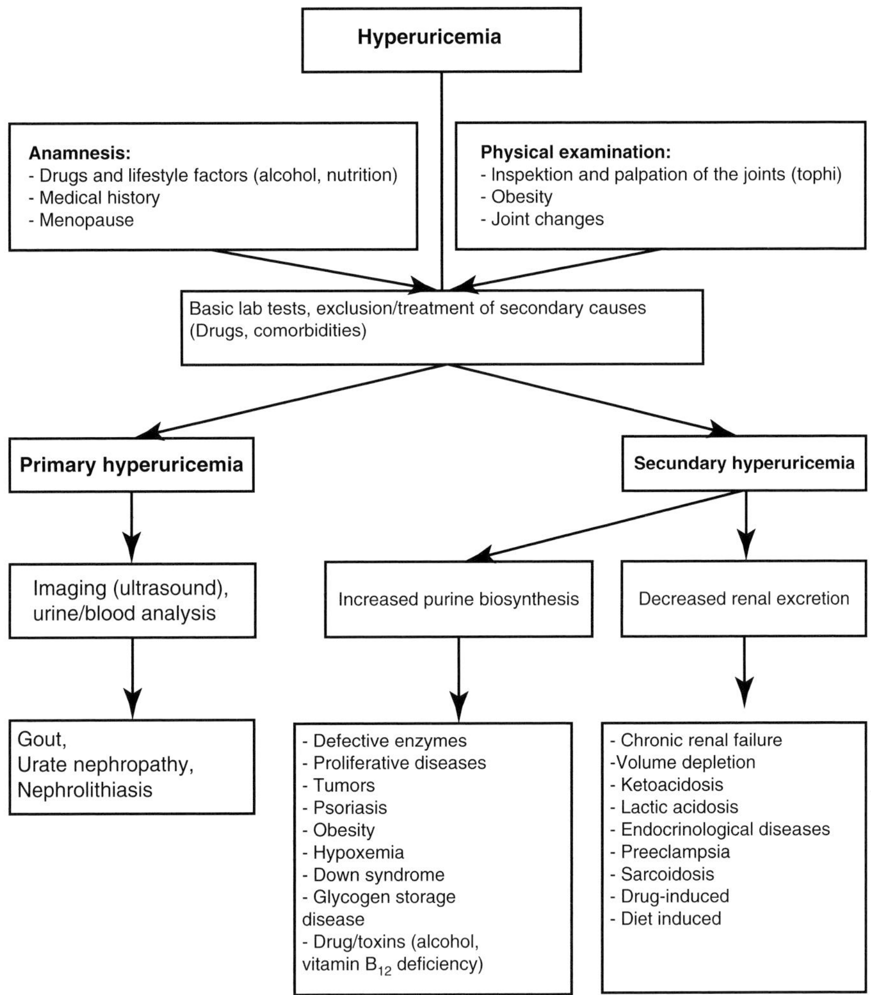

References

1. Brunkhorst R, Schölmerich J (editors). Differentialdiagnostik und Differentialtherapie. Urban & Fischer: München; 2010.
2. Jin M, et al. Uric acid, hyperuricemia and vascular disease. Front Biosci. 2012;17:656–69.
3. So A, Thorens B. Uric acid transport and disease. J Clin Invest. 2010;120(6):1791–9.

Acute Abdomen

24

Florian Imkamp

24.1 Definition

The acute abdomen refers to an acute abdominal pain with an unclear etiology of less than 24-h duration. It is a common emergent symptom in daily urology, and it can be caused by a wide variety of intra- and extra-abdominal organ malfunctions. Therefore, a detailed history, structured complain, and pain assessment as well as a systematic clinical examination are mandatory prior to further investigations.

24.2 History

The patient's history should be taken according to a structured scheme (Table 24.1). In patients complaining of an acute abdomen, history should cover history all of the following clinical fields: pain (Table 24.2), acute complaints in patients words, medical history, surgical history, drug history, social history, and family history. By current complaints and a detailed history, most of the common differential diagnosis (Table 24.3) can be ruled out, and further diagnostics initiated to confirm these diagnoses.

24.3 Diagnostics

24.3.1 Basic Clinical Examination

A detailed history is followed by an initial basic clinical examination to further elucidate the diagnosis and to localize the origin of the abdominal complaints (Fig. 24.1). Most common abdominal disorders are depicted in Table 24.3. To avoid

F. Imkamp
Department of Urology and Urologic Oncology, Hannover University
Medical School (MHH), Carl-Neuberg-Str. 1, Hannover 30625, Germany
e-mail: imkamp.florian@mh-hannover.de

A.S. Merseburger et al. (eds.), *Urology at a Glance*,
DOI 10.1007/978-3-642-54859-8_24, © Springer-Verlag Berlin Heidelberg 2014

Table 24.1 History assessment

History	
Present complaints	Acute complaints in patients own words
Medical history	Diabetes, heart, disease, cancers, inflammatory bowel disease, genitourinary disease
Surgical history	Previous abdominal surgery
Drug history	Documentation of all medications, anti-coagulant medications, drug-induced side effects
Social history	Diet, alcohol, drug abuse, home care
Family history	Hereditary diseases, cancers

Table 24.2 SOCRATES – mnemonic for pain assessment

Initial	Meaning
S	Site – Where is the pain or the most painful site
O	Onset – When did the pain start? Sudden or gradually? Progressive or regressive?
C	Character – What is the pain like? Sharp or dull? Cramp-like or stabbing?
R	Radiation – Does the pain radiate anywhere?
A	Associate – Are other symptoms associated?
T	Time course – Has the pain any time patterns?
E	Exacerbating/relieving factors – What changes the pain?
S	Severity – How strong is your pain?

interference of clinical examination, the following order of examinations is generally accepted.

24.3.1.1 Inspection

The initial glance at the patient might indicate the origin of abdominal pain. Restlessness and itinerancy under painful episodes can indicate acute colic pain; relieving postures and calmness indicate an inflammatory abdominal process involving the peritoneum.

24.3.1.2 Auscultation

The bowel sounds might indicate the underlying abdominal disorder: high-pitched or tinkling sounds indicate mechanical bowel obstructions; absence of bowel sounds might indicate peritonitis or paralytic ileus.

24.3.1.3 Palpation

Palpation starts distant from the point of maximum pain, to identify regions involved in the abdominal process. Rigid tension of abdominal muscles is usually associated with peritonitis and can be limited to a specific area or general due to an extensive peritonitis. Increased muscle tensing is a response to the area of abdominal pain.

Table 24.3 Acute abdomen – common localisation-dependent causes for abdominal symptoms

Area	Urological diagnoses	Male diagnoses	Female diagnoses	Non-gender specific diagnoses
Epigastic				Peptic ulcer Pancreatitis Perforating ulcer Coronary heart disease
Right upper quadrant				Gallstones Disseases of the hepatobiliary system
Right flank	Ureteric colic Renal infarction Pyelonephritis Kindey cyst rupture Renal trauma			
Right iliac fossa	Distal ureteric colic		Ovarian cyst torsion (Ectopic) pregnancy Miscarriage	Appendicitis Ceacal obstruction Chronic inflammatory bowel diseases
Suprapubic area	Cystitis Acute urinary retention	Testicular torsion	Miscarriage	
Left iliac fossa	Distal ureteric colic		Ovarian cyst torsion (Ectopic) pregnancy Misscarriage	Diverticulitis Perforating diverticulitis Constipation
Left flank	Ureteric colic Pyelonephritis Renal infarction Kindey cyst rupture Renal trauma			
Left upper quadrant				Small bowel obstruction Early appendicitis Gastroenteritis
Peri-umbilical				Gastroenteritis Small bowel obstruction Intestinal infarction Acute appendicitis

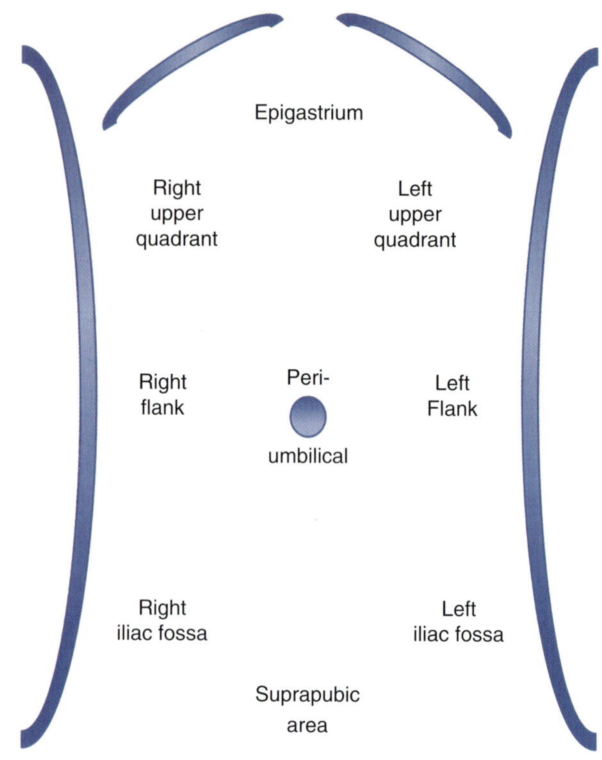

Fig. 24.1 Abdominal topography

24.3.1.4 Percussion

Lumps and bumps differentiate between enteric gas retentions and abdominal fluid collections (blood, ascites, purulence). Percussion can produce rebound tenderness.

24.3.1.5 Genital, Rectal, and Hernia Orifice Examination

These examinations are mandatory in acute abdomen patients.

24.3.2 Investigations

24.3.2.1 Blood Test

Full blood counts might indicate abnormalities, such as anemia or altered white cell counts, and are mandatory standard investigation. Electrolytes (sodium, potassium, calcium) and kidney values (creatinine, urea) are used to rule out renal malfunctions. Liver and biliary test (AST, ALT, AP, and gamma-GT) should indicate liver or biliary disorders. Pancreatic diseases are further examined by pancreatic enzymes (lipase, amylase). An acute abdomen is frequently followed by surgical procedures or other interventions. Therefore, blood coagulation test is indicated to rule out coagulopathies and to confirm sufficient liver function.

24.3.2.2 Urine Test

A urine dipstick test is performed to rule out urinary tract infections or hematuria. Disorders in dipstick test should be further assessed by urine microscopy or urine culture.

24.3.2.3 Ultrasound

Ultrasound is an important noninvasive investigation that should be performed prior to further imaging modalities. In emergency setting, it is used to rule out free fluids (blood, ascites) or free gas due to perforations in the abdominal cavity, renal or ureteral obstruction (renal masses, dilatation of renal pelvis, or ureter, stones), bladder abnormalities (urinary retention, stones, tumors), ovarian or uterus disorders (ovarian cyst, pregnancy, ectopic pregnancy), hepatobiliary diseases (gall stones, bile duct obstruction, tumors), and, if possible, intestinal disorders (distended bowel loops, impaired peristalsis).

24.3.2.4 Imaging

Erect chest x-ray might be useful to rule out thoracic disorders, influencing abdominal symptoms, such as lower lobe pneumonia or hiatal hernias. Moreover, it might show subphrenic gas due to perforation.

Abdominal x-ray can be used to identify free gas or distended bowel loops.

An abdominal CT scan with intravenous contrast media is the first choice of further imaging, if none of the abovementioned investigations identified the cause of the abdominal disorder.

24.4 Differential Diagnosis of Common Urologic Diseases

To focus on urologic diseases as causes for an acute abdomen, other intra- and extra-abdominal disorders have to be ruled out.

24.4.1 Ureteral Colic

The most common urologic cause is a ureteral colic, due to urinary obstruction caused by urinary calculi. Characteristically these patients complain of immediate onset, undulating flank or lower abdominal pain episodes mostly accompanied with variable peritoneal irritation leading to nausea and rarely to vomiting. Under acute colic episodes, patients appear restlessly wandering, without finding reliving postures.

Leading examination findings are flank pain due to palpation or percussion and clinical experience. The diagnosis is confirmed by urinary dipstick analysis, frequently revealing microscopic hematuria and basic kidney ultrasound examination, confirming ureteral or collecting system distention and renal or distal ureteral calculi. If diagnosis remains unclear, a low-dose CT scan of the abdomen is indicated as the gold standard of imaging modalities.

24.4.2 Acute Urinary Retention

Acute urinary retentions commonly appear as progressive blunt pain in the lower abdomen and imperative urgency. History frequently reveals previous voiding dysfunctions. Frequently a palpable mass in the lower abdomen is found in clinical examination, and the diagnosis is confirmed by ultrasound investigation. A chronic upper urinary tract distention due to bladder outlet obstruction with consecutive urinary congestion is ruled out by renal ultrasound.

24.4.3 Renal Infarction

Renal infarctions due to acute arterial embolism or to arterial dissection are infrequent events in urologic emergencies. Small renal infarctions commonly are asymptomatic, whereas patients with severe infarctions complain of acute-onset sharp flank pain that can be misinterpreted as acute ureteral colic. Mostly urinary dipstick is normal, and renal ultrasound shows a normal urinary tract configuration. Color duplex ultrasound of the kidney can prove renal infarction. Contrast-enhanced CT scan remains the diagnostic gold standard to determine the extent of renal infarction.

24.4.4 Urologic Trauma

Urologic traumas are described elsewhere. Nonetheless secondary to insignificant urologic traumas, a delayed acute abdomen can occur. Most common are retroperitoneal hemorrhages due to minor renal traumas. Expanding hematoma usually causes blunt flank pain and might be associated with clinical sign of hypovolemia or hypovolemic shock. Diagnosis is based on history, clinical examination, standard blood count, and renal ultrasound. If these investigations are suspicious for a kidney trauma, contrast-enhanced CT scan is indicated to further investigate the extent of the kidney injury.

24.4.5 Kidney Cyst Rupture

Kidney cyst ruptures can appear suddenly without any external influence or due to minor flank impacts. Patients complain of variable blunt flank pain episodes. Diagnosis is based on the following: patient's history, as many patients are aware of their kidney cysts; standard blood examinations; and ultrasound of the kidney, which occasionally demonstrates free fluid around the kidney. If diagnosis remains unclear, contrast-enhanced CT scan is indicated to further elucidate the complaints.

Oliguria/Anuria

25

Abdul-Rahman Kabbani

25.1 General Facts

While oliguria defined as a urinary output of less than 300–500 ml per 24 h, anuria is classified as an output below 50–100 ml per day. The incidence of oliguria is 18 % of medical–surgical ICU patients with normal renal function and 69 % of patients developing an acute kidney injury [1].

25.2 Symptoms, Classification and Grading

Anuria and oliguria are in themselves symptoms of various different diseases, which could be subdivided into prerenal, renal and postrenal categories. Among the prerenal conditions all causes of a reduced renal blood flow can be subsumed such as hypovolemia, sepis or low cardiac output. Renal disorders are associated with structural renal damage like in acute tubular necrosis, intoxications or nephritis. Topographically, the most common causes for a decreased urinary output are located postrenal, which include mechanical urinary obstruction (e.g. tumour, stone, prostatic hypertrophy, blocked urinary catheter, urethral stricture) and dysfunction of the bladder and/or sphincter (anticholinergics, postoperative retention). For this variety of causes, diagnostic studies should include urinalysis, full blood count, arterial blood analysis, renal function, inflammatory markers, estimation of fluid status and a renal ultrasonography for imaging. Depending on the original diseases, specific tests may be required like cystourethrography in bladder outlet obstructions.

A.-R. Kabbani
Department of Urology and Urological Oncology, Hannover University Medical School, Carl-Neuberg-Str. 1, Hannover 30625, Germany
e-mail: kabbaniar@gmail.com

A.S. Merseburger et al. (eds.), *Urology at a Glance*,
DOI 10.1007/978-3-642-54859-8_25, © Springer-Verlag Berlin Heidelberg 2014

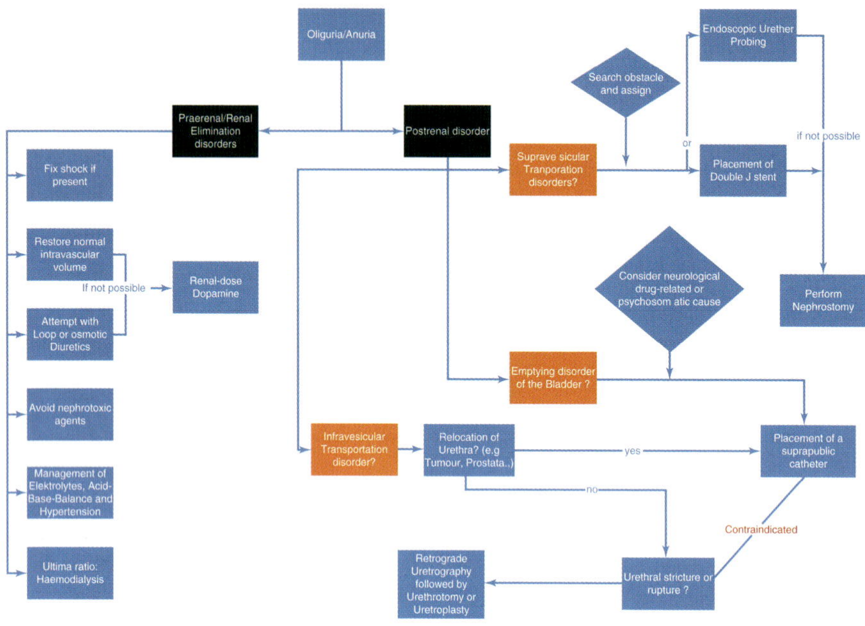

25.3 Therapy

The treatment is aimed at the origins of the oliguria. Therefore, renal and prerenal disorders can be initially addressed in same pathway, beginning with the relief of a potential shock and volume replacement. Acute tubular necrosis may be present with a volume overload and should be approached with fluid restrictions and intravenous loop or osmotic diuretics. Irrespondence to diuretics may be approached with renal-dosed dopamine [2]. In addition to the blood pressure, acid-base balance and electrolyte management (with focus on a sudden hyperkalemia), all nephrotoxic agents should be avoided. Dialysis is the ultima ratio if renal function is no longer sufficient in compensating electrolyte, blood pressure and/or toxic imbalances. On the other hand, it makes sense to divide the postrenal disorders in three subcategories as can be seen in the flowchart. Supravesical disorders are often associated with obstacles, which can be recoup by probing with ureter endoscope or by placement of a double J stent [3]. If both methods failed or are impossible to perform, a nephrostomy can be carried out. Neurological and/or psychosomatic diseases in addition to medication may induce a sphincter/bladder dysfunction. Symptomatically, this can be met by the placement of a suprapubic catheter. This approach also applies for any infravesicular disorder with a relocation of the urethra like in a prostatic hyperplasia. It should be noted that these techniques are contraindicated in urethral strictures and ruptures [4]. In fact, these kinds of diseases should be diagnosed by a retrograde urethrography and be followed by urethrotomy or urethroplasty.

Post-interventional workup includes the management of post-obstructive diuresis with the resultant polyuria and electrolyte imbalance [5].

25.4 Complications

Reduced urinary output is an important clinical criterion and staging hallmark for acute kidney injury (RIFLE and AKIN classification) [6]. On the other side, not all renal failures are associated with an oliguria [7]. Renal dysfunction may induce additionally cardiovascular (e.g. heart failure, pulmonary oedema, arrhythmia), haematological (e.g. anaemia), gastrointestinal (e.g. ileus, vomiting) and/or neurological complications (e.g. seizures, dizziness). Over the years, a non-fully recovered kidney can end in a chronic kidney disease. Furthermore, urinary obstruction predisposes to infection and may lead to a pyelonephritis or a urinary tract infection. The passage of endotoxins into the bloodstream as part of uraemia may also provoke a urosepsis [8].

References

1. Zaloga GP, Hughes SS. Oliguria in patients with normal renal function. Anesthesiology. 1990;72(4):598–602.
2. Flancbaum L, Choban PS, Dasta JF. Quantitative effects of low-dose dopamine on urine output in oliguric surgical intensive care unit patients. Crit Care Med. 1994;22(1):61–6.
3. RAMSAY J, et al. The effects of double J stenting on unobstructed ureters. An experimental and clinical study*. Br J Urol. 1985;57(6):630–4.
4. LUMEN N, et al. Etiology of urethral stricture disease in the 21st century. J Urol. 2009;182(3):983–7.
5. Vaughan ED, Jr, Gillenwater JY. Diagnosis, characterization and management of post-obstructive diuresis. J Urol. 1973;109(2):286–92. ISSN 0022–5347; 0022–5347.
6. Macedo E, et al. Defining urine output criterion for acute kidney injury in critically ill patients. Nephrol Dial Transplant. 2011;26(2):509–15.
7. Anderson RJ, et al. Nonoliguric acute renal failure. N Engl J Med. 1977;296(20):1134–8.
8. Haag-Weber M, Hörl W. Uremia and infection: mechanisms of impaired cellular host defense. Nephron. 1993;63(2):125–31.

Renal Colic

26

Stephan Kruck and Jens Bedke

26.1 Definition

Renal colic describes the pain arising from urinary tract obstruction. Symptoms are caused by the distension and spasm of the ureter, the pelvicalyceal system, and the renal capsule. The symptom generated by renal colic is primarily a sudden, sharp, severe loin pain in the lower back over the kidney, radiating forward into the groin, testes, or labia majora. Renal colic can be related to a variety of underlying clinical scenarios (calculi, tumors, strictures, lymphadenopathy, or anatomical abnormalities) and can occur at any point in the urinary tract. In accordance, symptoms are affected by the underlying intrinsic or occasionally extrinsic etiology. The respective etiologic causes lead to acute or chronic urinary tract obstruction, as a result of complete or partial blockade of urine drainage.

26.2 Medical History

A detailed medical history is mandatory to narrow down the underlying cause of an upper urinary tract obstruction for an efficient further diagnostic and therapeutic management. For each patient, not only the duration and type of symptoms but also personal (including smoking and exclusion for pregnancy), familial (familial stone disease or cancer syndromes), medical (including medications/allergies), and surgical history should be reviewed. Besides of that non-urologic diseases (acute appendicitis, gynecologic disorders, or abdominal aortic aneurysm) in particular with a detailed urologic medical history including the anamnesis of former urinary calculi, strictures in the whole urinary tract, urothelial carcinoma, urinary tract infections, voiding patterns, abdominal or retroperitoneal surgeries (including urinary diversion or renal transplantation), and presence of gross hematuria should be documented.

S. Kruck • J. Bedke (✉)
Department of Urology, Eberhard-Karls-University,
Hoppe-Seyler-Str. 3, 72076 Tuebingen, Germany
e-mail: stephan.kruck@gmail.com; bedke@live.com

A.S. Merseburger et al. (eds.), *Urology at a Glance*,
DOI 10.1007/978-3-642-54859-8_26,

26.3 Diagnostics

Initial assessment includes the documentation of vital signs, such as blood pressure, heart rate, respiration frequency, and the presence of fever. Acute ill patients due to a developed urosepsis have to be stabilized and monitored before any further diagnostic or therapeutic intervention can be performed. Besides a symptom-orientated basic physical examination, other factors like uremia or fluid overload, the presence of peritoneal signs, pulsating or solid abdominal masses, testicular disorders, premature labors, or labor pain in a parturient should not be neglected. For pregnant patients the welfare of the fetus should always be clarified. All patients should have a urine dipstick test, due to the high sensitivity of hematuria in patients with urolithiasis in about 90 % and to exclude a urinary tract infection. Blood investigations should be performed in any patient with renal colic, including a complete blood count and serum chemistry testing. Furthermore, all females of childbearing age should have a pregnancy test. In patients with fever and urinary tract infection, urine and blood cultures should be obtained before the administration of antibiotics. Lastly, known stone formers should have basic metabolic evaluation with at minimum serum calcium and urate analysis. Non-contrast CT (NCCT) has become the method of choice for investigating acute renal colic, a role formerly played by plain radiographs and excretory urography. Nevertheless, ultrasonography is a useful, cheap, and rapid available screening tool to evaluate the presence of urinary obstruction, especially important as first-line test in pediatric and pregnant patients.

26.4 Differential Diagnosis

Urogenital Urinary stones Acquired or congenital stricture Ureteropelvic or vesical junction obstruction Testicular torsion/trauma Retrocaval ureter Urinoma
Urinary tract infection (UTI) Upper UTI (pyelonephritis) Lower UTI (cystitis)/epididymo-orchitis Tuberculosis Abscess
Gynecologic disorders Endometriosis (Ectopic) pregnancy Ovarian torsion or rupture Ruptured ovarian cyst
Acute abdomen Appendicitis Diverticulitis Biliary colic Inflammatory bowel disease

(continued)

Vascular/renal diseases
Aortic and iliac aneurysms
Renal artery or vein thrombosis
Papillary necrosis
Cystic renal diseases
Parapelvic cysts
Renal artery aneurysm
Musculoskeletal system
Trauma
Degeneration
Retroperitoneal fibrosis
Cancer
Urothelial cancer
Renal carcinoma
Retroperitoneal malignancy
Iatrogenic
Ureteral trauma or ligation
Radiation therapy
Lymphocele

Renal Colic

• Vital Signs
• Stabilization / Analgesia
• Anamnesis (+ Risk Factors / Pregnancy)

• Physical examination
• Urine Test
• Blood Analysis

• Screening ultrasonography
(Only if rapidly available)
• Non-contrast CT
(Cave: pediatric and pregnant patients)

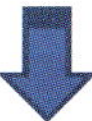

• Conformation
• Exclude Differential diagnosis (see table)

Fever

27

Iason D. Kyriazis, Panagiotis Kallidonis,
Vasilis Panagopoulos, and Evangelos N. Liatsikos

27.1 Definition

Fever is defined as any rise of body temperature above 37.8 °C (100 °F). It is not in the purposes of this chapter to describe in details the pathophysiology behind fever. Nevertheless, briefly, body temperature is regulated by the hypothalamus, which balances heat produced by metabolic activity with the heat lost from the skin and lungs to maintain a stable body temperature despite environmental variations. Febrile conditions stimulate the hypothalamic thermoregulatory center through exogenous or endogenous pyrogens. Many microbial products and toxins or even whole microorganisms can act as exogenous pyrogens. In addition, a number of endogenous pyrogens (e.g., interleukins 1 and 6, tumor necrosis factor, interferons, and others) also termed as pyrogenic cytokines are produced by human immune cells and endothelial cells during inflammation. As a response to pyrogens, the hypothalamic thermoregulatory center stimulates a systemic reaction including heat loss preservation in the periphery (vasoconstriction) and increase in heat production through raised metabolism and autonomic muscle activity (shivering). After pyrogenic stimulus has subsided, the hypothalamus increases heat loss through peripheral vasodilation and sweating until body temperature reaches normal levels [1].

27.2 Medical History and Clinical Examination

Although there are many febrile conditions that are not associated with infectious diseases, infection should be excluded in any patient presenting with fever. A history of a recent operation is indicative of postoperative fever of various etiologies and should be thoroughly investigated. Common postoperative febrile conditions are listed in Fig. 27.1. A low-grade fever in patients with a recent history of

I.D. Kyriazis (✉) • P. Kallidonis • V. Panagopoulos • E.N. Liatsikos
Department of Urology, University of Patras, Rion, Patras 26 504, Greece
e-mail: jkyriazis@gmail.com

A.S. Merseburger et al. (eds.), *Urology at a Glance*,
DOI 10.1007/978-3-642-54859-8_27, © Springer-Verlag Berlin Heidelberg 2014

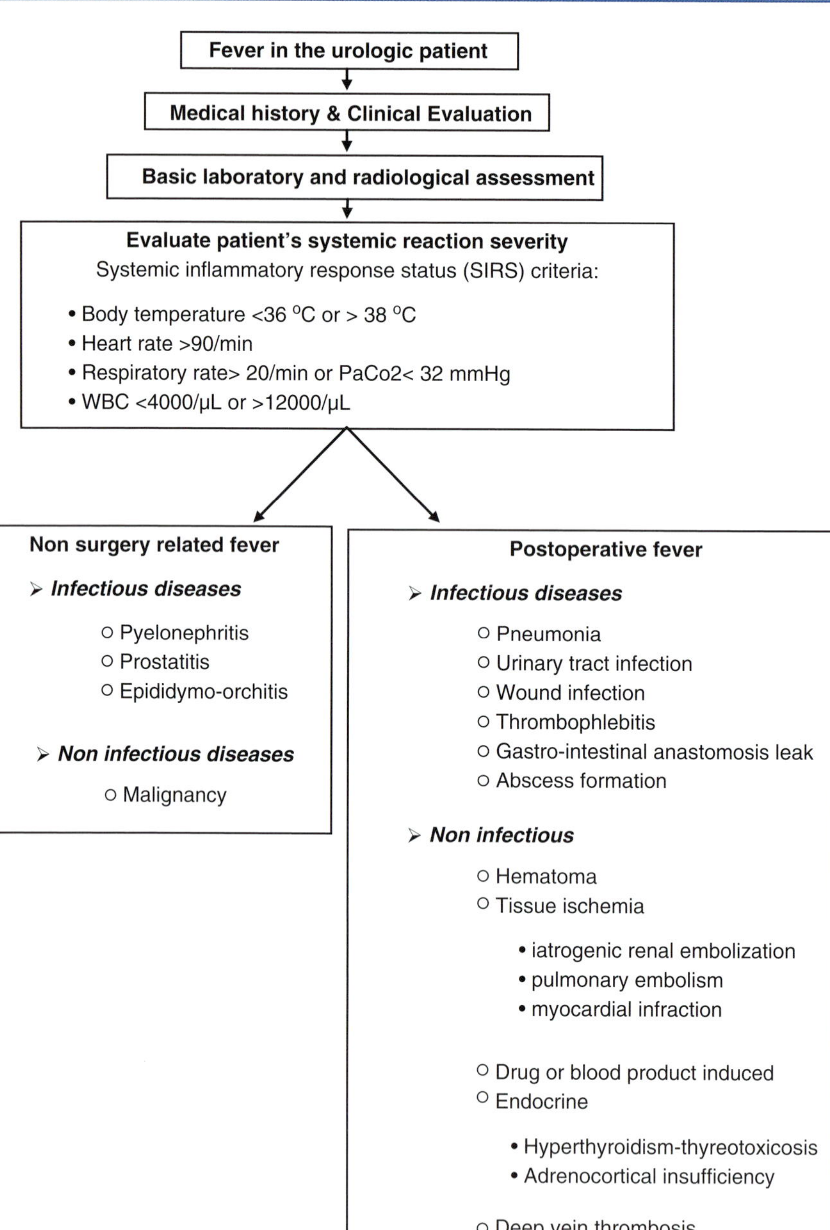

Fig. 27.1 Basic differential diagnosis of urologic origin fever

urinary tract instrumentation, urethral catheterization, or hosting foreign bodies (e.g., ureteral stents) is indicative of a possible urinary tract infection. Noninfectious febrile urological conditions could be associated with the presence of malignancy (neoplastic fever), with tissue ischemia (e.g., fever following renal embolization), with reactions to blood products or antibiotics (drug induced fever), and with other causes.

In case of fever of urological origin, clinical examination is usually enough to define the source of inflammation. Renal infection can induce high fever with shivering and is typically accompanied by loin pain and ipsilateral abdominal tenderness. Nevertheless, other febrile conditions mimicking the same symptomatology should be ruled out (e.g., ipsilateral lower lobe pneumonia, acute cholecystitis, and others). Acute prostatitis apart from high fever is regularly accompanied by severe dysuria and other lower urinary tract symptoms while pain in the lower abdomen or pain associated with bowel movements are usually present. A tender and swollen epididymis is indicative of epididymitis. An uncomplicated cystitis is rarely a cause of fever. In the case of postoperative fever, clinical examination must evaluate proper wound healing, exclude thrombophlebitis at sites of intravenous catheters, and rule out deep vein thrombosis. In addition, chest auscultation must be performed to reveal potential lung pathologies such as pneumonia or atelectasis [2].

27.3 Laboratory Investigation

Initial evaluation of a patient presenting with fever include:

- Vital signs
- Complete blood count
- Basic renal and liver biochemistry
- Inflammation markers (C-reactive protein, erythrocyte sedimentation rate)
- Urinalysis
- Chest x-ray
- Appropriate imaging (ultrasound, computer tomography)
- Urinary, blood, and stool cultures as indicated

An increase of white blood cells and especially neutrophil count increases the possibility of infectious diseases. A rise of inflammation markers could reinforce the latter and assist proper diagnosis. The assessment of renal biochemistry is necessary to exclude renal failure as a result of sepsis or obstructive uropathy and guide proper dosing of antibiotics. Liver biochemistry and chest x-ray are important to exclude non-urological febrile conditions. The presence of leucocytes in urinalysis is highly indicative of urinary tract infection. A urinary culture must be ordered before the initiation of an empirical antibiotic treatment. When upper urinary tract infection is suspected, appropriate imaging is necessary to exclude obstructive uropathy. In the septic patient, a computer tomography provides a fast assessment of intra-abdominal pathologies and rule out non-urological conditions. A scrotal ultrasound is mandatory in the evaluation of scrotal pain and the documentation of epididymo-orchitis.

Additional investigation in the case of postoperative fever should be guided by the presence of relevant symptoms. A febrile lower limb swelling should be investigated by duplex ultrasonography looking for deep vein thrombosis. A febrile diarrhea following prolonged antibiotic treatment should be evaluated including stool cultures for *Clostridium difficile* to rule out pseudomembranous colitis. Blood and urine cultures should be repeated in the febrile patient even after the initiation of antibiotic therapy to reveal potentially resistant pathogens to the administered antimicrobial agent. A chest x-ray should be ordered in any febrile postoperative patient with signs of cough or respiratory distress and if indicated to be supplemented by a contrast-enhanced spiral CT of the chest to exclude pulmonary embolism [3].

References

1. Dinarello CA. Infection, fever, and exogenous and endogenous pyrogens: some concepts have changed. J Endotoxin Res. 2004;10(4):201–22.
2. Hirschmann JV. Fever of unknown origin in adults. Clin Infect Dis. 1997;24(3):291–300.
3. High KP, Bradley SF, Gravenstein S, Mehr DR, Quagliarello VJ, Richards C, Yoshikawa TT. Clinical practice guideline for the evaluation of fever and infection in older adult residents of long-term care facilities: 2008 update by the Infectious Diseases Society of America. Clin Infect Dis. 2009;48(2):149–71.

Part II

From Diagnosis to Therapy

Acute Epididymitis

28

Florian Imkamp

28.1 General Facts

Acute epididymitis is a syndrome, consisting of pain, swelling, and inflammation of the epididymis of less than 6 weeks. It has to be distinguished from chronic epididymitis.

28.2 Etiology

In sexually active men younger than 35 years, epididymitis is usually caused by a spread of noncoliform and nongonococcal urethral infections. Two thirds are caused by *C. trachomatis* [1,4]. In men older than 35 years, urethral infections caused by bacteriuria due to obstructive urinary diseases are more common. Other pathogens, such as mycobacteria or noninfectious epididymitis, are rare.

28.3 Diagnosis

The clinical complex of pain, swelling, and inflammation of the epididymis as well as swelling and tenderness of the spermatic cord is pathognomonic. Clinical examination includes physical examination (palpation, inspection) and ultrasound

F. Imkamp
Department of Urology and Urological Oncology, Hannover University Medical School, Carl-Neuberg-Str. 1, 30625 Hannover, Germany
e-mail: imkamp.florian@mh-hannover.de

A.S. Merseburger et al. (eds.), *Urology at a Glance*,
DOI 10.1007/978-3-642-54859-8_28, © Springer-Verlag Berlin Heidelberg 2014

investigation. The microbiologic etiology is easily investigated by a Gram-stained urethral smear and MSU. If intracellular Gram-negative diplococci (*N. gonorrhoeae*) are ruled out and white blood cells are present, an infection with *C. trachomatis* is likely in two thirds of patients. Other pathogens can be isolated by microbiologic culture.

28.4 Differential Diagnosis

Generally, it is imperative to rule out an acute spermatic cord torsion immediately by all available clinical information and, in case of doubt, by surgical exploration.

28.5 Therapy

Therapy is based on clinical findings, ultrasound investigations, and anticipated pathogenic microorganisms. If ultrasound proves an acute abscess-forming epididymitis, surgical treatment with abscess drainage is required. Antibiotics are the therapy of choice in non-abscess-forming and in abscess-forming following surgical intervention. Few studies have shown that treatment with fluoroquinolones leads to sufficient tissue penetration [2]; therefore, fluoroquinolones with activity against *C. trachomatis* (ofloxacin or levofloxacin) are the drugs of choice. If infection with *C. trachomatis* is proven, treatment should be continued with doxycycline for two weeks and sexual partner therapy has to be taken into consideration [3]. The antibiotic treatment has to be adapted to the results of microbiologic culture (Figs. 28.1, 28.2, 28.3, and 28.4).

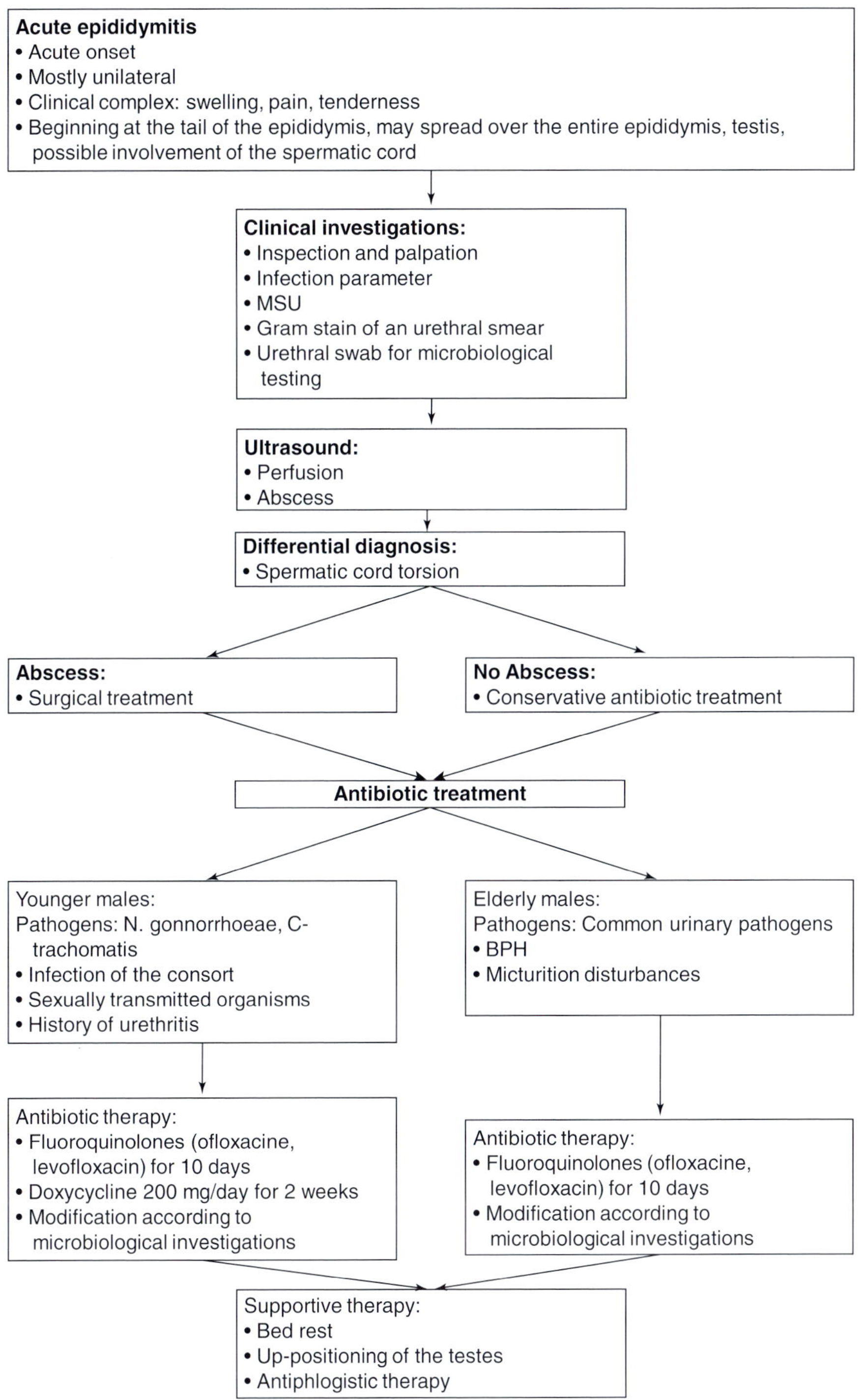

Fig. 28.1 Treatment algorithm of acute epididymitis

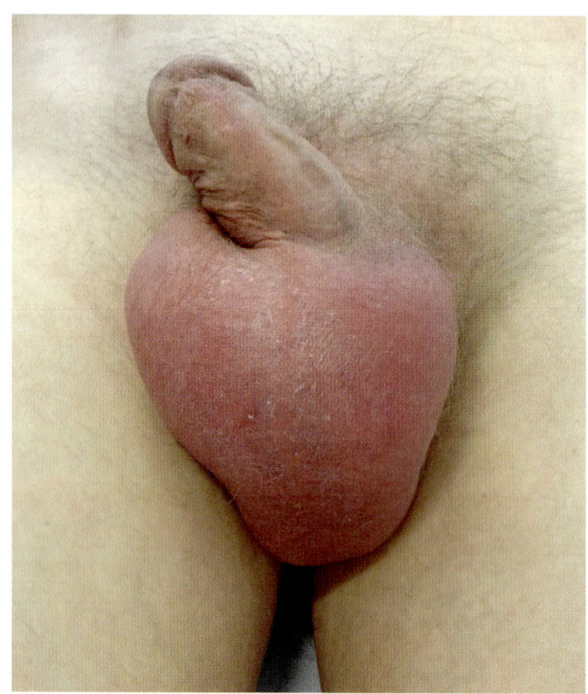

Fig. 28.2 Clinical aspect of acute epididymis

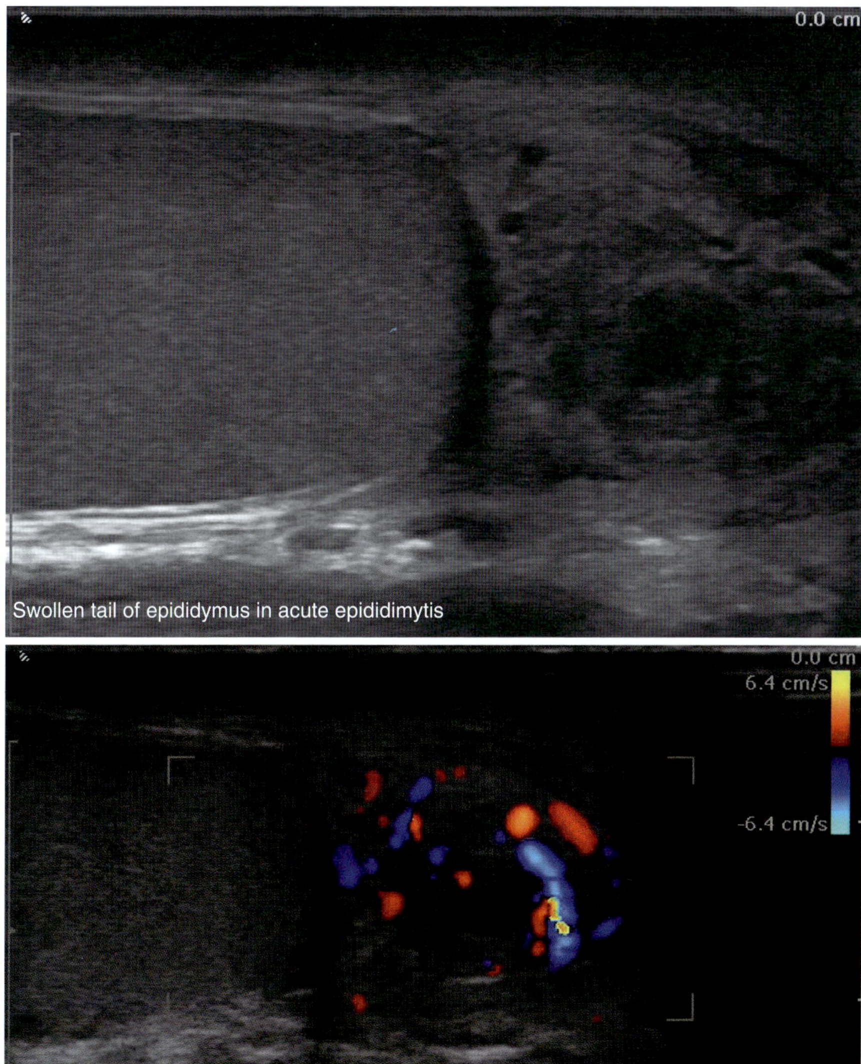

Fig. 28.3 Ultrasound findings in acute epididymitis

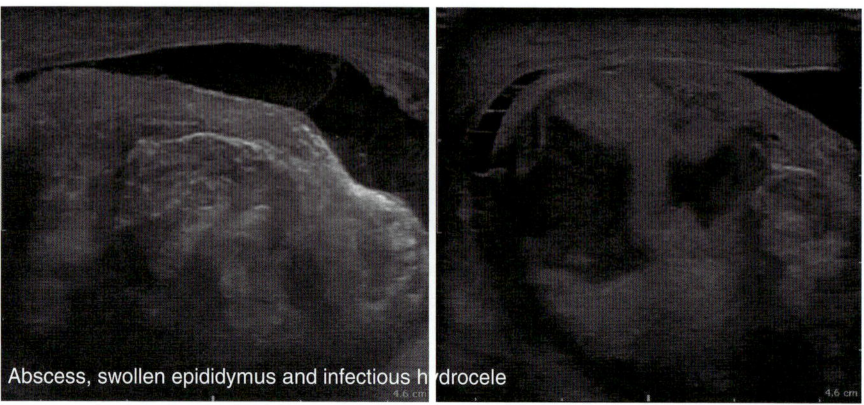

Fig. 28.4 Ultrasound findings in acute abscess-forming epididymo-orchitis

References

1. Berger RE. Urethritis and epididymitis. Semin Urol. 1983;1(2):138–45.
2. Ludwig M, Jantos CA, et al. Tissue penetration of sparfloxacin in a rat model of experimental Escherichia coli epididymitis. Infection. 1997;25(3):178–84.
3. Grabe M, Bjerklund-Johansen TE, Botto H, Wullt B, G. N. M. Çek, R.S. Pickard, P. Tenke, et al. Guidelines on urological infections. Uroweb. 2013. Available at http://www.uroweb.org/gls/pdf/19%20Urological%20infections_LR.pdf. ISBN 978-90-79754-65-6.
4. Weidner W, Schiefer HG, et al. Acute nongonococcal epididymitis. Aetiological and therapeutic aspects. Drugs. 1987;34 Suppl 1:111–7.

Orchitis

29

George Kedia and Rebecca Bongers

29.1 General Facts

Orchitis, the isolated inflammation of the testis, is an uncommon disease. The isolated inflammation of the epididymis, epididymitis, is relatively more common. Epidemiological data regarding the incidence and prevalence of these infections are lacking. In general, the aetiology of primary and secondary orchitis has been classified into nonspecific, specific and viral orchitis (Table 29.1). Viral orchitis, the most common type of primary haematogenous orchitis, is most often caused by mumps infection. According to older data, it does occur in 20–30 % of post-pubertal men with mumps infection [1]. Secondary orchitis usually occurs in connection with a nonspecific or specific epididymitis as "epididymoorchitis" and is usually bacterial in aetiology. In men aged 15–60 years, the incidence rate of epididymoorchitis have been reported as 21 per 10,000 patient-years in the UK [2]. The most common pathogens in men ≤35 years of age are sexually transmitted *Chlamydia trachomatis* or *Neisseria gonorrhoeae* infections. In boys younger than 14 years and in men older than 35 years, infection is generally caused by common urinary pathogens, such as *Escherichia coli* and other coliform bacteria, and often associated with urogenital malformations and bladder outlet obstruction. Specific granulomatous epididymoorchitis can occur by systemic infections such as tuberculosis, brucellosis, syphilis and fungal disease.

G. Kedia (✉) • R. Bongers
Department of Urology and Urological Oncology,
Hannover Medical School (MHH), Carl-Neuberg-Str. 1,
30625 Hannover, Germany
e-mail: kedia.george@mh-hannover.de; bongers.rebecca@mh-hannover.de

A.S. Merseburger et al. (eds.), *Urology at a Glance*,
DOI 10.1007/978-3-642-54859-8_29, © Springer-Verlag Berlin Heidelberg 2014

Table 29.1 Classification of orchitis

Forms of orchitis	Aetiology
Nonspecific epididymoorchitis	*Escherichia coli* Other enterobacteriaceae *Chlamydia trachomatis* *Neisseria gonorrhoeae* *Ureaplasma urealyticum* *Pseudomonas aeruginosa* *Proteus mirabilis* *Klebsiella pneumoniae* Staphylococci Streptococci
Nonspecific bacterial orchitis in children	Pneumococci *Salmonella* spp. *Klebsiella* spp. *Haemophilus influenzae*
Nonspecific granulomatous orchitis in adults	Idiopathic (*Autoimmune*)
Specific granulomatous orchitis	*Mycobacterium tuberculosis* *Treponema pallidum* *Brucella* spp. Intravesical Bacillus Calmette-Guerin (BCG) therapy
Viral orchitis	Mumps Mumps vaccine Coxsackie Mononucleosis Varicella Echovirus Lymphocytic choriomeningitis

29.2 Symptoms, Classification and Grading

Symptoms and clinical findings play a major role in diagnosing orchitis or epididymoorchitis. These infections are usually unilateral but can also occur bilaterally (e.g. by tuberculosis, brucellosis, mumps). Patients typically present with a gradual onset of scrotal pain and findings of scrotal erythema and swelling. According to the underlying aetiology, clinical manifestations may include dysuria, haematuria, urethral discharge, scrotal mass, scrotal fistula and associated systemic symptoms such as fatigue, malaise, myalgias, fever, chills, nausea and headache. In acute infectious process, physical examination reveals enlarged testis (and epididymis) with induration and tenderness. The spermatic cord may also be tender and swollen. Ultrasound examination usually shows homogeneously enlarged testis (and epididymis), a reactive hydrocele and oedematous scrotal skin (thickening), and is useful diagnostics for the detection of abscess formation (Fig. 29.1). In advanced cases, testis cannot

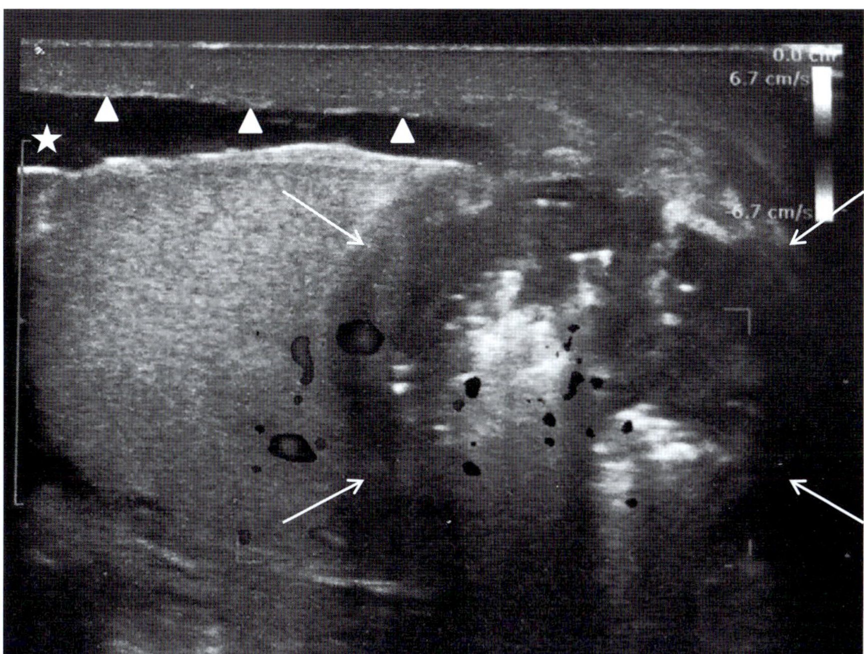

Fig. 29.1 A 57-year-old patient with abscess in the solitary right testis. A longitudinal sonographic image (obtained with a 12-MHz linear transducer) shows an abscess lesion in the lower testicular pole (*arrows*), a reactive hydrocele (*asterisk*) and scrotal skin thickening (*arrowheads*)

be isolated from epididymis. Multiple small hypoechoic nodules in an enlarged testis may occur by, e.g. tuberculous orchitis. Colour Doppler ultrasound of the testis (and epididymis) usually reveals hypervascularity of the involved tissue. The differential diagnosis of the orchitis or epididymoorchitis should include testicular torsion (especially in children and adults), isolated epididymitis, hernias, tumour, lymphoma and leukaemia.

Orchitis and epididymitis are classified as acute or chronic diseases according to the onset and clinical course. In acute phase, symptoms are present for <6 weeks and characterized by pain and swelling. Chronic infection is characterized by a ≥6 week history of symptoms of discomfort and/or pain in the scrotum, testicle or epididymis, generally without swelling.

29.3 Therapy

The management of bacterial epididymoorchitis is similar to that of epididymitis. Empiric antibacterial treatment should be initiated based on likely pathogens (Fig. 29.2). In addition, supportive treatment such as bed rest, scrotal elevation, intermittent use of cold packs and the use of nonsteroidal anti-inflammatory drugs

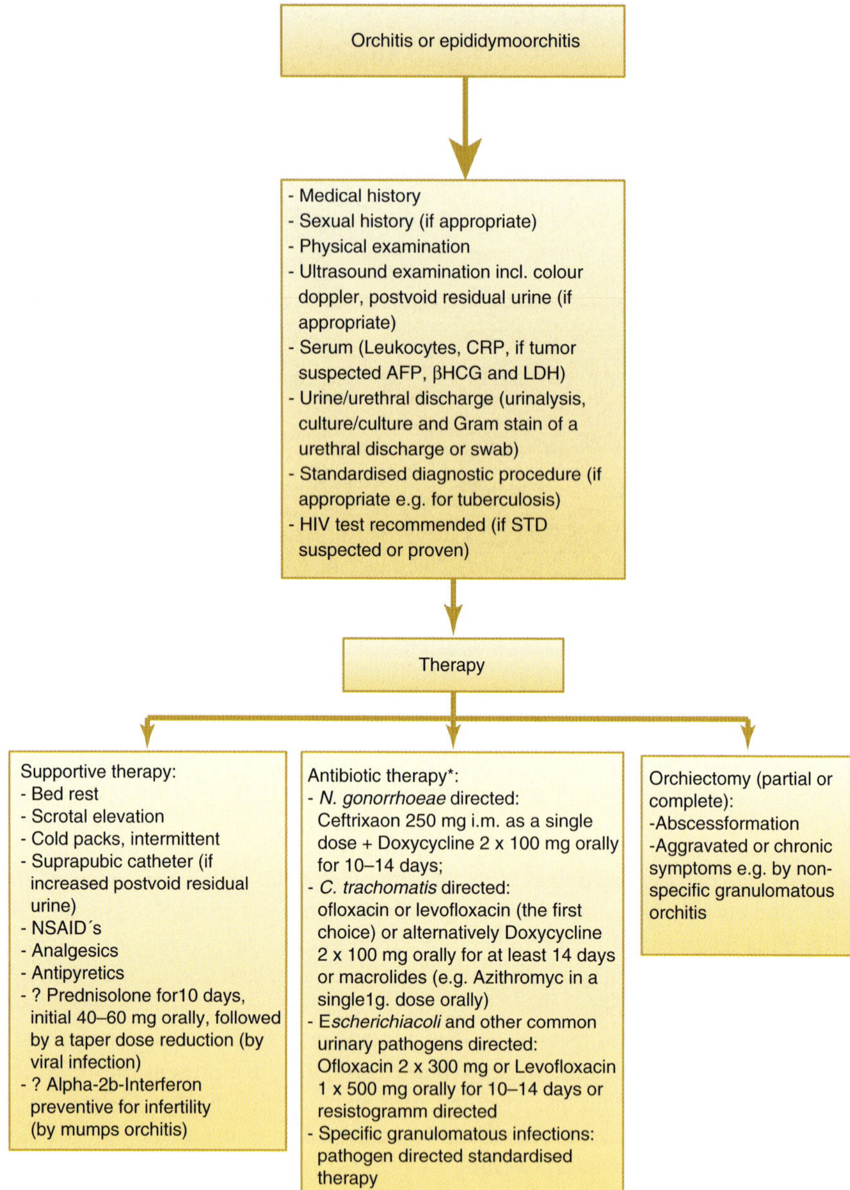

Fig. 29.2 Flow chart demonstrating the pathway from the diagnosis to therapy (*Grabe et al. [3], Centers for Disease Control and Prevention (CDC) [4])

(NSAIDs) are helpful in reducing the duration of the symptoms. In patients with sexually transmitted disease (STD), treatment of their female partners is recommended to prevent reinfection. For patients with severe infection, hospitalization and parenteral antibiotic therapy may be needed.

Antibacterial medications are not indicated for the treatment of viral orchitis. Systemic antiviral treatment is ineffective or not available. In patients with mumps orchitis and serological evidence of IgM antibodies, the use of α-2b interferon may be attempted to prevent testicular atrophy and infertility. In cases of specific granulomatous orchitis, the appropriate treatment is directed against causative pathogens. If the diagnosis remains unclear or testicular abscess or tumour is suspected, surgical exploration and treatment (partial or radical orchiectomy) are indicated. The flow chart (Fig. 29.2) demonstrates the pathway from the diagnosis to therapy.

29.4 Complications

Complications of orchitis or epididymoorchitis may include sepsis, abscess, loss of the testis, testicular atrophy, subfertility, infertility, sterility and testosterone deficiency.

References

1. Lambert B. The frequency of mumps and mumps orchitis. Acta Genet Stat Med. 1951;2 Suppl 1:1–166.
2. Nicholson A, Rait G, Murray-Thomas T, Hughes G, Mercer CH, Casell J. Management of epididymo-orchitis in primary care: results from a large UK primary care database. Br J Gen Pract. 2010;60:e407–22.
3. Grabe M, Bjerklund-Johansen TE, Botto H, Cek M, Naber KG, Pickard RS, Tenke P, Wagenlehner F, Wullt B. EAU guidelines on urological infections 2013. http://www.uroweb.org/guidelines/online-guidelines/.
4. Centers for Disease Control and Prevention (CDC). Sexually transmitted diseases treatment guidelines 2010. MMWR Recomm Rep. 2010;59:1–116.

Chronic Kidney Disease (CKD) 30

Marcus Hiß and Jan T. Kielstein

30.1 Definition

The first broad definition of chronic kidney disease was issued by a US American guideline (National Kidney Foundation. K/DOQI clinical practice guidelines for chronic kidney disease: evaluation, classification, and stratification. Kidney Disease Outcome Quality Initiative) [1]. It defines CKD as:

1. Kidney damage for >3 months as defined by structural or functional abnormalities of the kidney, with or without decreased glomerular filtration rate (GFR) manifest by either
   - Pathological abnormalities
   - Markers of kidney damage, including abnormalities in the composition of the blood or urine or abnormalities in imaging tests
2. GFR <60 ml/min /1.73 m^2 for >3 months, with or without kidney damage

A recent revision of this definition by the Kidney Disease Outcomes Quality Initiative (KDOQI) [2] took in account the epidemiological evidence underlining the importance of the reduction in GFR and proteinuria on hard endpoints such as all-cause and cardiovascular mortality and progression of CKD [3] and therefore recommended the following definition, summarized in Table 30.1. The presence of dialysis or transplantation is marked by "D" or "T," respectively.

CKD is a frequent finding in clinical medicine as the prevalence of CKD is about 14 % in industrialized countries [4], and it is known that these patients are more likely to die of cardiovascular diseases than to reach CKD 5 D, i.e., become dialysis dependent. Due to overwhelming and depressing epidemiological data, the American Heart Association listed CKD as a risk factor for cardiovascular disease [5]. The prevalence of CKD is rising. In the age group ≥80 years, 62.2 % of subjects have an eGFR <60 mL/min [6].

M. Hiß (✉) • J.T. Kielstein
Department of Nephrology and Hypertension, Hannover Medical School, Carl-Neuberg-Str. 1, Hannover 30625, Germany
e-mail: hiss.marcus@mh-hannover.de; kielstein@yahoo.com

A.S. Merseburger et al. (eds.), *Urology at a Glance*,
DOI 10.1007/978-3-642-54859-8_30, © Springer-Verlag Berlin Heidelberg 2014

Table 30.1 Classification of CKD according to the two dimension GFR and albuminuria and the corresponding cardiovascular risk as published in Kidney International Supplements [23] (with permission)

Prognosis of CKD by GFR and albuminuria categories: KDIGO 2012				Persistant albuminuria categories Description and range		
				A1	A2	A3
				Normal to mildly increased	Moderately increased	Severely increased
				<30 mg/g <3 mg/mmol	30–300 mg/g 3–30mg/mmol	>300 mg/g >30 mg/mmol
GFR categories (ml/min/ 1.73 m^2) Description and range	G1	Normal or high	≥90	Green	Yellow	Orange
	G2	Mildly decreased	60–89	Green	Yellow	Orange
	G3a	Mildly to moderately decreased	45–59	Yellow	Orange	Red
	G3b	Moderately to severely decreased	30–44	Orange	Red	Red
	G4	Severely decreased	15–29	Red	Red	Red
	G5	Kidney failure	<15	Red	Red	Red

Green low risk (if no other markers of kidney disease, no CKD), *Yellow* moderately increased risk, *Orange* high risk, *Red* very high risk)

30.2 Medical History

In terms of medical history, CKD is a rather silent disease, especially as no warning signals such as pain occur. Even in advanced kidney failure, there are no pathognomonic symptoms. One of the most overlooked warning signs is hypertension. There is a strong association between CKD and an elevated blood pressure whereby each can cause or aggravate the other [7]. Therefore, renal function has to be checked in every patient with hypertension. Documents like the "Mutterpass" maternal health passport can help gain access to reliable previous blood pressure readings. Less frequent but also rather often overlooked symptom is proteinuria, indicated by foamy urine. In severe proteinuria, marked edema can occur as part of the nephrotic syndrome (proteinuria >3 g/day, edema, hypoproteinemia, and hypercholesteremia), which are very often thought to be caused by heart failure. A sudden onset of edema, especially in young and middle-aged patients, should promptly result in a urine dipstick screening for proteinuria. Almost tragic is the fact that overt hematuria, a first class warning sign for the patients, is not followed up upon if urological evaluation excluded cancer or stones. Hematuria can be a warning sign of severe glomerular diseases!

Patients suffering from the two major diseases leading to CKD, i.e., diabetes and hypertension, should be regularly checked for GFR and (micro) albuminuria (>30 mg/day). According to the American Heart Association, renal function and proteinuria should be evaluated in every patient at increased risk for cardiovascular disease [8].

In systemic rheumatic diseases like systemic lupus and vasculitis determination of GFR and proteinuria should be part of the workup, which also includes a urine sediment [9]. The family history is unfortunately only of major importance for patients suffering from adult polycystic kidney disease [10]. A thorough medical history including medication is more important for acute kidney injury than for CKD, but it should be kept in mind that NSAID, ACE inhibitors, and ARBs can reduce glomerular perfusion. Many different classes of drugs can cause acute interstitial nephritis ranging from more frequent ones like antimicrobials (ampicillin, ciprofloxacin, methicillin, rifampicin, and sulfonamides) and nonsteroidal antiinflammatory drugs (acetylsalicylic acid, ibuprofen, naproxen) over proton pump inhibitors (omeprazole and pantoprazole) [11] to rarer causes like newer quinolones (moxifloxacin) [12] and/or iron-chelating agents (deferasirox) [13].

30.3 Diagnostics

30.3.1 The Measurement of Creatinine Alone Is Insufficient to Assess Renal Function!

The standard measure of kidney function is the measurement of GFR of its estimation (eGFR). This is hampered by the lack of reliable markers of GFR. The gold standard, inulin clearance, is cumbersome and expensive, reducing its utility in clinical practice. This is also true for estimations using the clearance of radioisotopes. Therefore, in clinical practice serum creatinine alone or in conjunction with a timed urine collection for creatinine clearance is typically used to assess renal function [14]. Reporting the serum creatinine alone makes no sense as creatinine itself has no notable toxicity. The creatinine measurement itself had not been standardized for a long period of time. This is important as the Jaffe determination method for serum creatinine has recently been replaced by the isotope dilution mass spectrometry technique (IDMS) which yields serum creatinine values that are 5–10 % lower on average.

Urine collection show considerable interindividual variability associated with muscle mass, protein intake, age, and sex. Moreover, obtaining accurate 24-h timed urine collections, although easy to perform in theory, seems to be impractical not only for infants and elderly patients. Therefore, formula-based estimates of GFR are currently used in clinical practice and mostly reported by the laboratory. Currently, the CKD-EPI method appears to be emerging as the method of choice for the staging CKD [15]. In terms of risk prediction (all-cause mortality and cardiovascular mortality), cystatin C alone or in conjunction with creatinine-based eGFR was superior to creatinine eGFR alone [16].

30.4 Therapy

Due to the large variety of underlying diseases leading to CKD, there is rarely a specific therapy with a few exceptions such as the use of the humanized murine complement inhibitor eculizumab for the treatment of atypical hemolytic uremic syndrome [17]. Immunosuppressive therapy represents the leading treatment strategy for immunological renal diseases, best epitomized by the use of steroids and cyclophosphamide for induction therapy of ANCA-associated vasculitis and lately the anti-CD20 agent rituximab [18].

Due to the paucity of specific treatments, the focus in treating patients with CKD had been to deliver optimal supportive care. Lately international clinical practice guidelines had been established by Kidney Disease: Improving Global Outcomes (KDIGO), an independent organization with the mission to improve care and outcomes of patients with kidney disease worldwide [19].

30.4.1 Blood Pressure

In general we should aim for a blood pressure <140/90 mmHg in CKD patients without albuminuria [7]. If the patients become albuminuric (albumin excretion rate of >30 mg/24 h), a lower target <130/80 mmHg is suggested. The use of a combination therapy is frequently required. Especially for albuminuric patients (albumin excretion rate of >30 mg/24 h), the use of agents blocking the renin-angiotensin-aldosterone system is recommended [7]. There is no marked difference in the recommendations for diabetics vs. nondiabetic patients.

30.4.2 Chronic Kidney Disease-Mineral and Bone Disorder (CKD-MBD)

Chronic kidney disease-mineral and bone disorder (CKD-MBD) is the triad of abnormalities in laboratory data, bone morphology, and vascular calcifications; thus, treating CKD-MBD is a cornerstone of care for CKD patients. Laboratory parameters such as phosphate, calcium, parathyroid hormone, vitamin D levels, and maybe the phosphatonin FGF-23 have to be measured on a regular basis below a GFR of 60 ml/min [20]. Also, assessment of bone status (by the best means available) should be used to guide treatment decisions. A mainstay of therapy and dietary education is aimed to reduce the phosphate load, as a high phosphate load has been shown to be associated with adverse outcome. Evidence that calcium load may influence progression of vascular calcification with effects on mortality should also be considered when choosing the type and dose of phosphate binder to be used [20].

30.4.3 Anemia

The treatment of anemia has dramatically changed over the last decade due to disappointing trials that could not prove the long lasting idea that a high hemoglobin level is beneficial in terms of retarding progression of CKD and improving mortality in patients on dialysis. Treatment of anemia should only be initiated when the hemoglobin levels is <10 g/dl. If absolute or functional iron deficiency is present, IV iron supplementation should be initiated. Therapy with erythrocytosis-stimulating agents (ESA) should be targeted to not exceed a hemoglobin level of 12 mg/dl. Restriction of IV iron is suggested if ferritin exceeds 500 ng/ml or TSAT is >30 % [21].

Preventive measures in CKD patients to avoid (iatrogenic) deterioration of renal function include the avoidance (reduction of volume) of contrast media as well as the avoidance of NSAIDs. Further, intense inhibition of the renin-angiotensin-aldosterone system should be done with care to avoid AKI and hyperkalemia, as recently seen in the dual blockade in patients with diabetic nephropathy using ACI-I and ARB [22].

References

1. National Kidney Foundation. K/DOQI clinical practice guidelines for chronic kidney disease: evaluation, classification, and stratification. Am J Kidney Dis. 2002;39:S1–266.
2. Levey AS, de Jong PE, Coresh J, El NM, Astor BC, Matsushita K, Gansevoort RT, Kasiske BL, Eckardt KU. The definition, classification, and prognosis of chronic kidney disease: a KDIGO Controversies Conference report. Kidney Int. 2011;80:17–28.
3. Matsushita K, Van d Velde M, Astor BC, Woodward M, Levey AS, de Jong PE, Coresh J, Gansevoort RT. Association of estimated glomerular filtration rate and albuminuria with all-cause and cardiovascular mortality in general population cohorts: a collaborative meta-analysis. Lancet. 2010;375:2073–81.
4. Coresh J, Selvin E, Stevens LA, Manzi J, Kusek JW, Eggers P, Van LF, Levey AS. Prevalence of chronic kidney disease in the United States. JAMA. 2007;298:2038–47.
5. Sarnak MJ, Levey AS, Schoolwerth AC, Coresh J, Culleton B, Hamm LL, McCullough PA, Kasiske BL, Kelepouris E, Klag MJ, Parfrey P, Pfeffer M, Raij L, Spinosa DJ, Wilson PW. Kidney disease as a risk factor for development of cardiovascular disease: a statement from the American Heart Association Councils on Kidney in Cardiovascular Disease, High Blood Pressure Research, Clinical Cardiology, and Epidemiology and Prevention. Circulation. 2003;108:2154–69.
6. Grams ME, Juraschek SP, Selvin E, Foster MC, Inker LA, Eckfeldt JH, Levey AS, Coresh J. Trends in the prevalence of reduced GFR in the United States: a comparison of creatinine- and cystatin C-based estimates. Am J Kidney Dis. 2013;62:253–60.
7. Wheeler DC, Becker GJ. Summary of KDIGO guideline. What do we really know about management of blood pressure in patients with chronic kidney disease? Kidney Int. 2013;83:377–83.
8. Brosius III FC, Hostetter TH, Kelepouris E, Mitsnefes MM, Moe SM, Moore MA, Pennathur S, Smith GL, Wilson PW. Detection of chronic kidney disease in patients with or at increased

risk of cardiovascular disease: a science advisory from the American Heart Association Kidney And Cardiovascular Disease Council; the Councils on High Blood Pressure Research, Cardiovascular Disease in the Young, and Epidemiology and Prevention; and the Quality of Care and Outcomes Research Interdisciplinary Working Group: developed in collaboration with the National Kidney Foundation. Circulation. 2006;114:1083–7.

9. Tesser Poloni JA, Bosan IB, Garigali G, Fogazzi GB. Urinary red blood cells: not only glomerular or nonglomerular. Nephron Clin Pract. 2012;120:c36–41.
10. Torres VE, Harris PC, Pirson Y. Autosomal dominant polycystic kidney disease. Lancet. 2007;369:1287–301.
11. Perazella MA, Markowitz GS. Drug-induced acute interstitial nephritis. Nat Rev Nephrol. 2010;6:461–70.
12. Chatzikyrkou C, Hamwi I, Clajus C, Becker J, Hafer C, Kielstein JT. Biopsy proven acute interstitial nephritis after treatment with moxifloxacin. BMC Nephrol. 2010;11:19.
13. Brosnahan G, Gokden N, Swaminathan S. Acute interstitial nephritis due to deferasirox: a case report. Nephrol Dial Transplant. 2008;23:3356–8.
14. Levey AS, Stevens LA, Hostetter T. Automatic reporting of estimated glomerular filtration rate – just what the doctor ordered. Clin Chem. 2006;52:2188–93.
15. Levey AS, Stevens LA, Schmid CH, Zhang YL, Castro III AF, Feldman HI, Kusek JW, Eggers P, Van LF, Greene T, Coresh J. A new equation to estimate glomerular filtration rate. Ann Intern Med. 2009;150:604–12.
16. Shlipak MG, Matsushita K, Arnlov J, Inker LA, Katz R, Polkinghorne KR, Rothenbacher D, Sarnak MJ, Astor BC, Coresh J, Levey AS, Gansevoort RT. Cystatin C versus creatinine in determining risk based on kidney function. N Engl J Med. 2013;369:932–43.
17. Legendre CM, Licht C, Muus P, Greenbaum LA, Babu S, Bedrosian C, Bingham C, Cohen DJ, Delmas Y, Douglas K, Eitner F, Feldkamp T, Fouque D, Furman RR, Gaber O, Herthelius M, Hourmant M, Karpman D, Lebranchu Y, Mariat C, Menne J, Moulin B, Nurnberger J, Ogawa M, Remuzzi G, Richard T, Sberro-Soussan R, Severino B, Sheerin NS, Trivelli A, Zimmerhackl LB, Goodship T, Loirat C. Terminal complement inhibitor eculizumab in atypical hemolytic-uremic syndrome. N Engl J Med. 2013;368:2169–81.
18. Stone JH, Merkel PA, Spiera R, Seo P, Langford CA, Hoffman GS, Kallenberg CG, St Clair EW, Turkiewicz A, Tchao NK, Webber L, Ding L, Sejismundo LP, Mieras K, Weitzenkamp D, Ikle D, Seyfert-Margolis V, Mueller M, Brunetta P, Allen NB, Fervenza FC, Geetha D, Keogh KA, Kissin EY, Monach PA, Peikert T, Stegeman C, Ytterberg SR, Specks U. Rituximab versus cyclophosphamide for ANCA-associated vasculitis. N Engl J Med. 2010;363:221–32.
19. Eckardt KU, Kasiske BL. Kidney disease: improving global outcomes. Nat Rev Nephrol. 2009;5:650–7.
20. Goldsmith DJ, Covic A, Fouque D, Locatelli F, Olgaard K, Rodriguez M, Spasovski G, Urena P, Zoccali C, London GM, Vanholder R. Endorsement of the Kidney Disease Improving Global Outcomes (KDIGO) Chronic Kidney Disease-Mineral and Bone Disorder (CKD-MBD) guidelines: a European Renal Best Practice (ERBP) commentary statement. Nephrol Dial Transplant. 2010;25:3823–31.
21. Locatelli F, Barany P, Covic A, De FA, Del VL, Goldsmith D, Horl W, London G, Vanholder R, Van BW. Kidney disease: improving global outcomes guidelines on anaemia management in chronic kidney disease: a European Renal Best Practice position statement. Nephrol Dial Transplant. 2013;28:1346–59.
22. Fried LF, Emanuele N, Zhang JH, Brophy M, Conner TA, Duckworth W, Leehey DJ, McCullough PA, O'Connor T, Palevsky PM, Reilly RF, Seliger SL, Warren SR, Watnick S, Peduzzi P, Guarino P. Combined angiotensin inhibition for the treatment of diabetic nephropathy. N Engl J Med. 2013;369:1892–903.
23. Kidney Disease: Improving Global Outcomes (KDIGO) CKD Work Group. KDIGO 2012 Clinical Practice Guideline for the Evaluation and Management of Chronic Kidney Disease. Kidney inter., Suppl. 2013;3:1–150.

Bladder Cancer

31

Mario W. Kramer, Hannes Cash, and Brant A. Inman

31.1 General Facts

Worldwide, approximately 330,000 new cases of bladder cancer (BC) are diagnosed each year and 130,000 people die annually of this disease. Median age at diagnosis is 70 years and men are at 3.8 times higher risk than women. In western countries, the lifetime risk of developing BC is 2.4 % and it is the fourth most common solid tumor in men. Exposures known to increase the risk of BC include tobacco smoke, occupational carcinogens, and schistosomiasis. Dietary factors that decrease BC risk include high water intake and cruciferous legume consumption.

31.2 Symptoms, Classification, and Grading

Presenting symptoms of BC include hematuria (75 %), irritative lower urinary tract symptoms (20 %), and pain (5 %, which is usually due to ureteral obstruction by tumor). In western countries, the most common histologic subtype of BC is

M.W. Kramer, MD (✉)
Department of Urology and Urologic Oncology, Hannover Medical School,
Carl-Neuberg-Str. 1, 30625 Hannover, Germany
e-mail: kramer.mario@mh-hannover.de

H. Cash, MD
Department of Urology, Charité University Medicine Berlin,
Campus Benjamin Franklin, Hindenburgdamm 30, 12200 Berlin, Germany
e-mail: hannes.cash@charite.de

B.A. Inman, MD MS FRCSC
Division of Urology, Department of Surgery, Duke University Medical Center,
DUMC 2812, Durham, NC 27710, USA
e-mail: brant.inman@duke.edu

A.S. Merseburger et al. (eds.), *Urology at a Glance*,
DOI 10.1007/978-3-642-54859-8_31,

Table 31.1 TNM classification of bladder cancer (2009)

T – Primary tumor			
Ta	Noninvasive papillary carcinoma		
Tis	Carcinoma in situ: "flat tumor"		
T1	Tumor invades subepithelial connective tissue		
T2	Tumor invades muscle		
T3	Tumor invades perivesical tissue		
T4	Tumor invades perivesical organs or pelvic/abdominal wall		
N – Regional lymph nodes			
N0	No regional lymph node metastasis		
N1	Metastasis in a single lymph node in the true pelvis		
N2	Metastasis in multiple lymph nodes in the true pelvis		
N3	Metastasis in common iliac lymph node(s)		
M – Distant metastasis			
M0	No distant metastasis		
M1	Distant metastasis		
Stage grouping	*TNM*	*5-year relative survival (%)*	*Median survival*
0	Ta or Tis	95	>10 years
I	T1	85	10 years
II	T2	65	5 years
III	T3 or T4a	45	2.5 years
IV	T4b or N+ or M1	15	10 months

urothelial carcinoma (90 %), with squamous cell carcinoma (5 %), adenocarcinoma (2 %), and small cell carcinoma (1 %) being less common. In areas where schistosomiasis is endemic, squamous cell carcinomas comprise 50 % of BCs.

Conventional white light cystoscopy remains the gold standard for diagnosing bladder cancer (sensitivity 90 %, specificity 90 %), though fluorescent cystoscopy is an alternative that is slightly more sensitive but less specific. Urine tests are also used in the diagnosis of bladder cancer though their precise role is unclear. Urine cytology has a sensitivity of 35 % (80 % for CIS) and specificity of 95 % for BC and remains the most frequently used urine test. Once a tumor is visualized at cystoscopy, the first step in diagnosis/treatment is transurethral resection (TURBT).

BC is staged using the TNM/AJCC system (Table 31.1). The TURBT procedure determines the preliminary T stage, while the N and M stages are determined by cross-sectional imaging of the abdomen/pelvis, chest imaging, and bone imaging. Brain imaging is only indicated if metastases are present elsewhere. The upper urinary tracts should be imaged at diagnosis (CT or MRI urography, retrograde or intravenous pyelography) since 5 % of patients will have ureteral or renal pelvic tumors. At diagnosis, 70 % of bladder tumors are non-muscle invasive (NMIBC; Ta, T1, or Tis), 20 % are muscle invasive (MIBC; T2, T3, or T4), and 10 % are metastatic (N+or M1). Median and relative survival rates are stage dependent (Table 31.1).

Table 31.2 1998 WHO/ISUP tumor grading system for urothelial carcinoma

Papillary urothelial neoplasm of low malignant potential (PUNLMP)
Low-grade papillary urothelial carcinoma
High-grade papillary urothelial carcinoma

BC grading is done using the WHO/ISUP system (Table 31.2). NMIBC is characterized by a very high local recurrence rate which ranges from 25 to 85 % depending on known risk factors. The risk of stage progression ranges from 5 to 35 % also depending on risk factors. The EORTC BC risk prediction tool quantifies these risk factors (www.eortc.com/tools/bladdercalculator).

31.3 Therapy

TURBT is the gold standard for the initial diagnosis/treatment of BC. Immediate postoperative instillation of intravesical chemotherapy (e.g., mitomycin C, epirubicin, doxorubicin) is indicated after TURBT for NMIBC since it lowers the recurrence rate by 35 %. Patients at intermediate or high risk of recurrence or progression should be treated with adjuvant intravesical chemotherapy or BCG (preferred for CIS and high-risk patients). These treatments should include an induction phase (weekly instillations for 6 weeks) and a maintenance phase lasting at least 1 year. A second look TURBT is performed 2–6 weeks later if the initial TURBT was incomplete, if a large tumor burden was present (size or multifocality), or if high-grade or T1 pathology was noted. Surveillance for recurrence consists of periodic cystoscopy and/or urine testing and imaging, the frequency of which is risk adapted. Patients with high-risk NMIBC that fail to respond to intravesical therapy should undergo radical cystectomy since survival decreases if these tumors progress to MIBC.

When MIBC is found at TURBT, more invasive therapies are needed to prevent metastasis and local progression. The gold standard therapy for MIBC is radical cystectomy (RC). In men, RC consists of resection of the bladder, prostate, and lymph nodes, while in women the uterus, fallopian tubes, and ovaries are also included. Urinary diversion options include ileal and colonic conduits, catheterizable cutaneous pouches, and neobladders. Bladder sparing chemoradiation therapy is an alternative to RC but is only administered to relatively asymptomatic patients with low tumor burden. Chemotherapy is a critical component of the management of MIBC and is best given neoadjuvantly to RC or concurrently with radiation. The two most active chemotherapy regimens are GC (gemcitabine, cisplatin) and MVAC (methotrexate, vinblastine, Adriamycin, cisplatin). These regimens increase survival by 5–10 % in MIBC patients and by 6 months in patients with metastases.

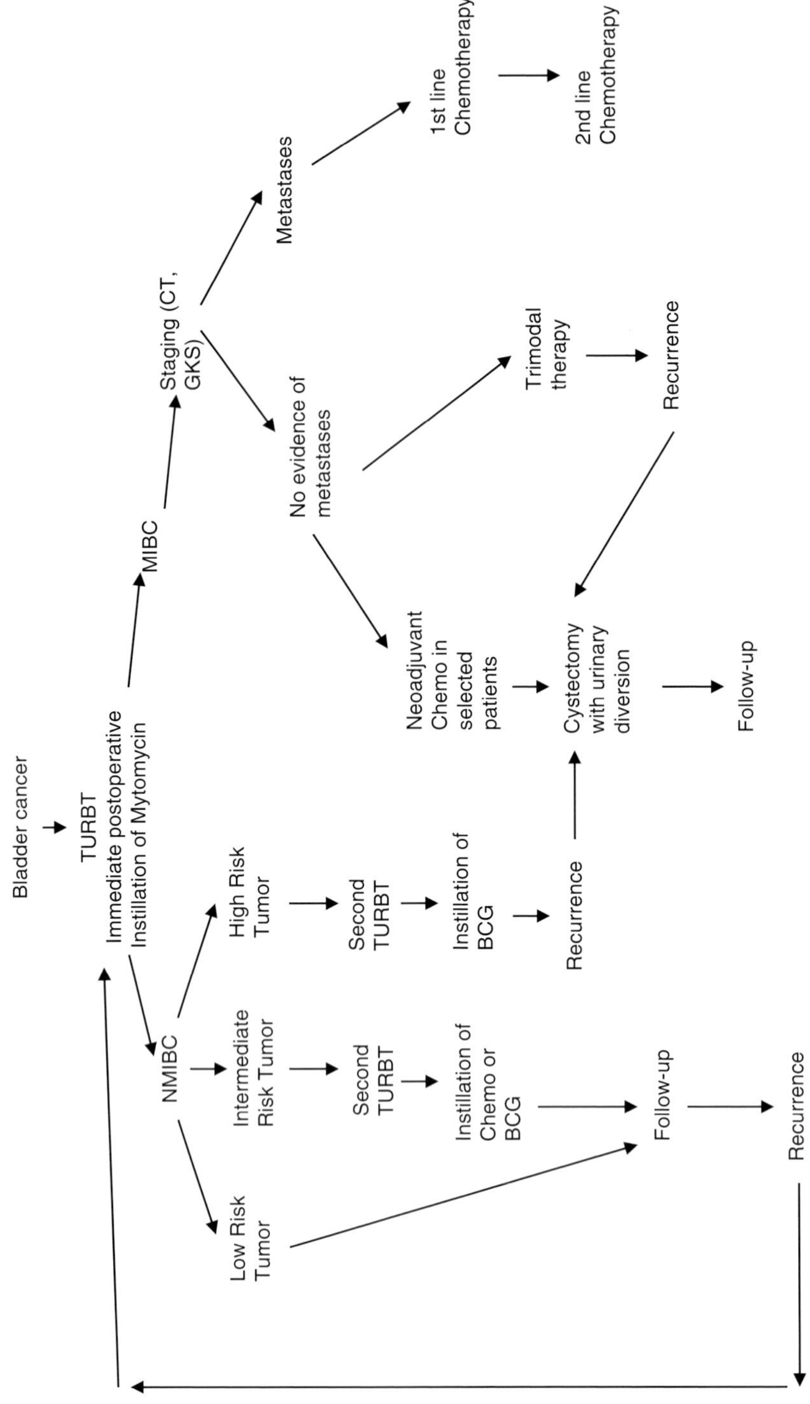
Bladder cancer
TURBT
Immediate postoperative
Instillation of Mytomycin
MIBC
Staging (CT,
GKS)
Metastases
1st line
Chemotherapy
2nd line
Chemotherapy
No evidence of
metastases
Trimodal
therapy
Recurrence
Neoadjuvant
Chemo in
selected
patients
Cystectomy
with urinary
diversion
Follow-up
NMIBC
High Risk
Tumor
Second
TURBT
Instillation of
BCG
Recurrence
Intermediate
Risk Tumor
Second
TURBT
Instillation of
Chemo or
BCG
Follow-up
Recurrence
Low Risk
Tumor

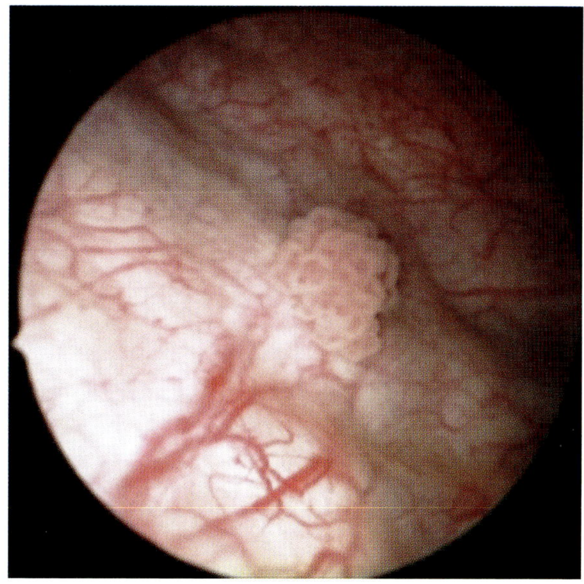

Fig. 31.1 Picture shows a non-muscle invasive bladder cancer under white light cystoscopy

31.4 Complications

TURBT is a minimally invasive procedure and serious complications are rare, but include bladder perforation and bleeding. Contrarily, RC is a very invasive procedure and perioperative mortality ranges from 1 to 5 % and is age and comorbidity dependent. While early postoperative complications occur in 25–50 % of RCs, most are minor and treatable. Late morbidity after RC is mainly associated with the urinary diversion (Fig. 31.1).

Urinary Tract Infection (UTI)

32

Mohammand Kabbani and Mario Kramer

32.1 General Facts

Urinary tract infections (UTIs) are one of the most common infections in modern medicine, ranking second after respiratory tract infections, causing more than seven million physicians' visits and 100,000 hospitalizations per year in the USA [1, 2]. UTIs are responsible for nearly 15 % of all community prescription antibiotics and are causes for more than one billion dollar costs per year to manage them [1, 3]. Women are in general more likely to be affected with UTIs. Almost half of all women will experience at least one UTI during their lifetime [3]. High prevalence of UTIs in conjunction with inappropriate and excessive antimicrobial treatment are risk factors of increasing antibiotic resistance. Since many clinical studies regarding treatment of UTIs have investigated women in large healthcare facilities in the USA, physicians should evaluate whether reviews and guidelines for UTI treatment are suitable to their local patients population. On the other side, inconsequent therapy of UTIs may result in potentially lethal urosepsis, renal abscess formation, and chronic pyelonephritis.

32.2 Symptoms, Classification

Typical symptoms of urinary tract infections are the onset of *frequency*, *dysuria*, and *urgency*. Without evidence of significant bacteriuria, these symptoms are defined as *acute urethral syndrome*. Urinary dipstick revealing positive nitrite

M. Kabbani, MD (✉) • M. Kramer MD
Department of Urology and Uro-Oncology, Hannover Medical School,
Carl-Neuberg-Str. 1, Hannover 30625, Germany
e-mail: mokkabbani@gmail.com; kramer.mario@mh-hannover.de

A.S. Merseburger et al. (eds.), *Urology at a Glance*,
DOI 10.1007/978-3-642-54859-8_32, © Springer-Verlag Berlin Heidelberg 2014

and/or leukocytes may indicate for UTI. *UTI* is defined by *significant bacteriuria* with more than *10^5 cfu/ml* from midstream urine, more than 10^2 cfu/ml from urine of urinary catheters, every evidence of bacteria from suprapubic catheter urine and pyuria (>10 white blood cells per high-power field [×400]). Asymptomatic bacteriuria is often seen in elderly and/or catheterized patients. The *acute onset of fever*, *chills*, *nausea* and *vomiting*, *abnormal fatigue*, *flank pain*, and *renal angle tenderness* refer to *acute pyelonephritis*. Urinary tract infections are defined by both clinical course and localization. *Upper urinary tract infections* are *pyelonephritis* and *ureteritis*, whereas *lower urinary tract infections* are *cystitis*, *urethritis*, and *prostatitis*. The *most common appearance of UTIs* is *uncomplicated cystitis among sexually active women. Complicating factors of UTIs* are *age* (<10 or >70 years), *pregnancy*, *urinary obstruction*, *anatomical abnormalities*, *vesicoureteral reflux*, *foreign bodies* (e.g., ureteral stents), *urinary catheterization*, *diabetes mellitus*, *immunosuppression*, *recurrent urinary tract infections*, and recently *undergone urologic surgery*. Chronic cystitis is defined by persistent cystitis or more than 3 cystitides per year. Recurrent urinary tract infections are defined by more than 2 UTIs per half year or more than 3 UTIs per year. Prostatitis is defined by the bacterial infection of the prostate in conjunction with fever, chills, lumbar and perineal pain, and lower urinary tract symptoms (frequency, urgency, dysuria, low urinary flow, and retention) (for further information look at Chap. 46).

32.3 Therapy

The therapy of UTIs should consider gender, complicating factors, and localization of the UTI. In addition to spectrum and efficacy, tolerability, and allergy, adverse effects and costs of antibiotics therapy should be evaluated for each patient. Local resistance rates for antibiotics are a big challenge in the treatment of UTIs. Healthy women with clear history and without pregnancy can be treated with 5 days of nitrofurantoin 100 mg 1-1-1; 3 days of co-trimoxazole (TMP-SMX) 960 mg 1-0-1 (caution: avoid if high local resistance rates are known); a single dose fosfomycin 3 g [4]. If the aforementioned antibiotics cannot be used, a 3 days treatment with ciprofloxacin 250–500 mg, 1-0-1 is an alternative (caution: fluoroquinolones should be preserved for complicated UTIs) [4]. β-Lactam agents, including amoxicillin-clavulanate in 3–7-day regimens are appropriate choices for therapy when other recommended agents cannot be used [4]. Amoxicillin or ampicillin as single agents is not recommended due to empirically known low efficacy.

Recurrent cystitis is most common in premenopausal young and healthy women. Micturition after sexual intercourse, sexual hygiene, high diuresis, and regular consumption of cranberry juice might help avoid reoccurrence. If these measures are not effective, antimicrobials taken at bedtime like nitrofurantoin 100 mg/day, TMP-SMX 40/200 mg/day (or 3×/week), and fosfomycin 3 g/10 days can be administered for 6 months. Ciprofloxacin 125 mg/day might be applied in cases of resistant pathogens. Alternatively, if recurrent cystitis is associated with sexual intercourse, post-intercourse prophylaxis might be considered [1]. In each individual case, complicating factors must be ruled out before given general recommendations.

In postmenopausal women with recurrent cystitis, local estrogen replacement therapy reduces the reoccurrence probability. During pregnancy, cephalosporins, amoxicillin, or nitrofurantoin can be administered. Asymptomatic bacteriuria in the absence of complicating factors usually does not require treatment. However, early screening and treatment after antibiotic sensitivity testing of asymptomatic bacteriuria during pregnancy is recommended due to the higher probability of pyelonephritis in pregnant women.

Women with complicating factors (see list) and acute cystitis or uncomplicated cystitis of the man (caution: exclude other risk factors) should be treated with at least 7 days oral antibiotics regimen of either fluoroquinolones, amoxicillin-clavulanate, cephalosporins, or TMP (urine culture should be taken *before* treatment). Usually outpatient management is sufficient. However, the onset of severe UTIs as seen in acute complicated pyelonephritis requires inpatient care. Therapy should be started with initial empirical intravenous antibiotics such as fluoroquinolones, amoxicillin-clavulanate, cephalosporins (3rd gen), or aminoglycoside for 1–3 days (urine culture and blood culture should be taken *before* treatment). Upon availability of the resistogram, an oral antimicrobial treatment for at least 2 weeks is possible. In case of a severe complicated UTI, combination therapy with aminoglycosides + ampicillins, aminoglycosides + cephalosporins, or piperacillin + BLI (beta-lactamase inhibitor) should be administered after initial therapy. Complicating factors *must* be evaluated.

32.4 Complications

Ascending infection of the lower urinary tract may lead to acute pyelonephritis. Epididymidis might follow UTI in men. The most feared complication is the potentially lethal urosepsis with additional signs of tachycardia and hypotension. Renal abscess formation may be induced by complicating risk factors and/or antimicrobial resistance. Chronic pyelonephritis after recurrent and not adequate treated acute pyelonephritis may lead to chronic kidney disease and on long term to renal failure.

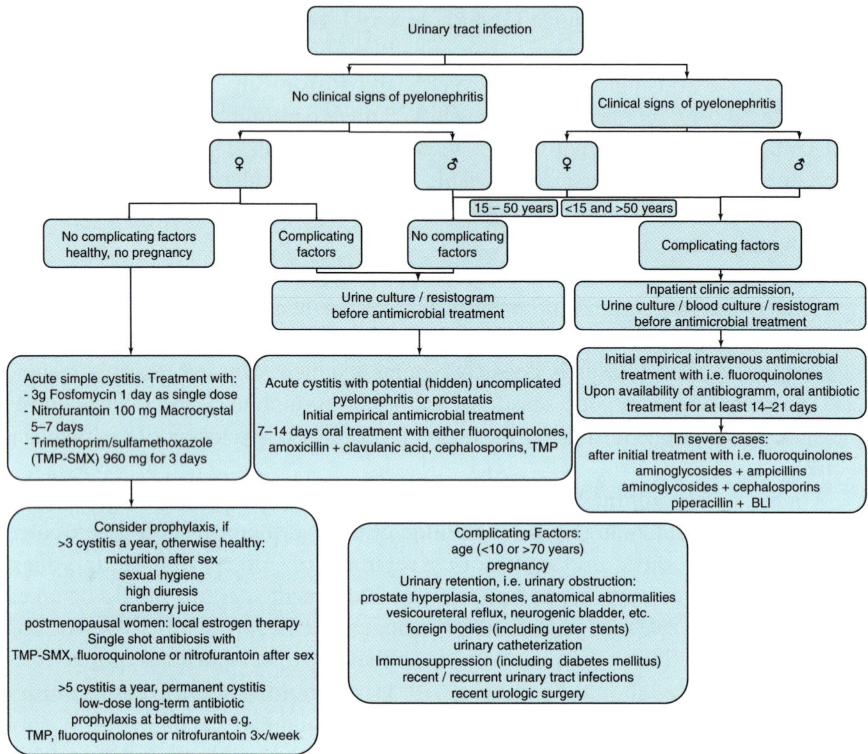

References

1. Grabe M, Bjerklund-Johansen TE, Botto H, Çek M, Naber KG, Pickard RS, Tenke P, Wagenlehner F, Wullt B. EAU guidelines on urological infections Uroweb 2013. Available at: http://www.uroweb.org/gls/pdf/18_Urological%20infections_LR.pdf. Accessed 6 June 2013.
2. Foxman B. Epidemiology of urinary tract infections: incidence, morbidity, and economic costs. Am J Med. 2002;113(Suppl 1A):5S–13.
3. Mazzulli T. Resistance trends in urinary tract pathogens and impact on management. J Urol. 2002;168(4 Pt 2):1720–2.
4. Gupta K, Hooton TM, Naber KG, Wullt B, Colgan R, Miller LG, Moran GJ, Nicolle LE, Raz R, Schaeffer AJ, Soper DE. International clinical practice guidelines for the treatment of acute uncomplicated cystitis and pyelonephritis in women: a 2010 update by the Infectious Diseases Society of America and the European Society for Microbiology and Infectious Diseases. Clin Infect Dis. 2011;52(5):e103–20.

Hyperparathyroidism

33

Bastian Amend and Karl-Dietrich Sievert

33.1 General Facts

An increased serum level of parathormone (PH) characterizes hyperparathyroidism. Different causes for hyperparathyroidism (HPT) are classified into primary, secondary, and tertiary hyperparathyroidism.

Primary HPT is defined as an autonomic secretion of PH; secondary HPT results from chronic kidney disease with hypocalcaemia, hyperphosphatemia, and reduced-activated vitamin D levels (endocrine renal insufficiency) or other reasons for vitamin D deficiency. Tertiary HPT is characterized by an inadequate PH secretion, in correlation to the serum calcium level in patients after long-term secondary HPT. Special forms of hyperparathyroidism include the paraneoplastic secretion of PH-like substances or genetic disorders including HPT (MEN 1 and MEN 2a or familiar hypocalciuric hypercalcemia) [1].

Epidemiological data is sparse but available data estimates a primary HPT incidence of approximately 21/100,000 persons, with a prevalence of 1–4/1,000 persons. Primary HPT is more frequent in females vs. males and appears as an age-related occurrence [2, 3]. Secondary HPT is strongly associated with the progression of chronic renal failure. About 80 % of the patients with a serum creatinine level of at least 5 mg/dl need treatment for secondary HPT and close follow-up [1].

33.2 Symptoms, Classification, and Grading

Increased serum PH levels lead to bone demineralization. In primary HPT patients, the traditional symptoms include bone pain (osteomalacia), nephrolithiasis and nephrocalcinosis (hypercalciuria), and abdominal pain (nausea, peptic/duodenal ulcer,

B. Amend (✉) • K.-D. Sievert
Department of Urology, Eberhard-Karls-University,
Hoppe-Seyler-Str. 3, Tuebingen 72076, Germany
e-mail: bastian.amend@med.uni-tuebingen.de; karl.sievert@med.uni-tuebingen.de

A.S. Merseburger et al. (eds.), *Urology at a Glance*,
DOI 10.1007/978-3-642-54859-8_33, © Springer-Verlag Berlin Heidelberg 2014

Table 33.1 Classification of hyperparathyroidism (HPT) and expected laboratory results

Primary HPT Causes: solitary adenoma, hyperplasia, or carcinoma (seldom) of the parathyroid gland(s) Calcium: serum ↑, urine ↑ Phosphate: serum ↓, urine ↑ Parathormone: ↑ Alkaline phosphatase: ↑ Normocalcemic primary HPT: some patient present with normal serum calcium
Secondary HPT Causes: renal insufficiency including endocrine function (activated vitamin D), malabsorption, chronic liver failure (vitamin D hydroxylation), cholestasis (reduced vitamin D absorption) Calcium: serum ↓ Phosphate: serum ↓/ normal (nonrenal), ↑ (renal) Parathormone: ↑ Alkaline phosphatase: ↑
Tertiary HPT Causes: disproportional high parathormone secretion based on a long-term secondary HPT Calcium: serum ↑ (increase although serum calcium was reduced during secondary HPT)

pancreatitis). Although these symptoms were regularly present in the past, laboratory testing and preventive medical checkups lead to a more and more asymptomatic patient population with HPT. In addition to the mentioned symptoms, neuromuscular and psychiatric signs may precipitate that a hypercalcemic crisis might occur.

Table 33.1 summarizes the typical laboratory findings and aspects of primary, secondary, and tertiary hyperparathyroidism [1].

33.3 Therapy

33.3.1 Primary HPT

Surgery with the removal of abnormal parathyroid tissue is characterized by a high cure rate of up to 98 % and should be recommended to all symptomatic patients. Asymptomatic patients should be counseled about the surgery and active surveillance, according to current recommendations of the Third International Workshop on the Management of Asymptomatic Primary Hyperparathyroidism (Table 33.2). If surgery is indicated, radiological imaging is helpful to advise the surgeon as to the disease's extent and surgical approach, especially with regard to ectopic parathyroid tissue. Ultrasounds, computed tomography, magnetic resonance imaging, and a delayed-phase sestamibi scan are considered beneficial to identify the location and number of autonomic glands [1–3]. In cases where there might be a single parathyroid gland that may cause autonomic parathormone excretion, minimal invasive surgery might be a valuable option.

Table 33.2 Recommendations according to the Third International Workshop on the Management of Asymptomatic Primary Hyperparathyroidism 2008 [2]

Criteria for surgery
Serum calcium level: >1.0 mg/dl (0.25 mmol/l) above upper limit of normal range
(Calculated) creatinine clearance: reduced to <60 ml/min
Bone mineral density: T score less than 2.5 at any site (lumbar spine, total hip, femoral neck, distal third of the radius) and/or previous fragility fractures
Age: <50 years
Surveillance without surgery
Serum calcium level: annually
(Calculated) creatinine clearance: annually
Bone mineral density: every 1–2 years (three sites)

If surgical removal of the parathyroid gland(s) is not feasible or the patient refuses surgery, the following recommendations of only symptomatic treatment might be helpful in some patients to reduce serum calcium: increased fluid intake, prescribing a prophylaxis of osteoporosis in postmenopausal women and cinacalcet (activator of the calcium-sensing receptor), and terminating thiazide diuretics or cardiac glycosides.

33.3.2 Secondary HPT

Treatment of nonrenal secondary HPT consists of an effective therapy that addresses the underlying disease and substitution of vitamin D (colecalciferol) and calcium [1]. Renal secondary HPT (renal osteodystrophy) is treated stepwise according to fundamental pathophysiology:

- Restriction of phosphate intake (0.8–1.0 g/day)
- Calcium intake of maximum 2 g/day
- Phosphate binders (aluminum-containing binders should be avoided with regard to possible aluminum-induced encephalopathy, anemia, and osteopathy; alternatives: calcium carbonate, calcium acetate, or calcium-free binders (sevelamer or lanthanum carbonate))
- Supplementation of vitamin D and activated vitamin D
- Cinacalcet (activates the calcium-sensing receptor of parathyroid tissue)
  Ineffective treatment of a secondary HPT will result in a tertiary HPT [1].

33.3.3 Tertiary HPT

Tertiary HPT requires surgical treatment with possible reimplantation of parathyroid tissue into the sternocleidomastoid or brachioradialis muscle.

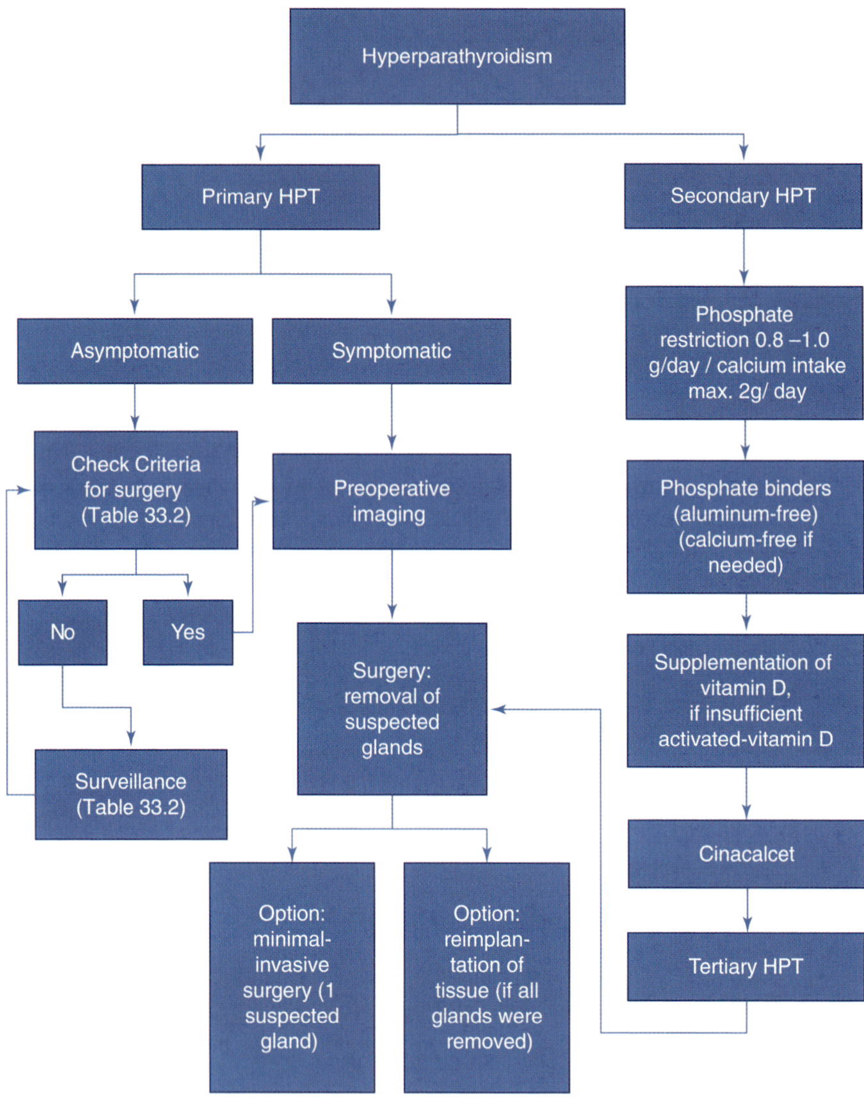

33.4 Complications

Untreated or insufficient treatment HPT might result in urolithiasis, osteopathy, gastrointestinal symptoms including ulcers and pancreatitis, muscle weakness, and other neuropsychiatric phenomena. Hypercalcemic crisis is associated with a case fatality rate of up to 50 % [1]. In experienced hands the complication rate of surgical treatment of HPT is reported to be low, between 1 and 3 % [2]. Specific risks of parathyroid surgery include laryngeal nerve palsy and postoperative hypocalcemia.

References

1. Herold G. Internal medicine. 1st ed. Gerd Herold: Cologne; 2011.
2. Marcocci C, Cetani F. Clinical practice. Primary hyperparathyroidism. N Engl J Med. 2011;365(25):2389–97.
3. Bollerslev J, Marcocci C, Sosa M, Nordenstrom J, Bouillon R, Mosekilde L. Current evidence for recommendation of surgery, medical treatment and vitamin D repletion in mild primary hyperparathyroidism. Eur J Endocrinol. 2011;165(6):851–64.

Adrenal Insufficiency

34

Axel Heidenreich and Andrea Thissen

34.1 Definition

Adrenal insufficiency is a rare endocrine disorder, characterized by an inappropriate secretion of adrenal hormones. It can be caused either by adrenal failure (Addison's disease, primary adrenal insufficiency) or by dysfunction of the integrity of the hypothalamic-pituitary-adrenal axis (secondary adrenal insufficiency). Primary adrenal insufficiency occurs with an estimated prevalence of 93–140 per million and is less frequently diagnosed than secondary adrenal insufficiency (prevalence of 150–280 per million) [1]. In the developed world, primary adrenal insufficiency most frequently stems from autoimmune adrenalitis, whereas in the developing world, infectious diseases such as tuberculosis or cytomegalovirus play a substantial etiological role. Pituitary adenomas and its treatment (surgical removal or radiation therapy) present the main causes of secondary adrenal insufficiency.

34.2 Medical History

Patients suffering from adrenal insufficiency often show nonspecific signs and symptoms such as persistent bodily and psychosocial impairments. Aspects regarding physical strength, lack of stamina, appetite, unspecific gastric pain and nausea, but also increased irritability or dizziness may be crucial for revealing the diagnosis. The intake of medication has to be enquired about, given that long-term steroid therapy; ketoconazole or etomidate are drugs that can cause adrenal insufficiency. Information about preexisting illnesses, infectious diseases (AIDS, tuberculosis), autoimmune disorders (autoimmune polyendocrine syndrome), cranial irradiation,

A. Heidenreich • A. Thissen (✉)
Department of Urology, RWTH University Aachen, Pauwelsstr. 30, Aachen 52074, Germany
e-mail: aheidenreich@ukaachen.de; anthissen@ukaachen.de

A.S. Merseburger et al. (eds.), *Urology at a Glance*,
DOI 10.1007/978-3-642-54859-8_34, © Springer-Verlag Berlin Heidelberg 2014

previous surgical interventions, or pregnancy/childbirth in women (autoimmune lymphocytic hypophysitis, Sheehan's syndrome) can be helpful in establishing the diagnosis of adrenal insufficiency. In about 5 % of patients, adrenal insufficiency can develop following unilateral radical nephrectomy for renal cell carcinoma despite an untouched contralateral adrenal gland so that the abovementioned clinical symptoms should be remembered.

34.3 Diagnostics

Since clinical signs of adrenal insufficiency are unspecific, a carefully performed physical examination is an indispensable part of the diagnostic pathway. The color of the skin and its turgor should be inspected. Skin darkening (hyperpigmentation) in chronic adrenal insufficiency often develops in palmar creases, elbow flexures, and areola mammae. It is due to elevated concentrations of proopiomelanocortin (POMC) as a byproduct of ACTH, which stimulates the synthesis of melanin in patients with primary adrenal insufficiency. On the other hand, deficiency of POMC in patients with secondary adrenal insufficiency results in alabaster-colored pale skin. Secondary adrenal insufficiency due to tumor masses in the sellar region with suprasellar extension can cause visual impairments, with bitemporal hemianopsia being the classical visual field defect [2]. As adrenal insufficiency may be subclinical, laboratory testing can confirm the diagnosis: a combination of low peripheral hormones with elevated adrenocorticotropic hormone (ACTH) level is suggestive of primary adrenal insufficiency, whereas secondary insufficiency becomes manifested with low peripheral hormones and inappropriate low pituitary hormones (see Fig. 34.1). Furthermore, hyponatremia and hyperkalemia can be observed in patients with primary adrenal insufficiency due to inappropriate secretion of mineralocorticoids, which stimulates the reabsorption of sodium and the excretion of potassium.

Due to diurnal rhythm of cortisol secretion, with highest concentrations in the early morning and lowest amounts around midnight, it is of particular importance to test morning serum cortisol level. If levels at 8 a.m. are repeatedly below 100 nmol/L, then adrenal insufficiency is highly likely, while values above 500 nmol/L exclude it [3]. Values between the upper and lower threshold require further dynamic testing, with insulin-induced hypoglycemia test (IHT) being the gold standard test for evaluating the HPA axis [3]. Hypoglycemia presents a strong stressor and stimulator of ACTH secretion. When cortisol response is greater than 500 nmol/l, adrenal insufficiency is ruled out. Yet it is worth noting that the performance of IHT requires absence of seizures and cardiovascular diseases and has to be undertaken only under close supervision at experienced centers. Alternatively, the standard 250-μg ACTH (1–24) stimulation test can be used to establish secondary adrenal insufficiency. Further imaging should be performed when tuberculous adrenalitis, acute adrenal hemorrhage, neoplasms of the adrenal gland, and pituitary adenomas are suspected (Fig. 34.2).

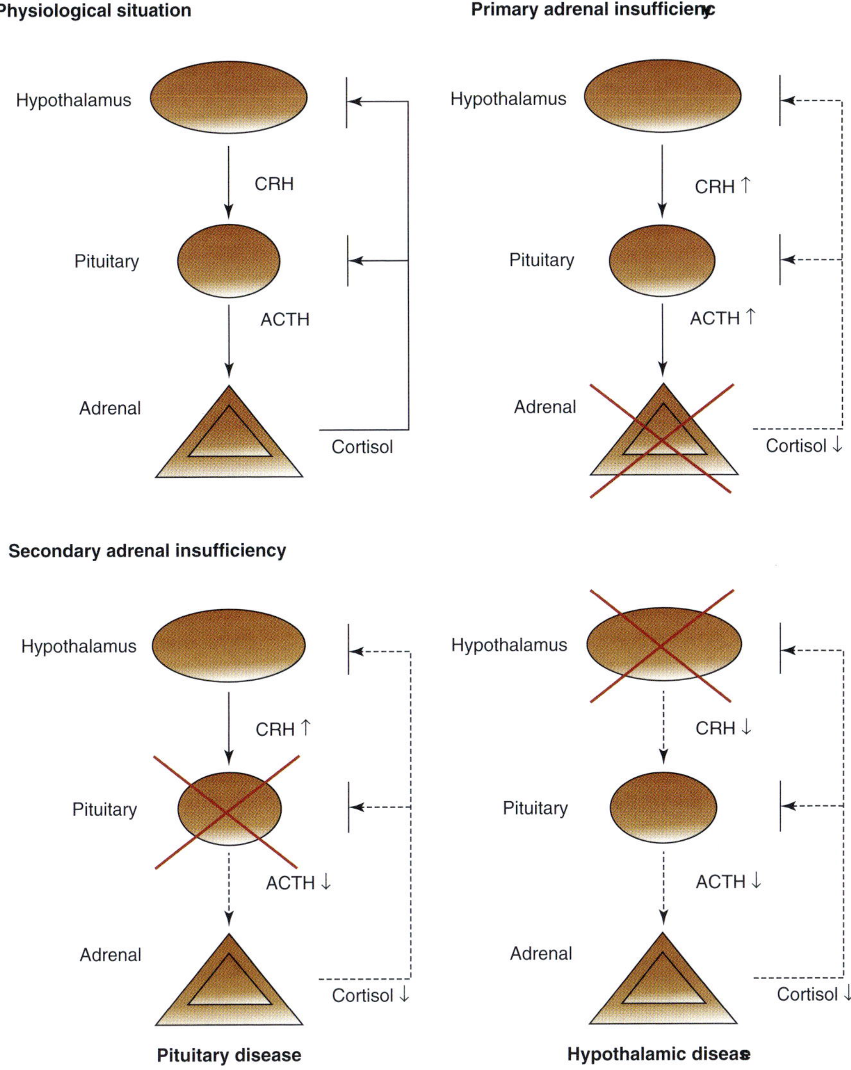

Fig. 34.1 Primary and secondary adrenal insufficiency. *CRH* corticotropin-releasing hormone [1]

34.3.1 Differential Diagnosis

- Hemochromatosis – hyperpigmentation
- Tumor cachexia – weight loss and weakness
- Depression – lack of stamina and fatigue

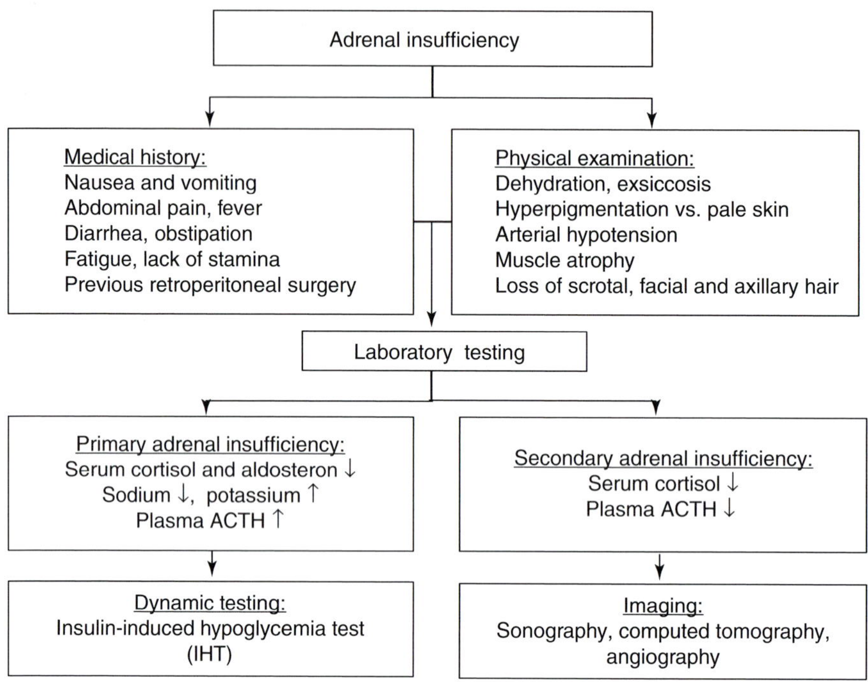

Fig. 34.2 Flow chart demonstrating pathway from symptoms to diagnosis

34.4 General Facts

The cortical layer of the adrenal gland comprises three different zones, with each zone producing and secreting its own hormones: glucocorticoids (zona fasciculata), mineralocorticoids (zona glomerulosa), and androgens (zona reticularis). Glucocorticoid secretion is under the control of corticotropin-releasing hormone, which activates pituitary corticotrophs to release anterior pituitary adrenocorticotropic hormone. Synthesis of mineralocorticoids is mainly regulated by the renin-angiotensin-aldosterone system (RAAS), which controls the blood volume and fluid/electrolyte balance. The production of mineralocorticoids is preserved in patients with secondary adrenal insufficiency.

Eighty to ninety percent of cases with primary adrenal insufficiency are due to autoimmune adrenalitis, which can develop isolated or as part of autoimmune polyendocrine syndrome [1]. Acute adrenal hemorrhage (e.g., in Waterhouse-Friderichsen syndrome), though uncommon, is another cause of primary adrenal insufficiency. Secondary adrenal insufficiency mostly results from pituitary adenomas or its surgical removal. Another important risk factor for secondary adrenal insufficiency is cranial irradiation in patients with malignant brain tumors, especially when involving the hypothalamic-pituitary axis. Long-term therapy with corticosteroids is an important iatrogenic factor for ACTH-receptor downregulation and consecutive adrenal atrophy. Autoimmune lymphocytic hypophysitis (inflammatory disorder involving pituitary gland and stalk) and Sheehan's syndrome (ischemic pituitary necrosis after severe postpartum hemorrhage) are rare but important causes of secondary adrenal insufficiency affecting women during pregnancy or after childbirth [4, 5].

34.5 Symptoms, Classification, and Grading

Chronic glucocorticoid deficiency leads to adynamia, fatigue, weight loss, gastric pain, vomiting, and fever. Shrunken orbits, hypotension, dehydration, and salt craving are due to mineralocorticoid deficiency. Androgen deficiency is related to loss of facial, scrotal, and axillary hair and impaired libido and well-being. A life-threatening and frequently underestimated event is acute adrenal crisis (Addisonian crisis), which regularly takes place in patients with diagnosed adrenal insufficiency under hormonal replacement therapy [6]. Severe hypotension, circulatory shock, acute abdominal pain, and coma are main signs of adrenal crisis. Nonetheless, affected patients can be misdiagnosed as having an acute abdomen. This leads not only to an unnecessary surgical intervention but also to the delay in the administration of life-saving glucocorticoid replacement therapy. The likelihood of Addisonian crisis is greater in patients suffering from primary adrenal insufficiency, particularly in instances of discontinuation of glucocorticoids or missing adjustment of the glucocorticoid dosage. Respiratory or gastrointestinal infections with fever, as well as surgical interventions carried out without sufficient steroid cover, may require parenteral administration of glucocorticoids and monitoring in intensive care unit [7].

34.6 Therapy

The therapy of primary adrenal insufficiency is simple when the correct diagnosis has been made. It mainly consists of the supplementation of deficient glucocorticoids and mineralocorticoids, usually for life, and leads to a spectacular improvement of the patient's condition. Physiological cortisol production varies between 5 and 10 mg/m^2 and corresponds to oral administration of hydrocortisone with a daily dose of 15–25 mg. Twice or thrice daily regimens are recommended [7]. The exact dose must be tailored to the patient's body weight and age. Mineralocorticoid replacement should be initiated at 100 ug of 9α-fludrocortisone once a day and has to be adapted to age, salt intake, or external factors such as humidity or outside temperature [7]. The administration of DHEA (dehydroepiandrosterone), taken as a single dose in the morning (25–50 mg), should be reserved for female patients with strongly impaired health-related quality of life, as reliable data about pharmaceutical quality control and safety are missing [7].

Primary adrenal insufficiency caused by infectious diseases has to be treated by antimicrobial agents, e.g., tuberculous adrenalitis requires the administration of antitubercular drugs. Treatment of secondary adrenal insufficiency depends on its causes. In case of

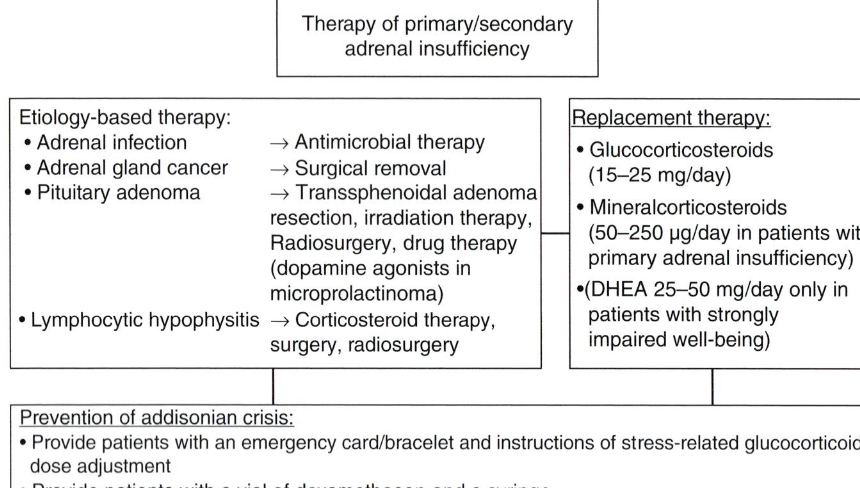

Fig. 34.3 Flow chart demonstrating pathway from diagnosis to therapy

pituitary tumor, endocrine function may be restored after surgical removal, depending on tumor size, accessibility, and surgical skills [2]. Patients with postoperatively persisting hypopituitarism have to receive pituitary hormone replacement therapy. Cancer survivors, who were treated by cranial irradiation, should be closely followed up, in view of the fact that neuroendocrine dysfunction presents a frequently diagnosed therapy-associated complication. Once adrenal insufficiency has been diagnosed, adequate hormone replacement has to be monitored regularly in order to anticipate possible complications of under- or overtreatment (e.g., weight gain, osteoporosis).

In case of adrenal crisis, emergency medical treatment is required, with parenteral administration of a glucocorticoid (e.g., dexamethasone), aggressive fluid resuscitation, and treatment of electrolyte imbalances being mandatory. An appropriate supplement therapy not only leads to a significant reduction of morbidity and mortality but also greatly enhances health-related quality of life of patients.

Several surgical interventions, for instance, bilateral adrenalectomy, require a stringent postoperative administration of a glucocorticoid replacement therapy. At the first postoperative day, 300 mg of hydrocortisone should be administered parenterally; at 2–3 days, the dose can be decreased to 200 mg. Thereafter, cortisol supplementation can be administered orally with 50 mg of prednisone (25–10–15 mg). It is important to reduce the dosage gradually until the abovementioned maintenance dose of hydrocortisone is reached.

Prevention of adrenal crisis is a mainstay in therapy of adrenal insufficiency and can be realized by providing patients with an emergency card/bracelet as well as with instructions of stress-related glucocorticoid dose adjustment (Fig. 34.3).

34.7 Complications

Since the synthetic production of glucocorticoids has been realized in 1952, mortality became a very rare endocrine complication in patients with adrenal insufficiency. Notwithstanding, in undiagnosed or untreated cases, death may still occur. Hence, it is crucial to make the correct diagnosis and promptly administrate therapy with life-saving glucocorticoids.

References

1. Arlt W, Allolio B. Adrenal insufficiency. Lancet. 2003;361(9372):1881–93.
2. Schneider HJ, Aimaretti G, Kreitschmann-Andermahr I, Stalla G-K, Ghigo E. Hypopituitarism. Lancet. 2007;369(9571):1461–70.
3. Petersenn S, Quabbe H-J, Schöfl C, Stalla GK, von Werder K, Buchfelder M. The rational use of pituitary stimulation tests. Dtsch Arztebl Int. 2010;107(25):437–43.
4. Laws ER, Vance ML, Jane JA. Hypophysitis. Pituitary. 2006;9(4):331–3.
5. Kelestimur F. Sheehan's syndrome. Pituitary. 2003;6(4):181–8.
6. White K, Arlt W. Adrenal crisis in treated addison's disease: a predictable but under-managed event. Eur J Endocrinol. 2010;162(1):115–20.
7. Arlt W. The approach to the adult with newly diagnosed adrenal insufficiency. J Clin Endocrinol Metab. 2009;94(4):1059–67.

Nephrotic Syndrome 35

Reinhard Brunkhorst

35.1 General Facts

Nephrotic syndrome is a complex of symptoms including proteinuria (>3.5 g/24 h), edema, hypoalbuminemia, and hypercholesterinemia. It is characterized by a damage of the capillary walls of the glomeruli, which alters their capacity to filter the substances transported in the blood.

35.2 Symptoms, Classification, and Grading

The lower serum oncotic pressure caused by the loss of protein by the kidneys can lead to complications in other organs and systems: puffiness around the eyes, pitting edema over the legs, pleural effusion, pulmonary edema, ascites, and anasarca. Disease laeding to nephrotic syndrome may either be limited to the kidney, called *primary* nephrotic syndrome (primary glomerulonephritis), or a condition that affects the kidney and other parts of the body, called *secondary* nephrotic syndrome.

Primary causes of nephrotic syndrome are different types of *glomerulonephritis* (*GN*) described by their histology: minimal change disease, focal segmental glomerulosclerosis (*FSGS*), membranous glomerulonephritis, and mesangial proliferative glomerulonephritis. Secondary causes of nephrotic syndrome are *glomerulopathies*, usually described by the underlying cause as diabetes mellitus, amyloidosis, and multiple myeloma.

R. Brunkhorst
Klinikum Oststadt-Heidehaus, Klinikum Region Hannover GmbH,
Klinik für Nieren-, Hochdruck- und Gefässerkrankungen,
Podbielskistr. 380, Hannover 30659, Germany
e-mail: sekretariat.brunkhorst.oststadt@klinikum-hannover.de

A.S. Merseburger et al. (eds.), *Urology at a Glance*,
DOI 10.1007/978-3-642-54859-8_35, © Springer-Verlag Berlin Heidelberg 2014

35.3 Therapy

The treatment of nephrotic syndrome can be symptomatic or can directly address the underlying disease of the kidney.

35.3.1 Symptomatic Treatment

The basic treatment of nephrotic syndrome consists of ACE inhibitors or sartans in order to reduce glomerular pressure and by this glomerular protein loss. In order to treat the fluid retention, water and sodium ingestion are restricted and diuretic drugs (loop diuretics and/or thiazides, aldosterone antagonists) are prescribed. In cases of severe hyperlipidemia, statins, fibrates, and resinous sequesters are recommended. Hypercoagulability is prophylactically treated with oral anticoagulants when serum albumin is <20 g/l, in order to avoid thromboembolic complications. Heparins are ineffective because of low AT III levels.

35.3.2 Treatment of Kidney Damage

Prednisone is usually prescribed at a dose of 60 mg/m^2 of body surface area/day in a first treatment for 4–8 weeks and then tapered. Frequent relapses are additionally treated by cyclophosphamide or nitrogen mustard or cyclosporine. Corticoids are indicated in *minimal change disease*, in recurring nephrotic syndrome. In *other types of glomerulonephritis*, a combined treatment of corticosteroids with immunossupressors is necessary. Besides cyclophosphamide (*IgA-GN*, *vasculitis-associated GN*), cyclosporine A and tacrolimus (*FSGS*) and chlorambucil (*membranous GN*) and as biological rituximab (*membranous GN*) have been successfully applied.

The glomerulopathies causing secondary nephrotic syndrome are treated by treatment of the underlying disease: diabetic nephropathy needs close monitoring of the diabetes treatment by insulin and blood pressure normalization. Multiple myeloma is treated with melphalan and steroids or thalidomide–dexamethasone, bortezomib-based regimens, and lenalidomide–dexamethasone. In younger patients, high-dose chemotherapy and autologous stem cell transplantation are recommended.

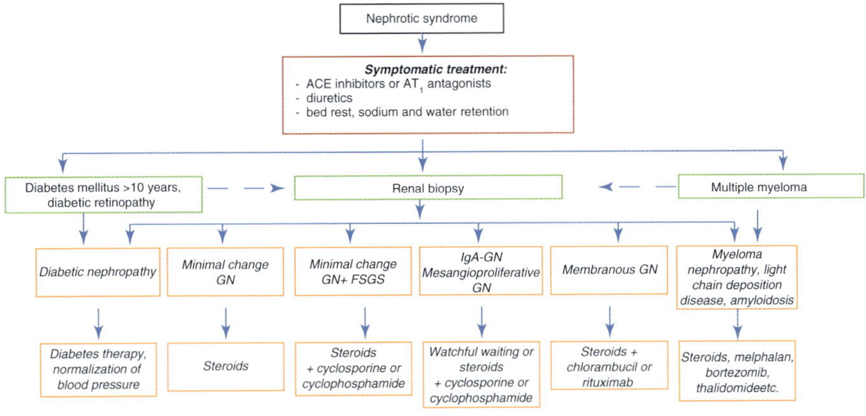

35.4 Complications

Nephrotic syndrome can be associated with a series of complications: *thromboembolic disorders* due to leakage of antithrombin III, *infections* caused by the loss of immunoglobulins, *acute kidney failure* due to hypovolemia, *pulmonary edema*, *hypothyroidism* by deficiency of the thyroglobulin transport protein thyroxin, *hypocalcaemia*, microcytic hypochromic *anemia* caused by iron deficiency, *protein malnutrition* by a negative nitrogen balance, and *growth retardation* in children (Figs. 35.1 and 35.2).

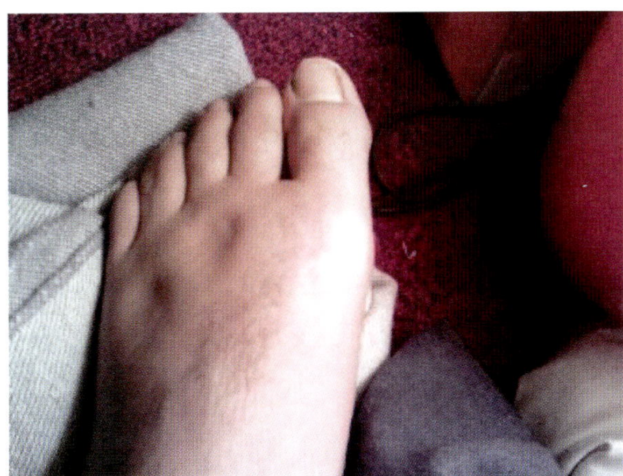

Fig. 35.1 Edema in nephrotic syndrome

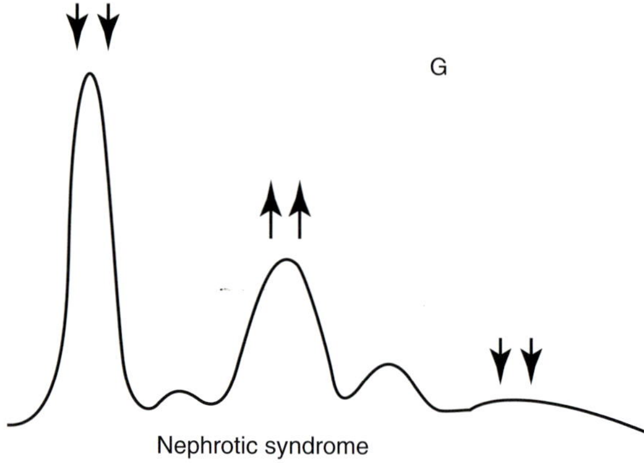

Fig. 35.2 Characteristic serum electrophoresis pattern in nephrotic syndrome: low albumin, increased β_2 and lowered γ-globulin peak

Pheochromocytoma

36

Jens Mani and Georg Bartsch

36.1 Key Points

A pheochromocytoma is a tumor of chromaffin cells, which secrete catecholamines, predominantly norepinephrine, as well as epinephrine, and rarely dopamine. The majority of pheochromocytomas are sporadic, but up to 25 % of cases are hereditary [1]. It may be associated with multiple endocrine neoplasia syndrome, type IIA and type IIB (also known as MEN IIA and MEN IIB), von Hippel-Lindau disease, neurofibromatosis type 1 (von Recklinghausen disease), phakomatosis, and paraganglioma syndromes.

Clinical signs and symptoms result from excessive catecholamine levels, the most common of these features is hypertension. The classic symptom triad of episodic headaches, tachycardia, and sweating may be present.

Diagnostic tests of choice are 24-h urine metanephrines and plasma fractionated metanephrines. Imaging studies should be performed after biochemical studies have confirmed the diagnosis of pheochromocytoma.

36.2 Background

Pheochromocytomas may occur in persons of any age. The peak incidence is between the third and the fifth decades of life, but approximately 10 % occur in children.

Tumors are normally located in the adrenal medulla, but approx. 10–20 % are located elsewhere – usually throughout the sympathetic chain in the thorax, abdomen, and pelvis.

J. Mani (✉) • G. Bartsch
Department of Urology, University Hospital Frankfurt,
Theodor-Stern-Kai 7, Frankfurt 60590, Germany
e-mail: jens.mani@kgu.de; georg.bartsch@kgu.de

A.S. Merseburger et al. (eds.), *Urology at a Glance*,
DOI 10.1007/978-3-642-54859-8_36, © Springer-Verlag Berlin Heidelberg 2014

About 10 % of pheochromocytomas are malignant; this goes up to 33 % in extra-adrenal pheochromocytomas. There are no reliable histopathological methods for distinguishing benign from malignant tumors. Instead, malignancy requires evidence of metastases at non-chromaffin sites distant from the primary tumor. The most common sites of metastasis are lymph nodes, bones, lungs, and liver. Malignant pheochromocytomas carry a very poor prognosis.

The pheochromocytoma "rule of 10": 10 % bilateral, 10 % malignant (higher in familial cases), 10 % extra-adrenal, and 10 % in children.

36.3 Therapy

Surgical resection of the tumor is the treatment of choice, along with preoperative management hypertension with full α-blockade (phenoxybenzamine, prazosin, doxazosin) for at least 2–3 weeks prior to surgery. In select cases, beta-blockers may be added after adequate alpha-blockade has been established in order to reduce tachycardia, a side effect of α-blockade [2]. That way permits the surgery to proceed while minimizing the likelihood of severe, life-threatening intraoperative hypertension, which might occur when the tumor is manipulated. Laparoscopic adrenalectomy is the procedure of choice today.

Hormone levels of norepinephrine and epinephrine return to normal after surgery.

In case of malignant pheochromocytoma, a multimodal treatment is required.

After aggressive surgery has been carried out, adjuvant treatment options include [3]:

- Combination chemotherapy: Chemotherapy with a combination of cyclophosphamide, vincristine, and dacarbazine provides partial remission and improvement of symptoms in up to 50 % of patients with malignant pheochromocytoma.
- External beam radiation therapy: Only in case of skeletal metastasis in order to prevent pathologic fractures.
- High-dose 131I-meta-iodobenzylguanidine (MIBG) radionuclide therapy: 131 I- MIBG is transported into the cell via the cell membrane norepinephrine transporter present on most neoplastic chromaffin cells. Overall, about 75 % of patients treated with 131 I-MIBG show improvement in symptoms, 50 % have reductions in hormonal activity, and 22 % show objective tumor responses.
- Somatostatin analogs: In patients with endocrine tumors expressing somatostatin receptors, targeted treatment with analogs of the natural ligand (e.g., octreotide, lanreotide) can lead to marked biochemical and, in part, radiological improvements.

For surgical follow-up, obtain plasma metanephrine levels yearly for 10 years. Ensure that blood pressure is under control. In patients with an underlying genetic mutation or malignant disease, lifelong follow-up is mandatory.

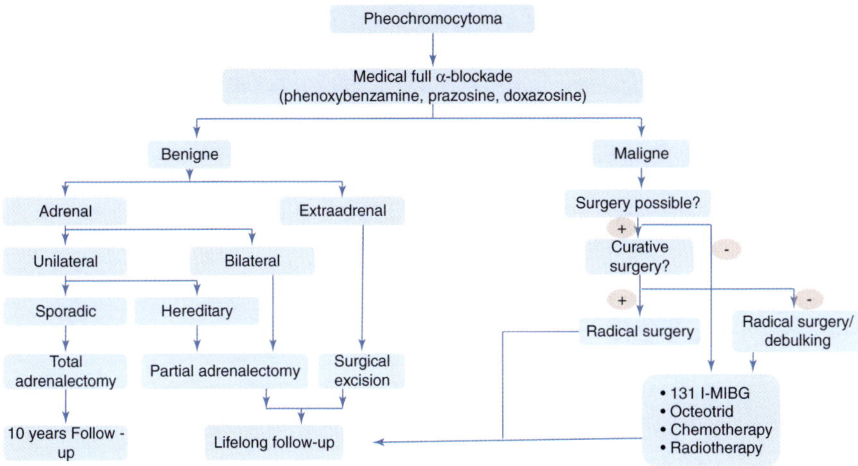

36.4 Complications

Untreated pheochromocytoma causes substantial morbidity and mortality, usually caused from a lethal hypertensive paroxysm. Cardiovascular complications may include hypertensive crisis (treatment: sodium nitroprusside, phentolamine, urapidil), cardiac arrest, sudden death, stroke, myocardial infarction, congestive heart failure, and renal insufficiency.

Complications of surgery for pheochromocytoma are primarily due to severe preoperative hypertension, high secretion tumors, or repeat intervention for recurrence. In case of bilateral adrenalectomy, adrenal insufficiency can occur.

In individuals with benign tumors, the 5-year survival rate after surgery is above 95 %. In case of malignant tumor, the 5-year survival rate after surgery is less than 50 %.

References

1. King KS, Pacak K. Familial pheochromocytomas and paragangliomas. Mol Cell Endocrinol. 2014;386:92–100.
2. Mazza A, Armigliato M, Marzola MC, Schiavon L, Montemurro D, Vescovo G, Zuin M, Chondrogiannis S, Ravenni R, Opocher G, Colletti PM, Rubello D. Anti-hypertensive treatment in pheochromocytoma and paraganglioma: current management and therapeutic features. Endocrine. 2014;45:469–78.
3. Jimenez C, Rohren E, Habra MA, Rich T, Jimenez P, Ayala-Ramirez M, Baudin E. Current and future treatments for malignant pheochromocytoma and sympathetic paraganglioma. Curr Oncol Rep. 2013;15(4):356–71.

Urinary Incontinence

37

Ngoc-Bich P. Le

37.1 General Facts

Urinary incontinence (UI) has been defined as "an involuntary loss of urine that is a social or hygienic problem and is objectively demonstrable." UI affects 30–50 % of elderly women and approximately 10 % of men of all ages [1]. UI negatively impacts a person's quality of life. Validated questionnaires have demonstrated that patients with UI have health-related quality of life scores comparable to those with multiple sclerosis. Even though UI may strongly impact their quality of life, many patients delay seeking treatment. Nearly half of patients are symptomatic for >3 years before seeking treatment [2]. Fifty-nine percent of patients do not seek treatment because they believe no effective treatment is available [2].

37.2 Symptoms, Classification, and Grading

UI may be due to a number of neurologic and non-neurologic causes. The presenting symptoms partially depend on the etiology. Presenting symptoms which are common to all types of UI include urinary leakage and dermatitis of the genital and perineal skin. The table below lists common causes of UI and their common presenting symptoms:

N.-B.P. Le, MD
Division of Urologic Surgery, Duke University Medical Center,
3707, Durham, NC 27710, USA
e-mail: nikki.le@duke.edu

A.S. Merseburger et al. (eds.), *Urology at a Glance*,
DOI 10.1007/978-3-642-54859-8_37, © Springer-Verlag Berlin Heidelberg 2014

Types of incontinence	Common presenting symptoms
Stress urinary incontinence (SUI)	Leakage with activities which increase intra-abdominal pressure including coughing, laughing, sneezing, exercise, and lifting
Urgency urinary incontinence (UUI)	Urgency, frequent low-volume voids, nocturia, enuresis Incontinence triggered by changes in position, washing hands, orgasm, walking to the bathroom, putting keys in the door Leakage can occur with "no warning"
Overflow incontinence	Delayed sensation of bladder fullness, infrequent voiding, incomplete bladder emptying Decreased force of stream Straining or Crede maneuver to facilitate voiding
Total incontinence	Continuous loss of urine without sensation of urgency and unrelated to activity Usually small volume, like dribbling or dripping faucet
Mixed incontinence	Any combination of the above symptoms

Severity of incontinence is addressed with a combination of objective and subjective metrics. Objective data are captured with pad weight, pad count, voiding diary, and valsalva leak point pressure on urodynamics. The most important measurements are level of bother and impact on quality of life. There are a number of validated questionnaires to evaluate the effect of UI on a patient's life, including the Urogenital Distress Inventory (UDI-6) and OAB-q.

37.3 Therapy and Complications

Treatment options are dependent on the type(s) of incontinence. However, there are generalized tenets which guide treatment. First of all, in the absence of medical sequelae, treatment of UI should be driven by degree of bother. If a patient is not bothered by UI, and if UI is not causing other medical problems like decubitus ulcers or osteomyelitis, then the risk/benefit ration of treatment would be unfavorable.

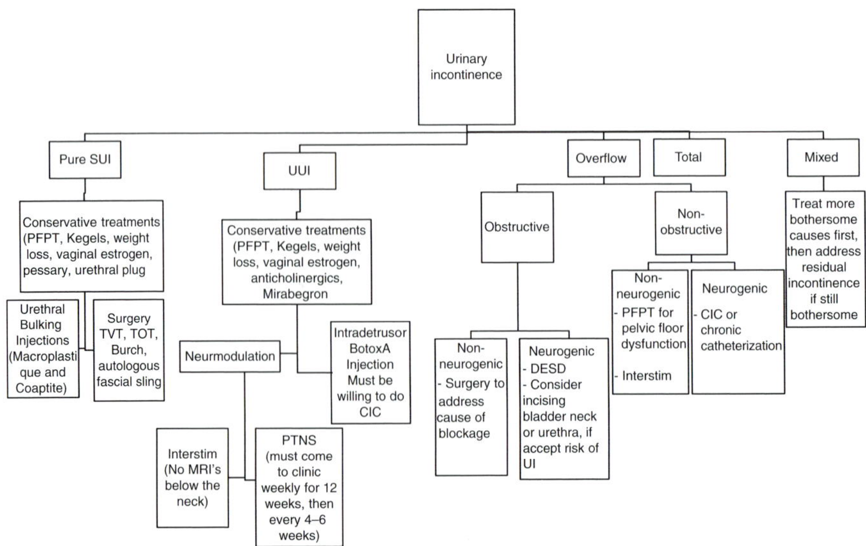

37.3.1 SUI

The first line of treatment for SUI includes conservative measures such as behavior modifications and pelvic floor exercises, with or without the aid of a pelvic floor physical therapist and biofeedback. Other non-procedural options to manage SUI include urethral inserts, anti-incontinence pessaries, and alpha-adrenergic medications. Injection of a urethral bulking agent is minimally invasive and can be performed in the clinic.

Nowadays, the most common surgeries for SUI are the tension-free retropubic (RP) and transobturator (TOT) midurethral slings. A randomized trial found that the RP and TOT groups had similar success rates (subjective cure RP 62 % vs TOT 55 %) and similar *total* complication rates (RP 37 % vs TOT 30 %, $p=0.07$) [3]. However, the *types* of complications differed between the groups. The retropubic group had higher rates of genitourinary events (13 % vs 8 %) and vascular/hematologic events (6 % vs 2 %) [3]. Conversely, the TOT group had higher rates of neurologic symptoms (9 % vs 4 %) [3]. Rates of mesh exposure rates (<2 %) and voiding dysfunction (<4 %) were similar [3]. Another study suggested that the TOT is less efficacious in patients with valsalva leak point pressure below 60 cmH_2O [4].

In certain situation, other SUI surgeries should be considered. If a patient has attenuated urethral, bladder, or vaginal tissue from a prior mesh excision or fistula surgery, one should consider an autologous fascial sling to avoid mesh erosion or extrusion. The Burch colposuspension was more widely used before the advent of the midurethral slings. However, the Burch procedure requires a transabdominal approach (open, laparoscopic, or robotic) and is now usually performed when other transabdominal procedures are performed concomitantly.

37.3.2 UUI

Conservative therapy for UUI also includes behavior modifications such as limiting fluid intake, avoiding caffeine and alcohol, and timed/scheduled voids. First-line therapy also includes pharmacotherapy with anticholinergic medications, or more recently, a beta-3-agonist. All of the anticholinergic medications have similar efficacy, but they differ in the side effects profile [5]. The most common side effects include dry mouth and constipation. In general, side effects are worse with the immediate release formulations and with oral administration (as opposed to transdermal) [6]. In 2012, Mirabegron, a beta-3-adrenoreceptor agonist, received FDA approval for the treatment of OAB. Mirabegron relaxes the smooth muscle of the bladder during the storage phase of the micturition cycle. It improves OAB symptoms without causing dry mouth and constipation. The most common side effects for Mirabegron are hypertension, UTI, headache, and nasal pharyngitis [7].

When UI is inadequately managed by pharmacotherapy, patients should be offered sacral neuromodulation (Interstim), percutaneous tibial nerve stimulation (PTNS), or intradetrusor injection of onaBotulinumtoxin A (Botox A). Interstim's mechanism of action is through the neuromodulation of somatosensory bladder afferents projecting into the pontine micturition center of the brainstem [8]. The process includes the insertion of an electrode into the S3 transforaminal space, followed by a trial phase to assess response, and implantation of the neurostimulator if there is significant improvement of symptoms. Interstim is a durable treatment option for UI as the failure rate at 2 years was only 2.9 % [9]. The most common side effects are pain at the stimulator or lead site, lead migration, and infection [10].

Another option for neuromodulation is via PTNS, whose mechanism is retrograde neuromodulation through the tibial nerve to the sacral nerve plexus. It requires 12×30 min weekly sessions. A study comparing PTNS to a sham treatment found that PTNS improves bladder symptoms (PTNS 55 % vs Sham 21 %) [11]. A follow-up study established that 77 % of patients who responded to the initial 12-week treatment maintained moderate or marked improvement of OAB symptoms at 3 years, but this required an average of 1.1 maintenance treatments a month [11].

Intradetrusor injection of Botox A prevents acetylcholine release at the neuromuscular junction and thereby decreasing detrusor hyperreflexia and increasing functional bladder capacity. A dose-range study performed by Denys et al. found that the 100 unit dose has the best safety-efficacy profile [12]. 65 % of patients receiving 100 units had significant improvement of their urgency and/or UI, and 55 % reported *complete continence.* A randomized, double-blind, double-placebo trial comparing Botox A 100 units to anticholinergic medications found that both groups had similar reductions in daily urgency incontinence episodes (–3.4), but different rates of complete continence (Botox A 27 % vs anticholinergics 13 %) [13]. Both groups reported similar improvements in quality of life. The most common side effects of Botox A injection include UTI (15–33 %) and urinary retention requiring self-catheterization (less than 11 %) [12–15].

37.3.3 Overflow Incontinence

Treatment of overflow incontinence hinges on addressing the underlying cause of urinary retention. In the neurogenic population, this can be due to detrusor sphincter dyssynergia or detrusor hypocontractility. In the idiopathic population, one should evaluate for and address any physical obstruction of the bladder outlet (e.g., obstructive benign prostatic hyperplasia, bladder neck contracture, or urethral stricture disease). In the case of idiopathic nonobstructive urinary retention, interstim sacral neuromodulation should be considered.

37.3.4 Total Incontinence

A history of continuous, unaware loss of urine raises the suspicion of a vesicovaginal, ureterovaginal, or urethrovaginal fistula. Fistulas should be repaired surgically. An ectopic ureter also requires surgical management. Patients who have been managed with chronic indwelling Foley catheters may develop urethral erosion and present with total incontinence from a patulous and incompetent urethra. Depending on the degree of erosion, these patients may require a bladder neck closure and urinary diversion.

References

1. Sandvik H, Hunskaar S, Vanvik A, et al. Diagnostic classification of female urinary incontinence: an epidemiological survey corrected for validity. J Clin Epidemiol. 1995;48(3):339–43.
2. Milsom I, Abrams P, Cardozo L, et al. How widespread are the symptoms of an overactive bladder and how are they managed? A population-based prevalence study. BJU Int. 2001;87(9):760–6.
3. Richter HE, Albo ME, Zycsynski HM, et al. Retropubic versus transobturator midurethral slings for stress incontinence. N Engl J Med. 2010;362(22):2066–76.
4. O'Connor RC, Nanigian DK, Lyon MB, et al. Early outcomes of mid-urethral slings for female stress urinary incontinence stratified by valsalva leak point pressure. Neurourol Urodyn. 2006;25(7):685–8.
5. Hartmann KE, McPheeters ML, Biller DH, et al. Treatment of overactive bladder in women. Evid Rep Technol Assess. 2009;187:1–120.
6. Gormley EA, Lightner DJ, Burgio KL, et al. Diagnosis and treatment of overactive bladder (non-neurogenic) in adults: AUA/SUFU guideline. J Urol. 2012;188(6 Suppl):2455–63.
7. Chapple CR, Kaplan SA, Mitcheson D, et al. Randomized double-blind, active-controlled phase 3 study to assess 12-month safety and efficacy of Mirabegron, a B(3)-adrenoceptor agonist, in overactive bladder. Eur Urol. 2013;63(2):296–305.
8. Leng WW, Chancellor MB. How sacral nerve stimulation neuromodulation works. Urol Clin North Am. 2005;32(1):11–8.
9. Leong RK, De Wachter SG, Nieman FH, et al. PNE versus 1st stage tined lead procedure: a direct comparison to select the most sensitive test method to identify patients suitable for sacral neuromodulation therapy. Neurourol Urodyn. 2011;30(7):1249–52.
10. Van Kerrebroeck PE, van Voskuilen AC, Heesakkers JP, et al. Results of sacral neuromodulation therapy for urinary voiding dysfunction: outcomes of a prospective, worldwide clinical study. J Urol. 2007;178(5):2029–34.
11. Peters KM, Carrico DJ, Perez-Marrero RA, et al. Randomized trial of percutaneous tibial nerve stimulation versus Sham efficacy in the treatment of overactive bladder syndrome: results from the SUmiT trial. J Urol. 2010;183(4):1438–43.
12. Denys P, Le Normand L, Ghout I, et al. Efficacy and safety of low doses of OnabotulinumtoxinA for the treatment of refractory idiopathic overactive bladder: a multicentre, double-blind, randomised, placebo-controlled dose-ranging study. Eur Urol. 2012;61(3):520–9.
13. Visco AG, Brubaker L, Ritcher HE, et al. Anticholinergic therapy vs. OnabotulinumtoxinA for urgency urinary incontinence. N Engl J Med. 2012;367(19):1803–13.
14. Chapple C, Sievert K-D, MacDiarmid S, et al. OnabotulinumtoxinA 100U significantly improves all idiopathic overactive bladder symptoms and quality of life in patients with overactive bladder and urinary incontinence: a randomized, double-blind, placebo-controlled trial. Eur Urol. 2013;64(2):249–56.
15. Nitti VW, Dmochowski R, Herschorn S, et al. OnabotulinumtoxinA for the treatment of patients with overactive bladder and urinary incontinence: results of a phase 3, randomized, placebo controlled trial. J Urol. 2013;189(6):2186–93.

Acute Urinary Retention

38

Thenappan Chandrasekar and Derya Tilki

38.1 General Facts

Acute urinary retention (AUR) is a painful urologic emergency specifically characterized by the sudden inability to urinate. It remains the most common urologic emergency managed by urologists worldwide and is a condition seen by all physicians regardless of their specialty. Population-based cohort studies in the United States and Belgium have put the incidence of AUR at 2.2–6.8 episodes per 1,000 man-years, but older studies have it as high as 130 episodes per 1,000 man-years [1–3, 5, 9, 11]. There is a significantly higher rate in the male population with benign prostatic hypertrophy (BPH). Due to the low occurrence rate in women, data on incidence is not readily available for the female population. Across numerous studies, the major risk factors for development of AUR in men are the following: age (age >70, RR 7.8), symptom severity (AUA symptom score >7, RR 3.2), prostate size (volume >30 mL, RR 3.0), and urinary flow rate (flow rate <12 mL/s, RR 3.9) [9, 13, 16]. Age is the predominant risk factor, with a nearly linear increase in incidence with age – up to 10 % of men over the age of 70 and almost one-third of men over the age of 80. While a variety of pathophysiologic mechanisms may contribute to the development of AUR, the three predominant mechanisms are outflow obstruction, neurologic impairment, and overdistension.

T. Chandrasekar, MD • D. Tilki, MD (✉)
Department of Urology, University of California, Davis, Medical Center,
4860 Y Street, Suite 3500, Sacramento, CA 95817, USA
e-mail: thenappan.chandrasekar@ucdmc.ucdavis.edu;
derya.tilki@ucdmc.ucdavis.edu, dtilki@me.com

A.S. Merseburger et al. (eds.), *Urology at a Glance*,
DOI 10.1007/978-3-642-54859-8_38, © Springer-Verlag Berlin Heidelberg 2014

38.2 Symptoms, Classification, and Grading

By definition, acute urinary retention is the inability to urinate – and this is often the main, if not only, presenting symptom. Regardless of other clinical signs or symptoms, if the patient states they are unable to urinate, they have urinary retention. Associated presenting symptoms may include lower abdominal or suprapubic discomfort, restlessness, or visible discomfort. If there are systemic signs such as fever, tachycardia, tachypnea, or hypotension, urinary tract infection superimposed on retention should be considered. Additionally, history should focus on symptom assessment to help determine the underlying etiology of AUR – with a focus on prostatitis symptoms (urgency, frequency, decreased flow rate, hesitancy, post-void dribbling, urinary incontinence) and gross hematuria (with or without clots prior to retention).

Evaluation of the patient should include a thorough history and physical examination. Patient history should include a genitourinary review of systems, neurologic symptoms, prior history of retention, malignancy, prior surgery (especially in the GU tract), radiation, or pelvic trauma. Complete medication review is also indicated as medications can often contribute to AUR. Physical examination should include low abdominal palpation, rectal examination, pelvic examination, and neurologic assessment. Laboratory results may not be too revealing, but a urinalysis and culture should be obtained following decompression. A complete blood count and basic metabolic panel may be warranted to evaluate for infection and renal function. Bedside ultrasound can be used to evaluate the bladder volume, and post-void residual bladder volumes are often used to assist clinical diagnosis.

Classification of acute urinary retention is not routine, either in practice or in the literature. However, the separation into spontaneous and precipitated AUR has clinical significance. The first study group to classify AUR was the PLESS trial [16]. Precipitated AUR is the inability to urinate after a triggering event, such as anesthesia, post-GU surgery, recent instrumentation, or ingestion of medications. In contrast, all other AUR episodes are considered spontaneous [15]. When classified accordingly, the long-term outcomes are noted to vary significantly – after spontaneous AUR, 15 % of patients had another episode of retention and 75 % proceeded to surgery; in contrast, after precipitated AUR, only 9 % had a recurrent episode, and only 26 % proceeded to surgery [16].

38.3 Therapy

The mainstay of management of acute urinary retention is bladder decompression to prevent permanent bladder injury and dysfunction, infection, and renal impairment. Bladder decompression can be achieved with suprapubic aspiration (popular among non-urologists), urethral catheterization (primary method), suprapubic catheterization, and clear intermittent urethral catheterization.

Urethral catheterization is the preferred method of decompression due to its simplicity and lower complication rates compared to suprapubic catheter placement.

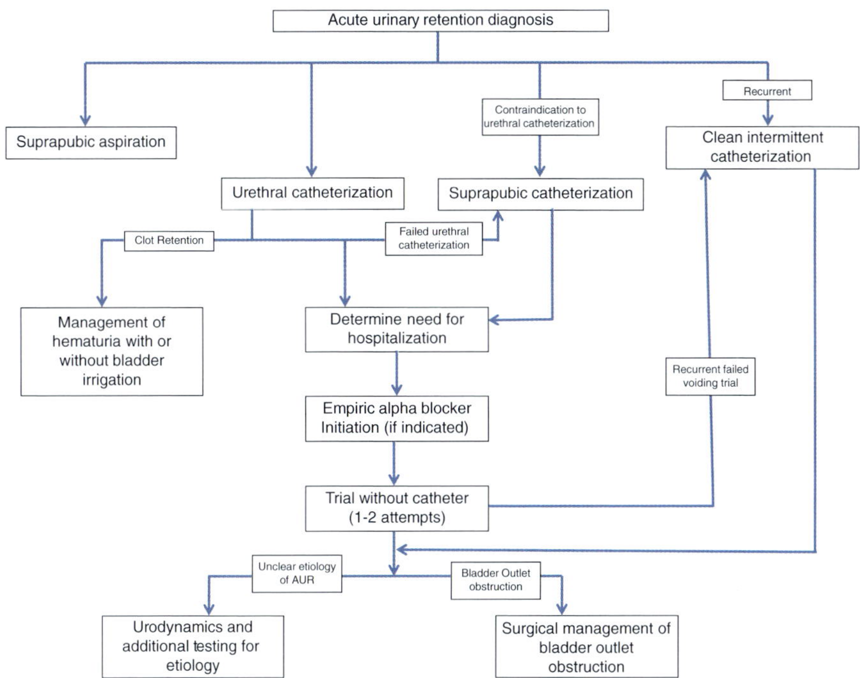

Fig. 38.1 Flowchart: management of acute urinary retention

However, in patients who have failed bedside catheter placement with or without endoscopic assistance OR have had recent urologic procedures (such as prostatectomy, TURP, urethral reconstruction), suprapubic catheter placement is indicated. Outcomes comparing urethral versus suprapubic catheterization have shown that suprapubic catheterization has fewer urinary tract infections and is more comfortable, but was associated with increased risk of complications with placement [7, 8]. However, if long-term drainage is expected, suprapubic catheterization may be preferred. There are no standardized guidelines or treatment algorithms for AUR. A suggested algorithm for initial management is included (Fig. 38.1).

Following decompression, the patient should be assessed for the need for inpatient hospitalization. Indications for hospital management include gross hematuria with clots that cannot be resolved in the initial setting, post-obstructive diuresis with salt-wasting and urine output >200 cc/h, evidence of urosepsis, obstruction related to malignancy, or spinal cord compression. Outside these instances, most AUR can be managed in the outpatient setting.

Trial without catheter (TWOC) (or voiding trial) is a part of the management algorithm of AUR, though it is not a definitive therapy. The recommended duration of catheter decompression varies based on source, but ranges from 2 to 14 days; success of TWOC will be affected by catheter duration, use of alpha-blocker, bladder volume at time of catheter placement, age of patient, and classification of AUR [6, 10].

In patients with suspected bladder outlet obstruction due to BPH, empiric treatment with alpha-blockers has been demonstrated to improve success of voiding trials [4, 12] and reduce risk of recurrent episodes. Of note, the use of 5-alpha-reductase inhibitors has not been shown to have a role in the management of AUR, as their time to full effectiveness is too long – however, they do have a role in long-term management of BPH. Surgical therapy is not a standard treatment option for patients with AUR, but is an important part of the algorithm of management for patients with BPH.

If the etiology is unclear, urodynamics testing with an experienced urologist should be the next step in management.

Special consideration: While bladder dysfunction is a common pathology in the female urologic patient, acute urinary retention is uncommon. Outlet obstruction due to anatomic distortion should be ruled out first with examination and potential endoscopic evaluation; if no anatomic abnormality is noted, bladder function should be evaluated using urodynamics. Clear intermittent catheterization is an important part of management of urinary retention in women [14].

38.4 Complications

Untreated or delayed treatment AUR may also lead to urinary tract infection due to urine stasis and renal impairment.

Relief of urinary tract obstruction can lead to a post-obstructive diuresis phenomenon, which is defined as a diuresis that persists after decompression of the bladder – however, this is primarily a problem with chronic, rather than acute, urinary retention. Recommendations include serial electrolyte monitoring and volume replacement.

Catheter placement may also be associated with hematuria, urethritis/cystitis, bacteremia, and sepsis. However, clinical significance of these complications is rare.

References

1. Ball AJ, Feneley RC, Abrams PH. The natural history of untreated prostatism. Br J Urol. 1981;53:613–6.
2. Barry MJ, Fowler FJ, Bin L, et al. The natural history of patients with benign prostatic hyperplasia as diagnosed by North American urologists. J Urol. 1997;157:10–5.
3. Birkhoff JD, Wiederhorn AR, Hamilton ML, Zinsser HH. Natural history of benign prostatic hypertrophy and acute urinary retention. Urology. 1976;7:48–52.
4. Chan P, Wong W, Chan L, Cheng C. Can terazosin relieve acute urinary retention and obviate the need for an indwelling urethral catheter? Br J Urol. 1996;77:7.
5. Craigen AA, Hickling JB, Saunders CR, Carpenter RG. Natural history of prostatic obstruction: a prospective survey. J R Coll Gen Pract. 1969;18:226–32.
6. Fitzpatrick JM, Kirby RS. Management of acute urinary retention. BJU Int. 2006;97(2):16.
7. Horgan AF, Prasad B, Waldron DJ, O'Sullivan DC. Acute urinary retention. Comparison of suprapubic and urethral catheterization. Br J Urol. 1992;81:712.
8. Ichsan J, Hunt DR. Suprapubic catheters: a comparison of suprapubic versus urethral catheters in the treatment of acute urinary retention. Aust N Z J Surg. 1987;57:33.

9. Jacobsen SJ, Jacobsen DJ, Girman CJ, et al. Natural history of prostatism: risk factors for acute urinary retention. J Urol. 1997;158:481–7.
10. Klarskov P, Andersen JT, Asmussen CF, et al. Symptoms and signs predictive of the voiding pattern after acute urinary retention in men. Scand J Urol Nephrol. 1987;21:23.
11. McConnell JD, Bruskewitz R, Walsh P, et al. The effect of finasteride on the risk of acute urinary retention and the need for surgical treatment among men with benign prostatic hyperplasia. Finasteride Long-Term Efficacy and Safety Study Group. N Engl J Med. 1998;338:557–63.
12. McNeill SA, Daruwala PD, Mitchell ID, et al. Sustained-release alfuzosin and trial without catheter after acute urinary retention: a prospective, placebo-controlled. BJU Int. 1999;84:622–7.
13. Meigs JB, Barry MJ, Giovannucci E, et al. Incidence rates and risk factors for acute urinary retention: the health professionals follow-up study. J Urol. 1999;162:376–82.
14. Ramsey S, Palmer M. The management of female urinary retention. Int Urol Nephrol. 2006;38:533.
15. Roehrborn CG. Acute urinary retention: risks and management. Rev Urol. 2005;7(4):S31–44.
16. Roehrborn CG, Bruskewitz R, Nickel GC, et al. Urinary retention in patients with BPH treated with finasteride or placebo over 4 years. Characterization of patients and ultimate outcomes. The PLESS Study Group. Eur Urol. 2000;37:528–36.

Renal Cell Carcinoma

39

Inga Peters, Maria Gabriel, Markus A. Kuczyk, and Axel S. Merseburger

39.1 General Facts

Renal cell cancer (RCC) accounts for approximately 2–3 % of all human malignancies and shows a worldwide increase of incidence rate of 2 % per year [1]. It primarily affects men and women at the age of 50–70 years with a twofold higher incidence rate in men. Clear cell carcinoma (ccRCC) is the most frequent histological subtype (~80–90 %) besides papillary (10–15 %) and chromophobe (4–5 %) subtype [2]. About 25–30 % of RCC patients present with a metastatic disease (mRCC) at the time of diagnosis. Patients with mRCC generally have a poor prognosis and the 5-year disease-specific survival for University of California Los Angeles integrated staging system (UISS) was 41 % in the low-risk group, 18 % in intermediate and 8 % in the high-risk group [3]. Aetiological risk factors for RCC seem to be smoking, hypertension and obesity [4]. The tumour node metastasis (TNM) staging system and the Fuhrman nuclear grade are commonly recommended for classification, diagnosis and prognosis of RCC patients (Table 39.1).

39.2 Symptoms, Classification and Grading

If a patient occurs with haematuria, flank pain and palpable abdominal mass, it is in all likelihood due to an already late stage renal cell cancer disease. Fortunately, nowadays about 50 % of renal masses are detected by using high-resolution imaging systems to investigate a range of non-specific symptoms. Paraneoplastic syndromes, which are summarised in Fig. 39.1, are frequently found (in about 30 %) to be associated with a RCC disease. Physical examination plays a minor role in diagnosing

I. Peters • M. Gabriel • M.A. Kuczyk • A.S. Merseburger (✉)
Department of Urology and Urologic Oncology, Medizinische Hochschule Hannover (MHH), Carl-Neuberg-Str. 1, Hannover 30625, Germany
e-mail: peters.inga@mh-hannover.de; kuczyk.markus@mh-hannover.de; merseburger.axel@mh-hannover.de

A.S. Merseburger et al. (eds.), *Urology at a Glance*,
DOI 10.1007/978-3-642-54859-8_39, © Springer-Verlag Berlin Heidelberg 2014

Table 39.1 TNM classification of kidney tumours

T – primary tumour	
T1a	Tumour ≤4 cm limited to the kidney
T1b	Tumour >4 cm but not more than 7 cm
T2a	Tumour >7 but not more that 10 cm
T2b	Tumour >10 cm, limited to the kidney
T3a	Tumour extends into renal vein or its segmental branches
T3b	Tumour grossly extends into vena cava below diaphragm
T4	Gerota fascia invasion, adrenal gland invasion
N – regional lymph nodes	
N1	Metastasis in a single regional lymph node
N2	Metastasis in more than one regional lymph node
M – distant metastasis	
M1	Distant metastasis

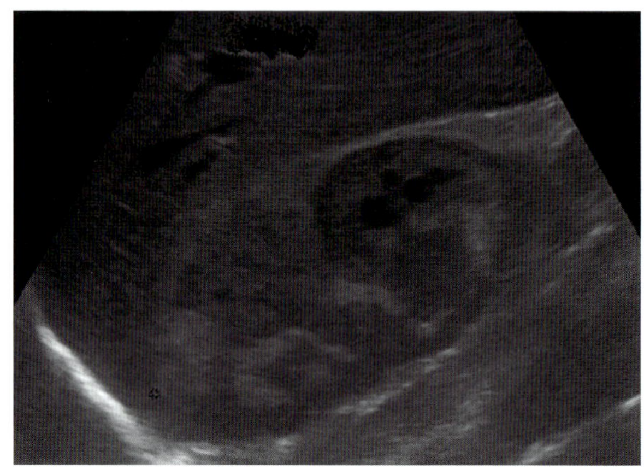

Fig. 39.1 Ultrasound image of a right kidney with suspicious lesion near the hilus

RCC, but in case of palpable abdominal mass, non-reducing varicocele, bilateral oedema of lower extremities or cervical lymphadenopathy, further radiological investigations should be urgently carried out. Generally, most renal tumours are diagnosed by abdominal ultrasound (US, see Fig. 39.1) or computer tomography (CT, Figs. 39.2 and 39.3). Renal cell carcinomas are classified according the TNM classification (2009) (Table 39.1).

39.3 Therapy

Clinical treatment mainly depends on staging criteria and co-morbidities of the patients. In fact, surgical treatment is the therapy of choice for a curative treatment. In localised tumours up to a diameter of 7 cm (*stage: T1a/b*), a nephron-sparing surgery (partial tumour resection) should be carried out [1]. In case of locally advanced

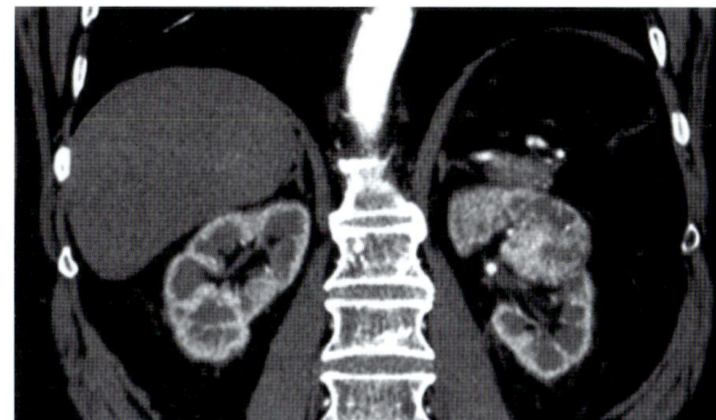

Fig. 39.2 CT image of the abdomen with central lesion in the left kidney

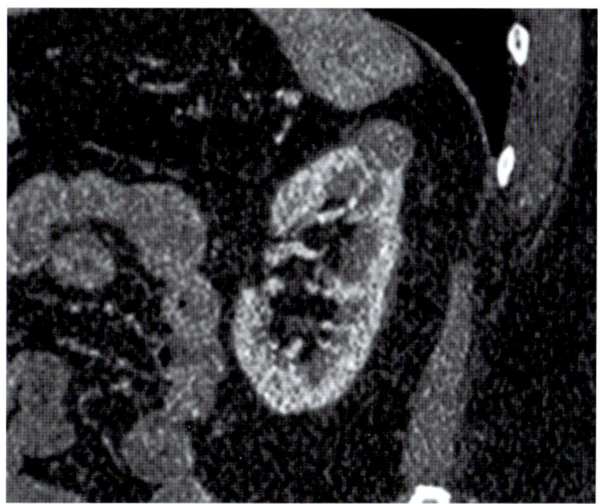

Fig. 39.3 CT image of a left kidney with small lesion in the upper pole

tumour growth, unfavourable location of the tumour or deterioration of patients' physical conditions, a laparoscopic radical nephrectomy should be performed. Oncological outcome data of patients undergoing nephron-sparing surgery is similar to patients treated with radical nephrectomy [5, 6], and in advantage the long-term renal function is significantly better in patients with nephron-sparing surgery [7]. Because nephron-sparing surgery has a faintly higher complication rate (i.e. postoperative bleeding) in contrast to radical nephrectomy, it should be carried out in specialised urological departments. Lymphadenectomy is only required for staging purposes, but does not improve the overall survival. In advanced tumours (*stage: T1b with centrally located tumour and T2-3a tumours*) where nephron-sparing surgery cannot be performed, laparoscopic radical nephrectomy (LRN) is the therapy of choice. Patients undergoing LRN have a shorter hospital stay and a faster convalescence compared to open radical nephrectomy. Patients with RCC including thrombosis of the renal vein and vena cave infradiaphragmal/vena cava supradiaphragmal (*stage: T3b/c*) or a local tumour infiltration into neighbouring organs (*stage: T4*) should be treated with an open radical nephrectomy. To determine the accurate

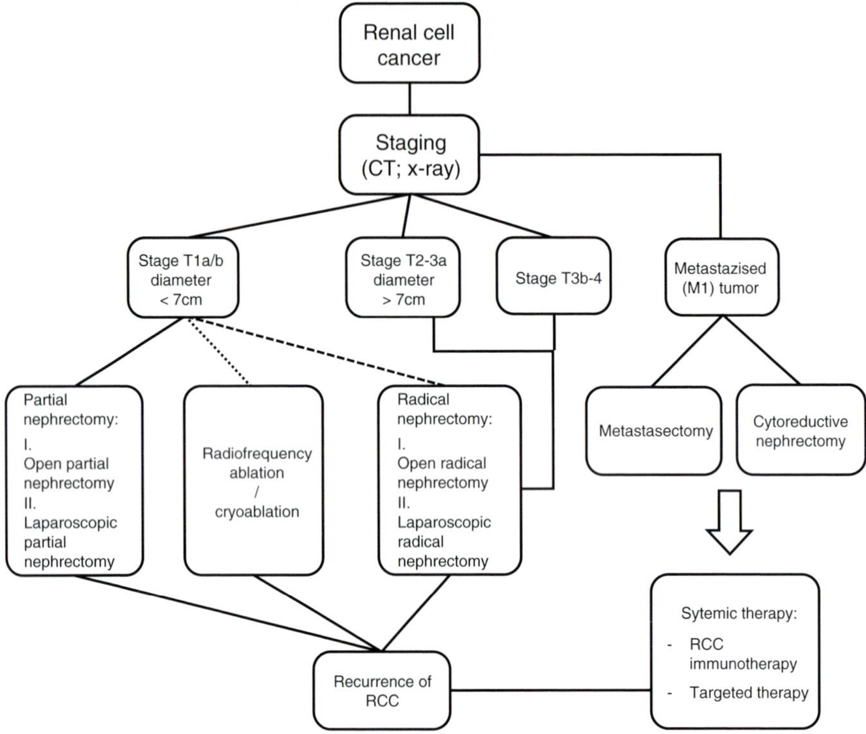

Fig. 39.4 Flow chart demonstrating the pathway from diagnosis to therapy

location and extension of the thrombus, it is necessary to investigate the patient with MRI or transoesophageal ultrasound preoperatively. In case of metastatic RCC disease (*M1*), a cytoreductive nephrectomy before systemic treatment should be discussed according to the risk status [8]. The benefit of metastasectomy has not been demonstrated as yet, but it should be considered previous to a systemic therapy if a complete resection of all lesions seems possible.

Radiofrequency ablation (RFA) and cryoablation are available ablative techniques. Both could be considered as an alternative treatment in patients with small renal masses (diameter of 2–4 cm) to surgical procedures in well-selected patients not fit for surgical resection. The flow chart demonstrates the way from diagnosis to therapy and its complications (Fig. 39.4).

39.4 Complications

In case of extensive tumour growth, flank pain, macrohaematuria and pulmonary embolisation due to tumour thrombus can occur. In case of inoperability, palliative embolisation of the kidney could cure acute bleeding. The most common paraneoplastic syndromes are hypertension, weight loss, anaemia, hypercalcaemia, abnormal liver function and polycythaemia. Only a few patients present with bone pain or persisting cough as a consequence of metastatic spread.

References

1. Ljungberg B, Cowan NC, Hanbury DC, Hora M, Kuczyk MA, Merseburger AS, Patard JJ, Mulders PF, Sinescu IC. EAU guidelines on renal cell carcinoma: the 2010 update. Eur Urol. 2010;58(3):398–406.
2. Bruder E, Passera O, Harms D, Leuschner I, Ladanyi M, Argani P, Eble JN, Struckmann K, Schraml P, Moch H. Morphologic and molecular characterization of renal cell carcinoma in children and young adults. Am J Surg Pathol. 2004;28(9):1117–32.
3. Bensalah K, Pantuck AJ, Crepel M, Verhoest G, Mejean A, Valeri A, Ficarra V, Pfister C, Ferriere JM, Soulie M, et al. Prognostic variables to predict cancer-related death in incidental renal tumours. BJU Int. 2008;102(10):1376–80.
4. Waalkes S, Rott H, Herrmann TR, Wegener G, Kramer MW, Merseburger AS, Schrader M, Hofmann R, Kuczyk MA, Schrader AJ. Does male sex influence the prognosis of patients with renal cancer? Onkologie. 2011;34(1–2):24–8.
5. Raz O, Mendlovic S, Shilo Y, Leibovici D, Sandbank J, Lindner A, Zisman A. Positive surgical margins with renal cell carcinoma have a limited influence on long-term oncological outcomes of nephron sparing surgery. Urology. 2010;75(2):277–80.
6. Marszalek M, Meixl H, Polajnar M, Rauchenwald M, Jeschke K, Madersbacher S. Laparoscopic and open partial nephrectomy: a matched-pair comparison of 200 patients. Eur Urol. 2009;55(5):1171–8.
7. McKiernan J, Simmons R, Katz J, Russo P. Natural history of chronic renal insufficiency after partial and radical nephrectomy. Urology. 2002;59(6):816–20.
8. Waalkes S, Kramer M, Herrmann TR, Schrader AJ, Kuczyk MA, Merseburger AS. Present state of target therapy for disseminated renal cell carcinoma. Immunotherapy. 2010;2(3):393–8.

Prostate Cancer

40

Michael R. Abern, Matvey Tsivian, and Judd W. Moul

40.1 Epidemiology

Prostate cancer is the second most common cancer in men worldwide [1]. In the USA alone, 239,000 men will be diagnosed with prostate cancer in 2013 and 30,000 will die of the disease. Overall, 1 in every 6 men in the USA will be diagnosed with prostate cancer during his lifetime, and over 2.6 million men are currently living with the diagnosis [2]. Well-established risk factors for the prostate cancer are increasing age, African ancestry, and family history in a first-degree relative.

40.2 Diagnosis and Staging

Since the 1990s prostate cancer detection has relied on serum prostate-specific antigen (PSA) testing and digital rectal examination (DRE). In this era of PSA-based screening, prostate cancer is commonly diagnosed in asymptomatic men with an elevated PSA or abnormal DRE by a transrectal ultrasound-guided needle biopsy. Occasionally, prostate cancer is diagnosed in tissue resected to relieve the symptoms of prostatic enlargement. Some patients may still present with the signs/symptoms of advanced disease such as hematuria, bone pain, or spinal cord compression; however, this is uncommon in the PSA screening era [3].

Adenocarcinoma is the most common type of prostate cancer comprising 90–95 % of incident cases. It is graded using the Gleason score classification, with which pathologists classify tumors based on the degree of loss of prostatic glandular architecture [4]. Gleason score of the biopsy, combined with clinical stage estimated by DRE or imaging, and serum PSA are commonly combined to stratify patients by risk of recurrence after therapy (Fig. 40.1). A commonly employed

M.R. Abern, MD (✉) • M. Tsivian, MD • J.W. Moul, MD
Division of Urology, Department of Surgery, Duke University Medical Center, DUMC 3707, Durham, NC 27710, USA
e-mail: joan.mcalexander@duke.edu; matvey.tsivian@duke.edu; judd.moul@duke.edu

A.S. Merseburger et al. (eds.), *Urology at a Glance*,
DOI 10.1007/978-3-642-54859-8_40,

Risk group	PSA (ng/ml)	Gleason sum	Clinical stage	Other
Very low	<10	≤6	T1c	<3 cores positive, ≤50 % tumor in any core, PSA density <0.15
Low	<10	≤6	≤T2a	
Intermediate	≥10 and <20	7	T2b	
High	≥ 20	≥8	≥T2c	Lymph node positive

Fig. 40.1 Risk stratification of clinically localized prostate cancer

schema developed by D'Amico separates men into low-, intermediate-, or high-risk prognostic categories [5]. Recently, a very low-risk group has been defined as a subset of low risk with low tumor volume on biopsy and low PSA per unit of prostate volume [6].

Staging for locally advanced tumors or metastatic disease to the pelvic lymph nodes or distant organs is based on imaging. Nuclear medicine bone scan is indicated for intermediate- to high-risk patients to detect metastases. Cross-sectional imaging using MRI or CT is indicated for men at high risk of lymph node involvement or to further stage suspected locally invasive prostate tumors [6]. Multiparametric MRI of the prostate is the most accurate for identification of tumors extending through the prostatic capsule and is increasingly used for therapeutic planning [7]. Currently, CT has low sensitivity (13 %) for lymph node metastases; however, bulky lymphadenopathy may be identified [8].

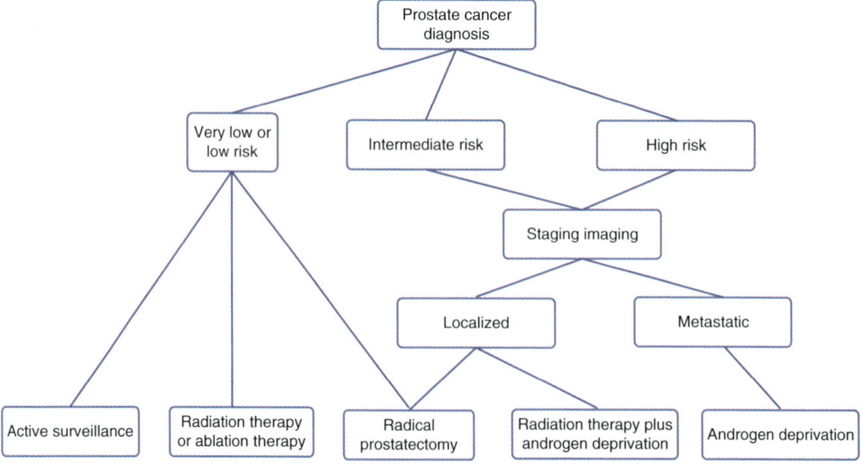

40.3 Therapy: Localized

Radical prostatectomy and radiation therapy are the mainstays of therapy for localized prostate cancer. Although a randomized head-to-head trial does not exist to compare the efficacy of radiation and surgery, observational data suggests that both modalities have excellent long-term cancer control with a slight advantage to radical prostatectomy [9, 10]. For intermediate- and high-risk disease, radiation therapy is combined with androgen deprivation therapy for optimal cancer control [11, 12]. In contrast, radical prostatectomy allows for more accurate tumor grading and staging based on the entire prostate and excised lymph nodes which can identify men who require subsequent therapy [13]. The ablation of prostate cancer using cryosurgery or high-frequency ultrasound is an alternative method for treating localized prostate cancer.

Recently, active surveillance has emerged as an alternative for men with low- or very low-risk prostate cancer. This entails serial PSA tests and prostate biopsies, and treatment if progression is detected. While safety of this approach has been proven for low-risk prostate cancer, it has been associated with inferior oncologic outcomes in men with intermediate- or high-risk disease [14, 15].

40.4 Therapy: Metastatic

Prostate cancer growth can be dramatically slowed by androgen deprivation, making this the mainstay for treatment of metastatic disease [16]. Androgen deprivation is achieved with luteinizing hormone releasing hormone agonists or antagonists, androgen receptor blockers, adrenolytic agents, or surgical castration with a goal to decrease serum testosterone below 20 ng/dl. Therapy is generally lifelong; however, the optimal dosing schedule (intermittent vs. continuous) is debatable [17].

While androgen deprivation will improve the symptoms of metastases and delay progression, prostate tumors eventually become castration resistant (CRPC) and grow independently of circulating androgens. Standard therapy for CRPC is cytotoxic chemotherapy with docetaxel or cabazitaxel with prednisone [18]. Recently, several new therapies have emerged for CRPC including immunotherapy and next-generation hormonal agents.

40.5 Quality of Life

Treatment for localized prostate cancer is associated with variable morbidity based on the modality. Radical prostatectomy may be associated with stress urinary incontinence and erectile dysfunction. Radiation therapy is associated with erectile dysfunction and radiation cystitis and proctitis. In addition, radiation therapy is associated with an increased risk of second pelvic malignancies [19]. Androgen deprivation therapy results in metabolic changes such as decreased insulin sensitivity, loss of lean muscle mass, cardiovascular events, and bone fractures [20]. Men on androgen deprivation should have careful monitoring of blood glucose and cholesterol, bone mineral density testing, and calcium and vitamin D supplementation. In addition, bisphosphonates and denosumab are employed to prevent pathologic bone fractures in high-risk men.

It is important to consider treatment morbidity in men with prostate cancer, especially those over the age of 65, as they have other illnesses and variable life expectancy. Many men with prostate cancer are likely to die of comorbid illnesses; therefore, age and these competing risks should be balanced with the side effects of treatment [21].

References

1. Haas GP, Delongchamps N, Brawley OW, Wang CY, de la Roza G. The worldwide epidemiology of prostate cancer: perspectives from autopsy studies. Can J Urol. 2008;15(1):3866–71.
2. SEER cancer statistics review, 1975–2010. http://seer.cancer.gov/csr/1975_2010/.
3. Scosyrev E, Wu G, Mohile S, Messing EM. Prostate-specific antigen screening for prostate cancer and the risk of overt metastatic disease at presentation: analysis of trends over time. Cancer. 2012;118(23):5768–76.
4. Gleason DF, Mellinger GT. Prediction of prognosis for prostatic adenocarcinoma by combined histological grading and clinical staging. J Urol. 1974;111(1):58–64.
5. D'Amico A, Whittington R, Malkowicz SB, et al. BIochemical outcome after radical prostatectomy, external beam radiation therapy, or interstitial radiation therapy for clinically localized prostate cancer. JAMA. 1998;280(11):969–74.
6. Mohler JL, Armstrong AJ, Bahnson RR, Boston B, Busby JE, D'Amico AV, Eastham JA, Enke CA, Farrington T, Higano CS, et al. Prostate cancer, version 3.2012: featured updates to the NCCN guidelines. J Natl Compr Canc Netw. 2012;10(9):1081–7.
7. Wang L, Akin O, Mazaheri Y, Ishill NM, Kuroiwa K, Zhang J, Hricak H. Are histopathological features of prostate cancer lesions associated with identification of extracapsular extension on magnetic resonance imaging? BJU Int. 2010;106(9):1303–8.
8. Briganti A, Abdollah F, Nini A, Suardi N, Gallina A, Capitanio U, Bianchi M, Tutolo M, Passoni NM, Salonia A, et al. Performance characteristics of computed tomography in detecting lymph node metastases in contemporary patients with prostate cancer treated with extended pelvic lymph node dissection. Eur Urol. 2012;61(6):1132–8. doi:10.1016/j.eururo.2011.11.008.
9. Cooperberg MR, Vickers AJ, Broering JM, Carroll PR. Comparative risk-adjusted mortality outcomes after primary surgery, radiotherapy, or androgen-deprivation therapy for localized prostate cancer. Cancer. 2010;116(22):5226–34.
10. Boorjian SA, Karnes RJ, Viterbo R, Rangel LJ, Bergstralh EJ, Horwitz EM, Blute ML, Buyyounouski MK. Long-term survival after radical prostatectomy versus external-beam radiotherapy for patients with high-risk prostate cancer. Cancer. 2011;117(13):2883–91.
11. Pilepich MV, Caplan R, Byhardt RW, Lawton CA, Gallagher MJ, Mesic JB, Hanks GE, Coughlin CT, Porter A, Shipley WU, et al. Phase III trial of androgen suppression using goserelin in unfavorable-prognosis carcinoma of the prostate treated with definitive radiotherapy: report of Radiation Therapy Oncology Group Protocol 85-31. J Clin Oncol. 1997;15(3): 1013–21.
12. Bolla M, Collette L, Blank L, Warde P, Dubois JB, Mirimanoff RO, Storme G, Bernier J, Kuten A, Sternberg C, et al. Long-term results with immediate androgen suppression and external irradiation in patients with locally advanced prostate cancer (an EORTC study): a phase III randomised trial. Lancet. 2002;360(9327):103–6.

13. Epstein JI, Feng Z, Trock BJ, Pierorazio PM. Upgrading and downgrading of prostate cancer from biopsy to radical prostatectomy: incidence and predictive factors using the modified Gleason grading system and factoring in tertiary grades. Eur Urol. 2012;61(5):1019–24.
14. Abern MR, Aronson WJ, Terris MK, Kane CJ, Presti Jr JC, Amling CL, Freedland SJ. Delayed radical prostatectomy for intermediate-risk prostate cancer is associated with biochemical recurrence: possible implications for active surveillance from the SEARCH database. Prostate. 2013;73(4):409–17.
15. Wilt TJ, Brawer MK, Jones KM, Barry MJ, Aronson WJ, Fox S, Gingrich JR, Wei JT, Gilhooly P, Grob BM, et al. Radical prostatectomy versus observation for localized prostate cancer. N Engl J Med. 2012;367(3):203–13. doi:10.1056/NEJMoa1113162.
16. Huggins C, Hodges CV. Studies on prostatic cancer. I. The effect of castration, of estrogen and of androgen injection on serum phosphatases in metastatic carcinoma of the prostate. Cancer Res. 1941;1(4):293–7.
17. Niraula S, Le LW, Tannock IF. Treatment of prostate cancer with intermittent versus continuous androgen deprivation: a systematic review of randomized trials. J Clin Oncol. 2013;31:2029–36.
18. Tannock IF, de Wit R, Berry WR, Horti J, Pluzanska A, Chi KN, Oudard S, Théodore C, James ND, Turesson I, et al. Docetaxel plus prednisone or mitoxantrone plus prednisone for advanced prostate cancer. N Engl J Med. 2004;351(15):1502–12.
19. Abern MR, Dude AM, Tsivian M, Coogan CL. The characteristics of bladder cancer after radiotherapy for prostate cancer. Urol Oncol. 2013;31:1628–34.
20. Levine GN, D'Amico AV, Berger P, Clark PE, Eckel RH, Keating NL, Milani RV, Sagalowsky AI, Smith MR, Zakai N. Androgen-deprivation therapy in prostate cancer and cardiovascular risk: a science advisory from the American Heart Association, American Cancer Society, and American Urological Association: endorsed by the American Society for Radiation Oncology. CA Cancer J Clin. 2010;60(3):194–201.
21. Briganti A, Spahn M, Joniau S, Gontero P, Bianchi M, Kneitz B, Chun FK, Sun M, Graefen M, Abdollah F, et al. Impact of age and comorbidities on long-term survival of patients with high-risk prostate cancer treated with radical prostatectomy: a multi-institutional competing-risks analysis. Eur Urol. 2013;63(4):693–701.

Non-neurogenic Male Lower Urinary Tract Symptoms (incl. Benign Prostatic Hyperplasia)

41

Maximilian Rom and Shahrokh Shariat

41.1 General Facts

In the past, lower urinary tract symptoms (LUTS) in men over 40 years were always attributed to the enlarged prostate. The common term which was used in the medical world was benign prostatic hyperplasia (BPH), which is merely a histological diagnosis. Benign prostatic enlargement (BPE) means an enlarged prostate, with or without symptoms, whereas benign prostatic obstruction (BPO) is a urodynamic term which can only be diagnosed after pressure-flow studies and is defined by bladder outlet obstruction (BOO) due to BPE (Table 41.1). We know that other factors other than prostate enlargement contribute to LUTS, such as overactive bladder (OAB), detrusor underactivity, and nocturnal polyuria.

The incidence of male LUTS/BPH increases with age and is closely related to the growth of the prostate. Prevalence numbers from 10 to 40 % in the fifth life decade [1, 2] and from 24 to 90 % in the ninth life decade are reported.

41.2 Symptoms, Classification, and Grading

Male LUTS are defined as storage and voiding symptoms in men over 40 years of age. They are divided into storage symptoms, such as nocturia, urgency and frequency, and voiding symptoms, such as weak stream, intermittency, and post-void residual urine (PVR). Most of these symptoms are summarized in the International Prostate Symptom Score (IPSS), which divides LUTS into a mild (IPSS 0–7), moderate (IPSS 8–19), and severe (IPSS 20–35) group. Together with post-void residual urine (PVR) and uroflowmetry, the IPSS is the central diagnostic tool for men with LUTS/BPH.

M. Rom, MD (✉) • S. Shariat
Department of Urology, Medical University of Vienna, Vienna General Hospital, Waehringer Guertel 18-20, Vienna 1090, Austria
e-mail: maximilian.rom82@gmail.com

A.S. Merseburger et al. (eds.), *Urology at a Glance*,
DOI 10.1007/978-3-642-54859-8_41, © Springer-Verlag Berlin Heidelberg 2014

Table 41.1 Terminology of male LUTS

BPH	Benign prostatic hyperplasia
BPE	Benign prostatic enlargement
BPO	Benign prostatic obstruction
BOO	Bladder outlet obstruction
LUTS	Lower urinary tract symptoms

It is known that male LUTS/BPH is a progressive disease which can eventually lead to acute urinary retention and/or the need for deobstructive surgery. Patients who present with a prostate volume of 30 ml or more, a Qmax of less than 12 ml/s, PSA of 1.4 ng/ml or more, and higher age have an increased risk of progression [3, 4].

41.3 Therapy

In patients suggestive of LUTS, lifestyle modifications can really make a difference. These include a moderate fluid intake, reduction of alcohol and caffeine, physical activity, and micturition training. Behavioral treatment and watchful waiting is suitable for men with mild symptoms.

Men with moderate to severe LUTS should be offered an α-blocker. By relaxation of the smooth muscle in the bladder neck and the prostate, alpha-blockers can increase the flowrate by 15–30 % and a reduction in the IPSS by 30–45 % [5]. Side effects include orthostasis, low blood pressure, and retrograde ejaculation.

5-α-Reductase inhibitors are recommended for patients with moderate to severe LUTS and an enlarged prostate. They can inhibit disease progression and thus the risk of acute urinary retention and the need for surgery [6].

A combination treatment of α-blockers and 5-α-reductase inhibitors can reliably prevent dynamic and mechanic progression of the disease and should be given to men with moderate to severe LUTS with enlarged prostates and a reduced Qmax [7, 8].

If the patient suffers mainly from storage symptoms like urgency and increased daytime frequency, antimuscarinic medication hast to be considered. If such a treatment is started, it is very important to ensure that no significant PVR is present, because the therapy could worsen the retention. Antimuscarinic medication can also be combined with alpha-blockers [9].

PDE-5 inhibitors can also reduce moderate to severe LUTS and short-term studies provide proof of the symptom benefit with minimal side effects [10].

Desmopressin can be used for the treatment of nocturia based on a polyuric background and only if more than 33 % of a patients urine is produced during sleep [11].

Phytotherapy can also be effective and there is a wide spectrum of different drugs.

Several surgical approaches are used to treat BPH. Indications for surgery are listed in Table 41.2.

Open prostatectomy is very effective but has a significant morbidity profile, with a blood transfusion rate of 7–14 % and an incidence of urinary incontinence up to 10 %. It is still recommended for prostates with a volume of more than 80 ml, if there is no Holmium laser available [12].

Transurethral resection of the prostate (TURP) is the current surgical standard for prostates sized from 30 to 80 ml and moderate to severe LUTS/BPH. The indications for

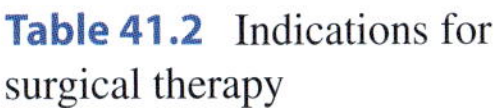

Table 41.2 Indications for surgical therapy

Bothersome LUTS refractory to conservative management (most frequent indication)
Recurrent/refractory urinary retention
Overflow incontinence
Bladder stones or diverticula
Treatment-resistant macrohematuria due to BPH/BPE
Dilatation of upper urinary tract due to BPO with or without renal insufficiency

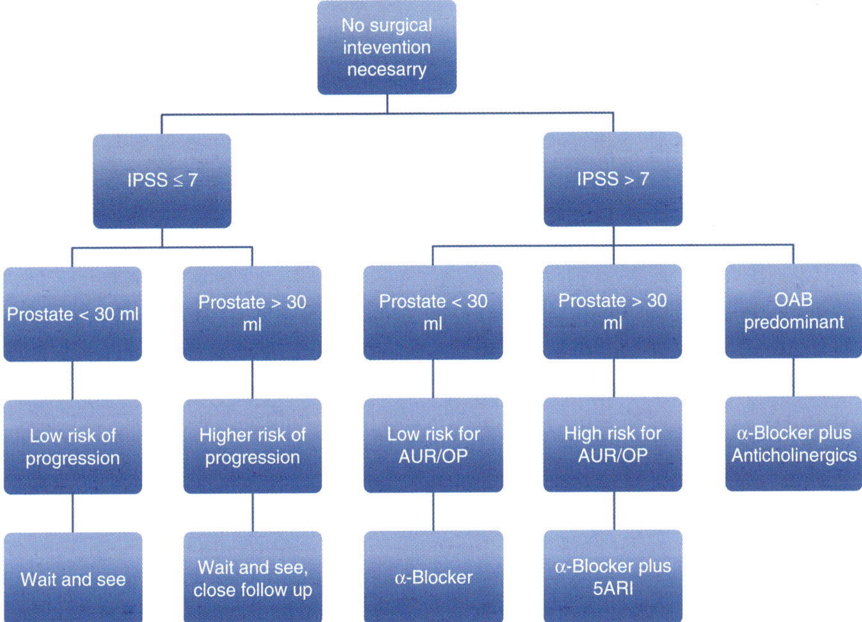

Fig. 41.1 Treatment algorithm of male lower urinary tract symptoms (LUTS) using medical and/or conservative treatment options [10]

surgery are listed in Table 41.2. TURP achieves a mean decrease in LUTS of 70 % and a mean increase in Qmax by 125 % after TURP [13]. Bipolar TURP is a well-investigated alternative to monopolar TURP. It has better safety and there is no difference in efficacy after 12 months. However, there are no long-term data available yet [14].

The Holmium laser resection of the prostate (HOLEP) is highly effective even in large prostates and the safety is confirmed by long-term studies. Photoselective vaporization of the prostate shows great intraoperative safety and should be considered for men receiving anticoagulant medication [15].

Transurethral needle ablation of the prostate (TUNA) is an alternative to TURP but has significant re-treatment rates and less improvement of symptoms. Transurethral microwave therapy (TUMT) is an outpatient procedure with low morbidity. It achieves improvement comparable to TURP but is also lacking durability [16, 17] (Figs. 41.1 and 41.2).

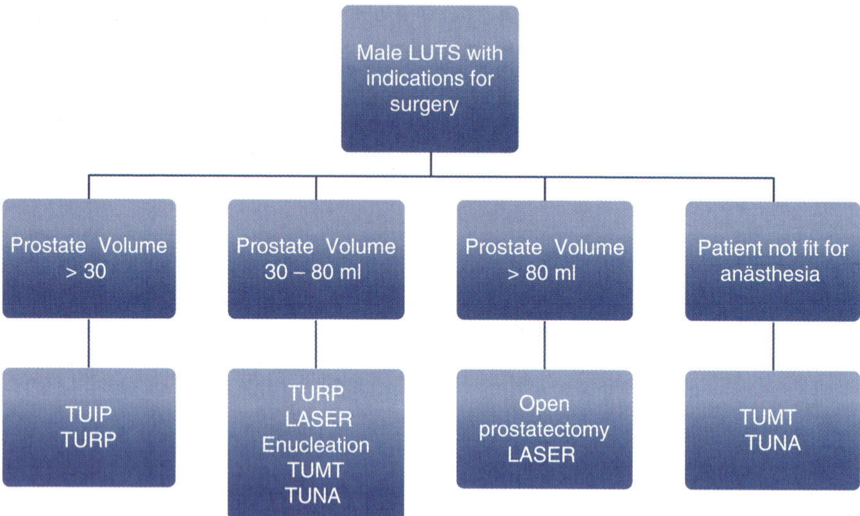

Fig. 41.2 Treatment algorithm of bothersome lower urinary tract symptoms (LUTS) refractory to conservative/medical treatment or in cases of absolute operation indications [10]

41.4 Complications

Typical complications of LUTS/BPH are acute urinary retention, the need for surgery, but also prostatitis and renal failure due to obstruction. As mentioned above, the risk of a progression of the disease can be predicted in early stages of the disease, and it is crucial to identify the respective risk factors. Affected patients must receive therapy in order to avoid complications.

References

1. Berry SJ, Coffey DS, Walsh PC, Ewing LL. The development of human benign prostatic hyperplasia with age. J Urol. 1984;132(3):474–9.
2. Verhamme KM, Dieleman JP, Bleumink GS, van der Lei J, Sturkenboom MC, Artibani W, Begaud B, Berges R, Borkowski A, Chappel CR, Costello A, Dobronski P, Farmer RD, Jiménez Cruz F, Jonas U, MacRae K, Pientka L, Rutten FF, van Schayck CP, Speakman MJ, Sturkenboom MC, Tiellac P, Tubaro A, Vallencien G, Vela Navarrete R, Triumph Pan European Expert Panel. Incidence and prevalence of lower urinary tract symptoms suggestive of benign prostatic hyperplasia in primary care–the Triumph project. Eur Urol. 2002;42(4):323–8.
3. Roehrborn CG, Malice M, Cook TJ, Girman CJ. Clinical predictors of spontaneous acute urinary retention in men with LUTS and clinical BPH: a comprehensive analysis of the pooled placebo groups of several large clinical trials. Urology. 2001;58(2):210–6.
4. Marberger MJ, Andersen JT, Nickel JC, Malice MP, Gabriel M, Pappas F, Meehan A, Stoner E, Waldstreicher J. Prostate volume and serum prostate-specific antigen as predictors of acute urinary retention. Combined experience from three large multinational placebo-controlled trials. Eur Urol. 2000;38(5):563–8.

5. Michel MC, Mehlburger L, Bressel HU, Goepel M. Comparison of tamsulosin efficacy in subgroups of patients with lower urinary tract symptoms. Prostate Cancer Prostatic Dis. 1998;1:332–5.
6. McConnell JD, Bruskewitz R, Walsh P, Andriole G, Lieber M, Holtgrewe HL, Albertsen P, Roehrborn CG, Nickel JC, Wang DZ, Taylor AM, Waldstreicher J. The effect of finasteride on the risk of acute urinary retention and the need for surgical treatment among men with benign prostatic hyperplasia. Finasteride Long-Term Efficacy and Safety Study Group. N Engl J Med. 1998;338(9):557–63.
7. Kaplan SA, Lee JY, Meehan AG, Kusek JW, MTOPS Research Group. Long-term treatment with finasteride improves clinical progression of benign prostatic hyperplasia in men with an enlarged versus a smaller prostate: data from the MTOPS trial. J Urol. 2011;185(4):1369–73. doi:10.1016/j.juro.2010.11.060. Epub 2011 Feb 22.
8. Roehrborn CG, Siami P, Barkin J, Damião R, Becher E, Miñana B, Mirone V, Castro R, Wilson T, Montorsi F, CombAT Study Group. The influence of baseline parameters on changes in international prostate symptom score with dutasteride, tamsulosin, and combination therapy among men with symptomatic benign prostatic hyperplasia and an enlarged prostate: 2-year data from the CombAT study. Eur Urol. 2009;55(2):461–71. doi:10.1016/j.eururo.2008.10.037. Epub 2008 Nov 6.
9. Kaplan SA, Roehrborn CG, Rovner ES, Carlsson M, Bavendam T, Guan Z. Tolterodine and tamsulosin for treatment of men with lower urinary tract symptoms and overactive bladder: a randomized controlled trial. JAMA. 2006;296(19):2319–28.
10. Oelke M, Giuliano F, Mirone V, et al. Monotherapy with tadalafil or tamsulosin similarly improved lower urinary tract symptoms suggestive of benign prostatic hyperplasia in an international, randomised, parallel, placebo-controlled clinical trial. Eur Urol. 2012;61:917–25.
11. Van Kerrebroeck PE, Dmochowski R, FitzGerald MP, Hashim H, Norgaard JP, Robinson D, Weiss JP. Nocturia research: current status and future perspectives. Neurourol Urodyn. 2010;29(4):623–8.
12. Oelke M, Bachmann A, Descazeaud A, Emberton M, Gravas S, Michel MC, N'dow J, Nordling J, de la Rosette JJ. EAU guidelines on the treatment and follow-up of non-neurogenic male lower urinary tract symptoms including benign prostatic obstruction. Eur Urol. 2013;64(1):118–40.
13. Madersbacher S, Marberger M. Is transurethral resection of the prostate still justified? Br J Urol. 1999;83:227–37.
14. Mamoulakis C, Ubbink DT, de la Rosette JJ. Bipolar versus mono- polar transurethral resection of the prostate: a systematic review and meta-analysis of randomized controlled trials. Eur Urol. 2009;56:798–809.
15. Westenberg A, Gilling P, Kennett K, Frampton C, Fraundorfer M. Holmium laser resection of the prostate versus transurethral resection of the prostate: results of a randomized trial with 4-year minimum long-term followup. J Urol. 2004;172:616–9.
16. Rosario DJ, Phillips JT, Chapple CR. Durability and cost-effectiveness of transurethral needle ablation of the prostate as an alternative to transurethral resection of the prostate when alpha-adrenergic antagonist therapy fails. J Urol. 2007;177(3):1047–51.
17. Hoffman RM, Monga M, Elliott SP, et al. Microwave thermotherapy for benign prostatic hyperplasia. Cochrane Database Syst Rev. 2012:9:CD004135.

Urolithiasis

42

Nicholas J. Kuntz and Michael E. Lipkin

42.1 General Facts

Stone disease is a common and costly health problem, and its prevalence in on the rise. In the United States between 2007 and 2010, the overall prevalence was reported to be 8.8 % [1]. This increase is likely due to similar trends in the obesity epidemic [1–4] and associated conditions like the metabolic syndrome [5, 6]. There are numerous other risk factors associated with metabolic stone formation, and these include genetic causes (gout, primary hyperoxaluria, cystinuria), gastrointestinal related (inflammatory bowel disease, previous bowel resection), and medication use (topiramate and tenofovir). Despite these risk factors, stone formation and recurrence can often be prevented with simple dietary and lifestyle modifications such as adequate hydration and low salt and low animal protein intake.

42.2 Symptoms, Classification, and Grading

Renal colic is the hallmark presenting symptom during an acute stone episode. This is characterized by acute, severe, intermittent flank pain, with associated nausea and emesis. Radiation to the groin (testicles or penis in males, vaginal pain in females), lower abdomen, and suprapubic region is not uncommon and may indicate progression of the stone into the distal ureter. Physical examination should be focused on hemodynamic stability, general appearance, and findings that may aid in future surgical intervention. Routine laboratory evaluation may reveal gross or microscopic hematuria, elevated creatinine, and leukocytosis (nonspecific marker of inflammation or stress). Imaging is an important diagnostic tool as symptoms can

N.J. Kuntz, MD (✉) • M.E. Lipkin, MD
Division of Urologic Surgery, Duke University Medical Center,
3707, Durham, NC 27710, USA
e-mail: nicholas.kuntz@duke.edu; michael.lipkin@duke.edu

A.S. Merseburger et al. (eds.), *Urology at a Glance*,
DOI 10.1007/978-3-642-54859-8_42,

Table 42.1 Common imaging modalities for urolithiasis

Imaging modality	Indications	Advantage	Efficacy	Limitations
Ultrasound	First line for pediatrics and pregnant women	No radiation exposure	*Renal stones:*	Not as sensitive or specific compared to NCCT
			29–81 % sensitivity	Overestimate the size of stones
			82–90 % specificity *Ureteral stones* 11–93 % sensitivity	Decreased effectiveness in obese patients
			87–100 % specificity	
Computed tomography	Study of choice	Fast, accurate and can evaluate other solid organs	95–100 % sensitivity	Higher cost
			92–98 % specificity	Exposure to ionizing radiation
Plain film (KUB)	Prior to SWL or to follow a radiopaque ureteral stone.	Low cost	*Combined with ultrasound*	Limited utility for radiolucent stones
		Low radiation	96 % sensitivity 91 % specificity	
Intravenous pyelogram	Rarely used as first-line evaluation	Useful to define complex collecting system	52–64% sensitivity	Required administration of contrast (risk of contrast induced nephropathy)
		Evaluates renal function and obstruction	92–94 % specificity	Contrast allergies
Magnetic resonance imaging	Limited role in primary stone evaluation	No radiation exposure	*Ureteral stones:*	High cost
	Second line in pregnant patients		93 % specificity 95 % specificity	Time consuming Stones not directly visualized

often be nonspecific and may overlap with other non-urologic diagnoses. The ideal imaging modality must take into consideration the patient-, facility-, and system-specific factors, such as radiation exposure and cost. Specific indications and limitations of various imaging modalities used for the evaluation of stones are listed in Table 42.1.

There are two broad stone categories based on the mineral composition: calcium stones and non-calcium stones. These are summarized in Table 42.2 along with important clinical characteristics and imaging properties. Although the stone composition may not be known during the initial workup and evaluation process, imaging and clinical characteristics may still influence the optimal management strategy. A common clinical scenario of urolithiasis, from diagnosis to treatment, is demonstrated in Fig. 42.1.

Table 42.2 Stone classification

	Composition	Clinical characteristic	X-ray characteristics	Urine pH
Calcium stones	Calcium oxalate	Most common stone composition in adults and pediatrics	Radiopaque	Variable
	Calcium phosphate	Primary stone composition in renal tubular acidosis	Radiopaque	Alkaline
Non-calcium stones	Uric acid	Usually associated with normal serum and urinary uric acid levels	Radiolucent	Acidic
	Ammonium acid urate	Associated with laxative abuse and low urinary phosphate	Radiolucent	Variable
	Cystine	Hard stone Caused by cystinuria	Radiopaque	Acidic
	Magnesium ammonium phosphate	AKA struvite Composition of many large stones especially in setting of UTI with urease splitting organism	Radiopaque	Alkaline
	Matrix	Associated with proteus UTI	Radiolucent	

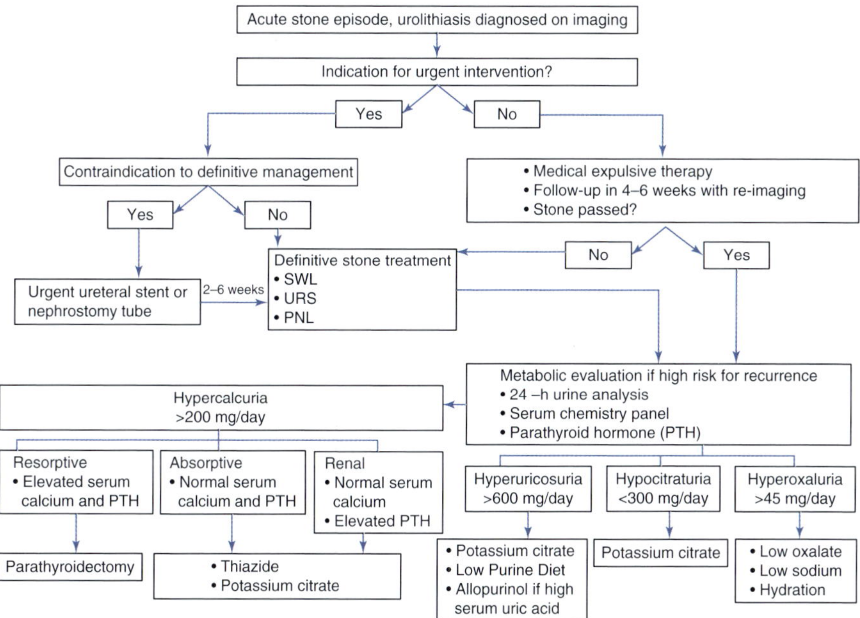

Fig. 42.1 Management of urolithiasis from diagnosis to therapy

42.3 Therapy

Fortunately, today there are many good surgical options available for the treatment of stone disease, as well as guidelines for their implementation. Despite this, there remains some debate on the best treatment based on the clinical scenario, as there are many factors to consider including success rates, cost, morbidity, and patient preference. The common surgical options include shockwave lithotripsy (SWL), ureteroscopy (URS), and percutaneous nephrolithotomy (PNL). These are listed in Table 42.3,

Table 42.3 Surgical treatments for urolithiasis

	Recommendation for use	Advantages	Limitations	Contraindications
SWL	First-line treatment for intrarenal stones <2 cm	Lower complications compared to URS	Hard stones	Absolute
	An acceptable first-line option for ureteral stones	Does not require general anesthesia	Lower pole stones	Active infection
		Does not routinely require a ureteral stent		Bleeding diathesis
				Pregnancy
				Distal obstruction
				Relative
				Stone burden >2 cm
				Hard stones
				Renal artery or aortic aneurysms
URS	First-line treatment for ureteral stones	High success rates for mid and distal ureteral stones	Higher complication rate	Untreated urinary tract infection
	Preferred for radiolucent stones, obese patients, hard stones, or absolute indication for anticoagulation	Safe in pregnancy	Stent pain	Inability to obtain retrograde access (urinary diversion)
PNL	First-line treatment for most staghorn stones	Superior stone-free rate for large renal stone	Requires general anesthesia	Irreversible coagulopathy
	First-line therapy for renal calculi >2 cm and for lower pole stones >1.5 cm		Higher morbidity and complications	Untreated urinary tract infection
	Failed SWL, urinary diversions, horseshoe kidneys			Inability to tolerate anesthesia
MET	<10-mm ureteral stone	Noninvasive	Temporary burden for patients	Bilateral obstructing stones or unilateral stone in a solitary kidney
	Controlled symptoms	Reserves costly and potentially morbid intervention for those who need it		Infection
	No evidence of infection			Intractable pain, nausea, or emesis
				Acute kidney injury

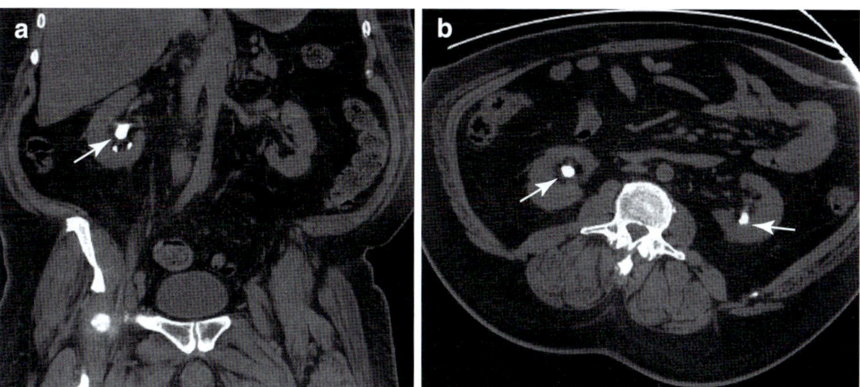

Fig. 42.2 Bilateral renal stones on CT scan indicated with white *arrows*. Coronal (**a**) and transverse (**b**) cuts

along with common indications for use, advantages, and limitations. Surgical interventions, including URS and PNL, have increased over the past several years [7]. Higher stone complexity and inherent limitations of SWL in obese patients have likely contributed to this trend; however, improved technology, less invasive surgical techniques, and superior stone-free outcomes are certainly at play as well.

Despite the high success rates and low morbidity associated with surgical interventions, there is still a role for medical therapy for the prevention of stone disease, and these are outlined in Fig. 42.1. In addition, medical expulsive therapy (MET) has gained wide acceptance recently for the acute management of ureteral stones and is included in the 2007 AUA guidelines for the management of ureteral stones [8]. MET is the practice of prescribing a medication to facilitate stone passage, in addition to routine pain control, aggressive hydration, and trial of spontaneous passage. Alpha blockers have become the preferred medication owning to higher stone passage rates, shorter time to pass, and less analgesia use compared to calcium channel blockers in randomized prospective trials [9].

42.4 Complications

Complications from urolithiasis include pain, infection/sepsis, calyceal rupture, abscess formation, pyonephrosis, xanthogranulomatous pyelonephritis, and loss of renal unit. Additionally, surgical interventions carry intrinsic complications as well. SWL causes symptomatic perirenal hematoma in up to 4 % of patients [10] with a transfusion rate as high as 31 % [11]. Complications unique to ureteroscopy include ureteral stricture, perforation, and avulsion. Fortunately, these are rarely encountered in the age of modern endoscopy. Bleeding and infection are the most common complications following PNL including a 5.7 % transfusion rate in one large multinational study [12]. In the case of delayed hemorrhage, patients may require angiography with selective arterial embolization of a bleeding arteriovenous fistula or pseudo-aneurysm. Other complications unique to PNL include pneumothorax, hydrothorax, or hemothorax and can be as high as 35 % if access is obtained above the 11th rib [13, 14]. If symptomatic, these patients may require a chest tube, nephrostomy tube or both. Colonic and splenic injuries have been reported but are rare. Lastly, steinstrasse is a well-known complication following SWL, URS, or PNL. This phenomenon is characterized by ureteral obstruction due to the accumulation of stone fragments and is directly related to the pre-treatment stone size. Although burdensome for patients, most episodes can be managed conservatively with MET. More aggressive options include SWL of the lead fragment, URS with laser lithotripsy, or placement of a nephrostomy tube.

References

1. Scales Jr CD, Smith AC, Hanley JM, Saigal CS. Prevalence of kidney stones in the United States. Eur Urol. 2012;62(1):160–5.
2. Taylor EN, Stampfer MJ, Curhan GC. Obesity, weight gain, and the risk of kidney stones. JAMA. 2005;293(4):455–62.
3. Nowfar S, Palazzi-Churas K, Chang DC, Sur RL. The relationship of obesity and gender prevalence changes in United States inpatient nephrolithiasis. Urology. 2011;78(5):1029–33.
4. Semins MJ, Shore AD, Makary MA, Magnuson T, Johns R, Matlaga BR. The association of increasing body mass index and kidney stone disease. J Urol. 2010;183(2):571–5.
5. Jeong IG, Kang T, Bang JK, Park J, Kim W, Hwang SS, et al. Association between metabolic syndrome and the presence of kidney stones in a screened population. Am J Kidney Dis. 2011;58(3):383–8.
6. Kohjimoto Y, Sasaki Y, Iguchi M, Matsumura N, Inagaki T, Hara I. Association of metabolic syndrome traits and severity of kidney stones: results from a nationwide survey on urolithiasis in Japan. Am J Kidney Dis. 2013;61(6):923–9.
7. Morris DS, Wei JT, Taub DA, Dunn RL, Wolf JS, Hollenbeck BK. Temporal trends in the use of percutaneous nephrolithotomy. J Urol. 2006;175(5):1731–6.
8. Preminger GM, Tiselius HG, Assimos DG, Alken P, Buck C, Gallucci M, et al. 2007 guideline for the management of ureteral calculi. J Urol. 2007;178(6):2418–34.
9. Ye Z, Yang H, Li H, Zhang X, Deng Y, Zeng G, et al. A multicentre, prospective, randomized trial: comparative efficacy of tamsulosin and nifedipine in medical expulsive therapy for distal ureteric stones with renal colic. BJU Int. 2011;108(2):276–9.
10. Dhar NB, Thornton J, Karafa MT, Streem SB. A multivariate analysis of risk factors associated with subcapsular hematoma formation following electromagnetic shock wave lithotripsy. J Urol. 2004;172(6 Pt 1):2271–4.
11. Collado Serra A, Huguet Perez J, Monreal Garcia de Vicuna F, Rousaud Baron A, Izquierdo de la Torre F, Vicente Rodriguez J. Renal hematoma as a complication of extracorporeal shock wave lithotripsy. Scand J Urol Nephrol. 1999;33(3):171–5.
12. de la Rosette J, Assimos D, Desai M, Gutierrez J, Lingeman J, Scarpa R, et al. The Clinical Research Office of the Endourological Society Percutaneous Nephrolithotomy Global Study: indications, complications, and outcomes in 5803 patients. J Endourol. 2011;25(1):11–7.
13. Aron M, Goel R, Kesarwani PK, Seth A, Gupta NP. Upper pole access for complex lower pole renal calculi. BJU Int. 2004;94(6):849–52. discussion 52.
14. Stening SG, Bourne S. Supracostal percutaneous nephrolithotomy for upper pole calyceal calculi. J Endourol. 1998;12(4):359–62.

Pyelonephritis

43

Michael Froehner

43.1 General Facts

Urinary tract infections belong to the most common infectious diseases. Hospital-acquired urinary tract infections associated with catheterization represent an increasingly important health problem. Bacteria usually reach the upper urinary tract by ascension via the urethra, partially promoted by endoscopic interventions or catheterization; lymphatic spread and hematogenic spread are less common. The development of bacterial resistance requires attention, particularly the resistance to fluoroquinolones and cephalosporins due to the overuse of these substances [1].

43.2 Symptoms, Classification, and Grading

Fever, flank pain and tenderness, nausea, and vomiting are typical symptoms of pyelonephritis. Symptoms of cystitis (dysuria, urgency, hematuria) may also be present [1, 2]. Urine analysis shows signs of urinary tract infection (increased leukocyte and erythrocyte count, partially accompanied by nitrites). 10^4 or more colony-forming units per mL is considered a clinically relevant bacteriuria [1]. Besides the clinical history (presence of catheters, history of interventions, urinary diversion, renal insufficiency, diabetes mellitus, immunodeficiency), complicating factors may be revealed by abdominal ultrasound (residual urine, ureteral obstruction, stone disease) or by computed tomography (CT) scan or magnetic resonance imaging (MRI) [1].

M. Froehner
Department of Urology, University Hospital "Carl Gustav Carus",
Dresden University of Technology, Fetscherstrasse 74, Dresden D-01304, Germany
e-mail: michael.froehner@uniklinikum-dresden.de

A.S. Merseburger et al. (eds.), *Urology at a Glance*,
DOI 10.1007/978-3-642-54859-8_43, © Springer-Verlag Berlin Heidelberg 2014

Pyelonephritis may be classified as uncomplicated or complicated [1, 2]. Complicated pyelonephritis may be subdivided into cases where the complicating factor may be eliminated (for instance, by removal of a stone or by instrumental urinary diversion) and those where such elimination is not possible (for instance, presence of permanent catheters) [1]. Further classification of pyelonephritis may be made by the grade of clinical severity. Fever, shivering, and circulatory failure indicate a systemic inflammatory response syndrome (SIRS) which may lead to organ dysfunction and subsequent failure [1]. SIRS is defined as systemic inflammatory response fulfilling two or more of the following criteria: temperature >38 or <36 °C, heart rate >90 beats per minute, respiratory rate >20 breaths per minute or $PaCO_2$ <32 mmHg, white blood cell count >12 or <4 GPt/L, or >10 % immature (band) leukocyte forms [3]. Sepsis is considered a SIRS related to infection. Severe sepsis is defined as a sepsis associated with organ dysfunction [3].

43.3 Therapy

Antibiotic treatment, fluid substitution, and – if required – circulatory support are essential parts of pyelonephritis treatment. Figure 43.1 gives an algorithm to treatment of pyelonephritis and its acute complications. Table 43.1 shows antibiotic treatment options. Ureteral obstruction may require immediate urinary diversion by transurethral ureteral stent or percutaneous nephrostomy placement; the latter should

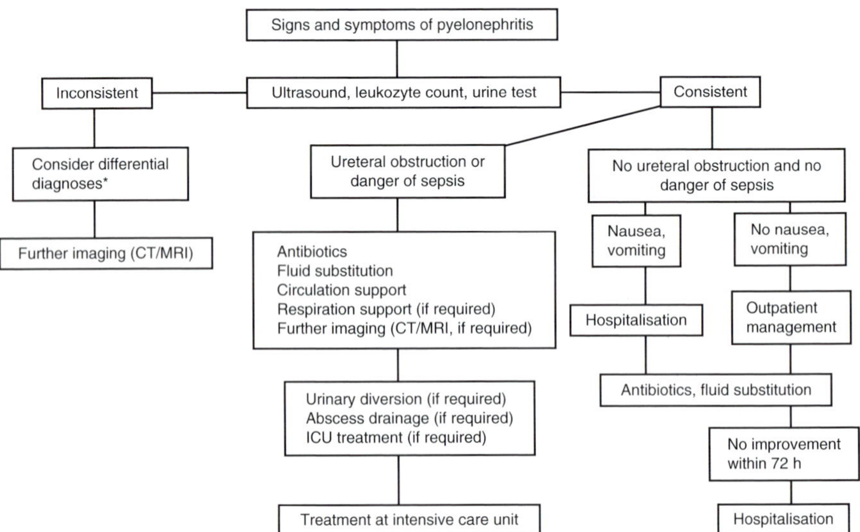

Fig. 43.1 Flow chart demonstrating the pathway from diagnosis to therapy. *An example for a possible differential diagnosis is given in Fig. 43.2

Table 43.1 Antibiotic treatment options for pyelonephritis

	Mild or moderate cases	Severe cases
First-line treatment	Oral fluoroquinolone	Parenteral fluoroquinolone[a] Third-generation parenteral cephalosporin[b] Aminopenicillin plus a β-lactamase inhibitor[c]
Alternative	Third-generation oral cephalosporin	Parenteral aminoglycoside or carbapenem[a]
Duration (days)	7–10	14–21

Adapted from Grabe et al. [1]
[a]When expected *E. coli* fluoroquinolone resistance rates below 10 %
[b]When expected extended spectrum beta-lactamase-producing *E. coli* rates below 10 %
[c]When susceptible Gram-positive pathogens are expected

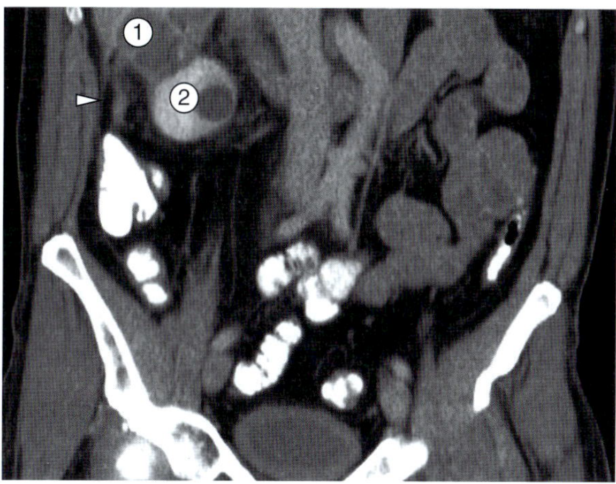

Fig. 43.2 Contrast medium-enhanced coronary CT scan revealing a retrocecal appendicitis and subhepatic abscess (initially misinterpreted as pyelonephritis) in a 49-year-old man (*1*, abscess; *2*, kidney; *arrowhead*, appendix vermiformis)

be preferred in more severe cases. Intrarenal or perinephritic abscesses require immediate percutaneous or open surgical drainage or – in very severe cases – emergency nephrectomy. Disseminated intravascular coagulation may require substitution of platelets or plasma components and/or the application of recombinant human activated protein C [4].

43.4 Complications

Intrarenal or perinephritic abscesses (Figs. 43.3 and 43.4) and SIRS are relatively rare but potentially life-threatening complications of pyelonephritis. In these cases, immediate diagnosis and percutaneous or open surgical intervention with subsequent intensive care unit treatment are essential. Disseminated intravascular coagulation may lead to severe bleeding and organ failure. The development of renal scars in the absence of complicating factors of pyelonephritis is controversially discussed [1].

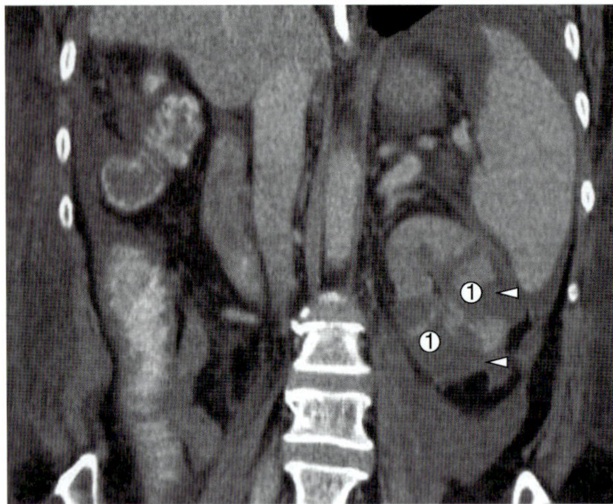

Fig. 43.3 Multiple intrarenal abscesses (*1*) with perirenal protrusion (*arrowheads*) in a nonobstructed kidney causing septic shock, disseminated intravascular coagulation, and multiorgan failure requiring emergency nephrectomy in a 58-year-old man with liver cirrhosis and diabetes mellitus (contrast medium-enhanced coronary CT scan)

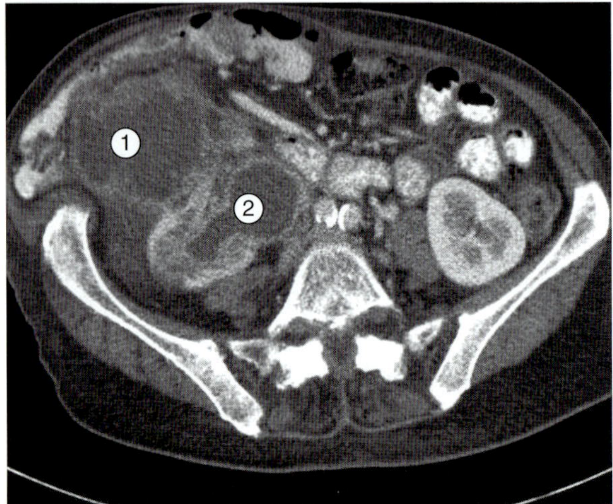

Fig. 43.4 Large perinephritic abscess (*1*) subsequently treated by nephrectomy in an 80-year-old woman with a largely indolent clinical course (contrast medium-enhanced axial CT scan; (*2*) hydronephrotic and atrophic kidney)

References

1. Grabe M, Bjerklund-Johansen TE, Botto H, Çek M, Naber KG, Pickard RS, Tenke P, Wagenlehner F, Wullt B. Guidelines on urological infections. Available at: http://www.uroweb.org/gls/pdf/18_Urological%20infections_LR.pdf. Accessed 15 Sept 2013.
2. Deutsche Gesellschaft für Urologie: S-3 Leitlinie AWMF-Register-Nr. 043/044: Harnwegsinfektionen. Epidemiologie, Diagnostik, Therapie und Management unkomplizierter bakterieller ambulant erworbener Harnwegsinfektionen bei erwachsenen Patienten. [S3 guideline AWMF register no. 043/044: Urinary tract infections. Epidemiology, diagnostics, therapy and management of uncomplicated non-hospital-acquired urinary tract infections in adults. Guideline in German.] Available at: http://www.awmf.org/uploads/tx_szleitlinien/043-044l_S3_Harnwegsinfektionen.pdf. Accessed 15 Sept 2013.

3. Bone RC, Balk RA, Cerra FB, Dellinger RP, Fein AM, Knaus WA, Schein RM, Sibbald WJ. Definitions for sepsis and organ failure and guidelines for the use of innovative therapies in sepsis. The ACCP/SCCM Consensus Conference Committee. American College of Chest Physicians/Society of Critical Care Medicine. Chest. 1992;101:1644–55.
4. Levi M, Toh CH, Thachil J, Watson HG. Guidelines for the diagnosis and management of disseminated intravascular coagulation. British Committee for Standards in Haematology. Br J Haematol. 2009;145:24–33.

Peyronie's Disease

44

Georgios Hatzichristodoulou and Sven Lahme

44.1 From Symptoms to Diagnosis

44.1.1 Definition

Peyronie's disease (PD) is an acquired benign disease that affects the tunica albuginea of the penis leading to fibrous plaques. The major and most characteristic symptom in affected patients is penile deviation, which may lead to inability for sexual intercourse [1–3]. The prevalence of PD is 3–9 % of adult men, with males between 40 and 70 years being affected predominantly. However, PD also occurs in the younger population under 30 years [2, 4]. The etiology of PD is unknown, but some hypotheses exist. The disease is considered a wound-healing disorder that occurs in genetically susceptible males following repeated penile microtraumata. These microtraumata usually occur during sexual intercourse, without being noticed by the patient. However, PD has a multifactorial background including unregulated deposition of collagen and overexpression of transforming growth factor-β-1, which finally lead to the formation of characteristic penile plaques. Common comorbidities and risk factors for developing PD are diabetes mellitus, hypertension, hyperlipidemia, hypogonadism, smoking, and excessive consumption of alcohol. Dupuytren's disease is an associated collagen disease, affecting 9–39 % of PD patients [2, 5, 6].

G. Hatzichristodoulou (✉)
Department of Urology, Technical University of Munich, Rechts der Isar Medical Center, Ismaninger Str. 22, Munich 81675, Germany
e-mail: georgios.hatzichristodoulou@lrz.tum.de

S. Lahme
Department of Urology, Siloah St. Trudpert Hospital, Wilferdinger Str. 67, Pforzheim 75179, Germany

A.S. Merseburger et al. (eds.), *Urology at a Glance*,
DOI 10.1007/978-3-642-54859-8_44, © Springer-Verlag Berlin Heidelberg 2014

44.1.2 Medical History

History taking is essential in patients suffering from PD. It should address duration of the disease, which symptoms were initially present, and whether or how they have changed since the onset. The patient should address the most bothersome symptoms and be asked about their possible spontaneous improvement or progression, especially regarding pain and penile deviation. Any recognized penile trauma should be mentioned by the patient. In this regard history of penile fracture is important, as a remarkable number of patients experience penile deviation following penile fracture [7]. Impairment of sexual intercourse, mainly due to penile deviation, is of utmost importance, regarding further therapeutic considerations. Any preexisting concomitant medical conditions, especially erectile dysfunction (ED), diabetes mellitus, or Dupuytren's disease should be pointed out. Special attention should be paid to ED and penile shortening beginning at the same time of PD, as these conditions are very frequent among PD patients. Family history of PD or Dupuytren's disease is also useful, as these conditions are more common in the same family. Previous treatments for PD and their effects on the disease (successful or not) should be asked in order to plan the further treatment. Psychosocial assessment including depression and psychological distress can be evaluated by a team-based approach [2, 8].

44.1.3 Diagnostics

Penile pain is best assessed by a visual analog scale, ranging from 0 (no pain) to 10 (strong pain). Erectile function should be assessed by the short version of the International Index of Erectile Function questionnaire (IIEF-5). Currently, a PD-specific questionnaire is under investigation, which can serve as a diagnostic tool for the assessment of treatment success [9]. Physical examination with palpation of the stretched flaccid penis should be performed in order to detect penile plaques. Other concomitant medical abnormalities such as phimosis or short frenulum can be inspected simultaneously. Sonography is an easy and widely available imaging modality and should be performed to assess plaque formation, especially calcifications which can occur in about 30 % of patients, either in the stable or acute phase of the disease (Fig. 44.1) [1, 2]. Sonography should be done by a 7.5-MHz linear transducer allowing high-resolution imaging. In this regard it should be noted that accurate measurement of plaque size is impossible with any imaging or mechanical modality and therefore not indicated. Magnetic resonance imaging (MRI) provides high-resolution imaging of the tunica albuginea, but this does not add useful information regarding further therapeutic steps. Moreover, MRI is an expensive imaging modality. Its use in PD should be restricted to scientific studies. In conclusion, MRI is not recommended in the diagnostic of PD [1, 2]. The assessment of penile deviation is the most important part of clinical evaluation. This is best done by measuring the deviation angle by a goniometer after artificial erection using intracavernosal alprostadil (prostaglandin E1). This allows the best possible objective assessment of deviation. A successful erection can be determined objectively by the Erection

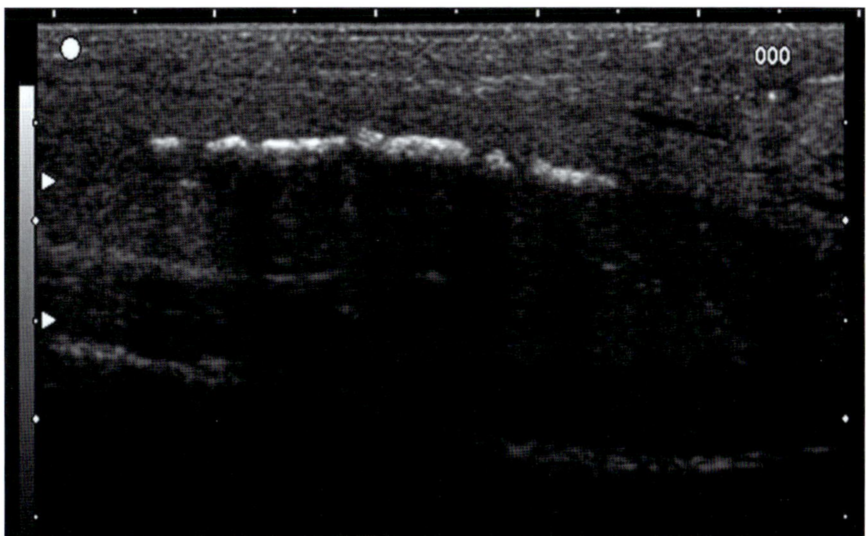

Fig. 44.1 Extensive plaque calcification of tunica albuginea in sonography (longitudinal aspect)

Hardness Score, ranging from 1 (Penis larger, but not hard) to 4 (Penis completely hard and fully rigid). When indicated, color duplex imaging can be performed simultaneously for detailed evaluation of erectile function. Photographic documentation of curvature is recommended in order to assess the development of deviation in the further disease course. It is also important to measure penile length during erection (from symphysis to glans), and pay attention to deformities such as hourglass narrowing.

44.1.4 Differential Diagnosis

The most common differential diagnosis, especially in younger patients, is congenital penile deviation which is caused by asymmetric development of the cavernous bodies leading to penile deviation [10]. In contrast to PD, deviation during erection in patients with congenital penile deviation is usually ventral or lateral. Discrimination to PD is easily done by history taking and clinical examination. The onset of penile deviation in patients with congenital deviation is in the adolescence when first erections occurred and persists in later life. Penile plaques are missing, and affected patients do not complain of penile pain or ED. However, like in PD, penile deviation can lead to inability for sexual intercourse and in these cases requires surgical therapy. Another differential diagnosis is penile cancer, which usually begins at the glans, the prepuce, or the penile skin and shows a tumorous growth. In suspected cases, biopsy and histopathological assessment should be performed. Penile Mondor's disease is a rare condition which can mimic PD. This condition is characterized by a thrombosis of the superficial dorsal penile vein, which might lead to penile pain in affected individuals [11]. Penile deviation and plaques of the tunica albuginea are missing in these patients. The cause of this benign disease is unknown. Therapy consists of anti-inflammatory medication and in exceptional cases surgical resection of the thrombus.

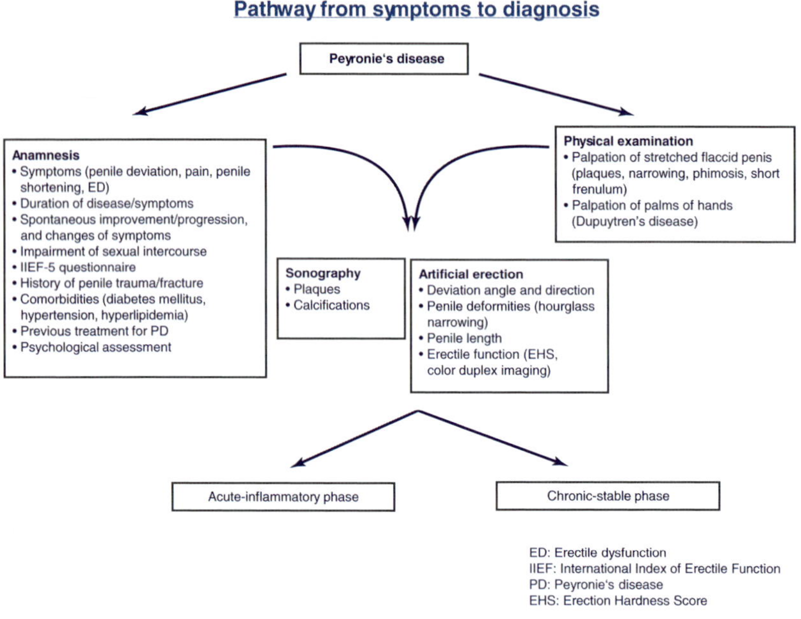

44.2 From Diagnosis to Therapy

44.2.1 General Facts

Due to lack of exact pathophysiologic knowledge, there is no causal therapy for PD. Several nonsurgical and surgical treatment options have been investigated in the past, but no one therapy can relieve all symptoms associated with PD. Patients suffering from PD should be counseled that all therapeutic options available today are symptomatic, i.e., they can relieve symptoms associated with the disease. However, there is no healing of the disease. This aspect is especially important in the surgical treatment of penile deviation as there is risk of recurrence of deviation in about 10 % of cases [2]. Therefore, surgical treatment of deviation should only be performed in the stable phase of the disease (see below) in order to minimize the risk of recurrence.

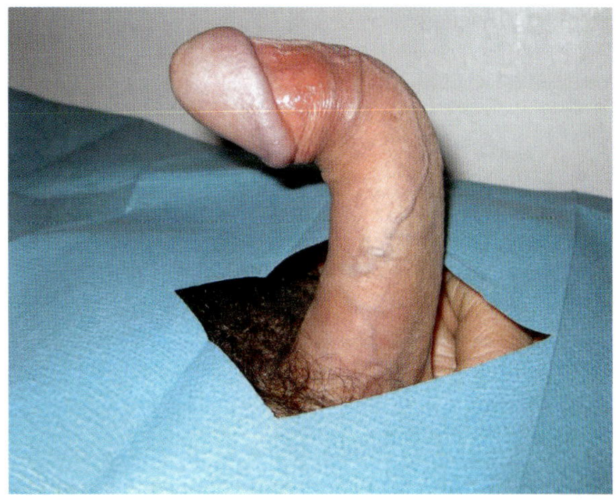

Fig. 44.2 Penile deviation (90° dorsal) during artificial erection

44.2.2 Symptoms and Classification

Peyronie's disease usually proceeds in an acute-inflammatory phase continued by a chronic-stable phase. The first, acute phase is characterized by plaque formation, penile pain, and progression of penile deviation. This phase usually last for about 12–18 months; however, its duration is variable. Penile pain at erection is more common than pain during the flaccid state of the penis. In the second, chronic phase of the disease, pain typically resolves, plaques remain stable, and penile deviation stabilizes and is the main symptom. According to the natural history of PD, 89 % of patients will be pain-free after a mean of 18 months without any treatment, when the inflammatory phase ends. In contrast, penile deviation improves in only 12 %, while it worsens in 48 % of patients [3]. Penile deviation may lead to inability for sexual intercourse (Fig. 44.2) [1–3]. Spontaneous improvement or even resolution of PD is rare. Another important symptom of the disease is penile shortening, which occurs in almost all patients as a result of scar formation and shrinking of the penile connective tissue. Moreover, PD is associated with ED in up to 58 % of men [1]. The disease can also result in psychological distress, depression, or anxiety [8]. One should keep in mind that the abovementioned symptoms associated with PD may change during the disease course. Penile deformities such as hourglass narrowing can develop as result of plaque formation/narrowing of the cavernous bodies (Fig. 44.3).

44.2.3 Therapy

Generally, therapy of PD can be subdivided in nonsurgical and surgical treatment options. Nonsurgical treatment is performed in the acute phase of the disease (disease duration <12–18 months), while patients in the stable phase usually undergo surgical therapy, providing the correct indication.

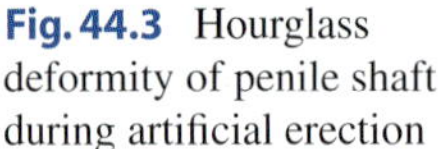

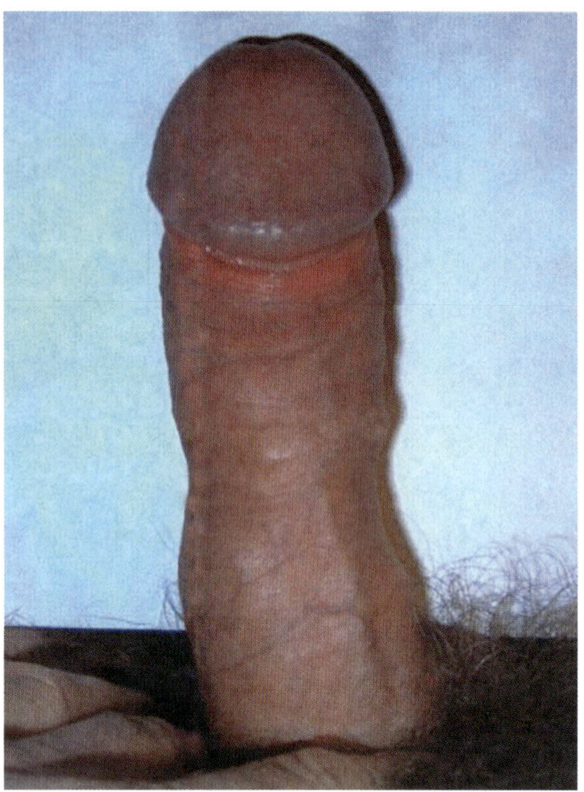

Fig. 44.3 Hourglass deformity of penile shaft during artificial erection

44.2.3.1 Nonsurgical (Conservative) Therapy

Various nonsurgical treatment modalities have been proposed and investigated in the past. However, only limited evidence exists and supports its use in PD. This is mainly attributed to lack of pathophysiologic knowledge of the disease and also due to lack of well-designed controlled trials. However, for lack of numerous alternatives, these nonsurgical treatment options are being used in clinical practice. In the following, only the most important and widely used treatment modalities are described.

Medical (Oral) Therapy

Vitamin E. Vitamin E is the most common medical therapy used in PD. It has an antioxidant effect and could be effective in the acute phase of the disease by reducing oxygen-free radicals. Its benefit is uncertain, but because of lack of serious side effects and low costs, this therapy is widely used.

Potassium Paraaminobenzoate. The other very common applied drug is potassium paraaminobenzoate (Potaba) which has an anti-inflammatory and antifibrotic effect and may prevent further progression of the disease. However, it does not improve penile deviation. Potaba has several side effects including gastrointestinal complaints such as diarrhea or gastric spasms, which are reasons for discontinuation [1, 2, 12–14].

Phosphodiesterase-Type-5 Inhibitors. Recently, phosphodiesterase-type-5 (PDE-5) inhibitors have been tested in the treatment of PD. These drugs offer an antifibrotic effect and thus may have a potential benefit by reducing progression of the disease or possibly by reducing penile deviation. However, so far only limited experience is available [15].

Other Medications. Further drugs and agents which are used for the oral treatment of PD include pentoxifylline, colchicine, tamoxifen, and carnitine. However, due to controversial results and only limited controlled trials available, these medications cannot be recommended [1, 2].

Electromotive Drug Administration (Iontophoresis)

Electromotive drug administration (EMDA) uses an external electric force to induce transport of ionic molecules through tissue layers. In PD, this mechanism is utilized for transdermal medications, such as verapamil or dexamethason, to reach the tunica albuginea and thus the plaques. This treatment is less invasive than intralesional therapy (see below) and therefore preferred by patients. Results of EMDA in the treatment of PD are controversial; however, recent data have shown an effect in regard to pain reduction [16].

Extracorporeal Shockwave Therapy

Extracorporeal shockwave therapy (ESWT) can be performed in patients with predominant penile pain for rapid pain relief. The analgetic effect has been shown in a recent controlled study. However, patients should be counseled that this therapy is for pain only and that penile deviation may worsen after ESWT [17]. Moreover, ESWT cannot reduce penile deviation and therefore cannot replace surgical therapy of penile deviation in PD. The exact mode of action of ESWT is still unknown.

Intralesional Therapy

Intralesional therapy represents the direct injection of medications into the PD plaques of the tunica albuginea. This allows the application of a high concentration of the drug at the plaques, which is much higher than by oral/systemic administration. Intralesional therapy can be applied with several medications, such as corticosteroids, collagenase, verapamil, and interferons. A possible benefit in regard to reduction of penile deviation has recently been shown for collagenase [18]. Importantly, when interferons are used, side effects like myalgia, fever, or flu-like symptoms can occur, which in turn may require treatment. Of note, because of repeated injections and thus traumata to the tunica albuginea during this treatment modality, there is risk of scar formation and worsening of penile deviation.

Penile Traction Devices

Recently, penile traction devices have been proposed as a novel conservative treatment option for PD. Penile deviation may be reduced by mechanical stretching of the

Table 44.1 Indications for surgical therapy of Peyronie's disease

Indications
Disease duration at least 12 months
Stable phase of disease (at least 6 months)
Stable penile deviation
No penile pain
Penile deviation leading to inability for sexual intercourse
Failed conservative therapy

penis and subsequent mechanically induced changes of the penile connective tissue [19]. Only preliminary results exist on this issue.

Radiation Therapy

Radiation has been used for the empirical treatment of PD in the past. However, due to controversial results in clinical studies, today it is not recommended [20]. Radiation should not be performed any more in PD.

44.2.3.2 Surgical Therapy

Surgical therapy is the gold standard to correct penile deviation in stable PD. Indications for surgical therapy are summarized in Table 44.1. Surgical therapy is subdivided in three main procedures: (1) plication techniques, (2) grafting procedures with partial plaque excision or incision followed by defect closure with various grafts, and (3) correction of deviation with simultaneous penile prosthesis implantation in patients with ED not responding to medical therapy [21, 22].

Plication Techniques

Plication techniques result in penile straightening by shortening the convex side of deviation. The most applied plication technique is the Nesbit procedure [23]. The main adverse effect associated with plication techniques is shortening of erect penile length. The more severe the deviation is, the more pronounced will penile shortening be postoperatively. Generally, plication techniques are applied when deviations are <60°, because penile curvatures >60° will exacerbate penile shortening after plication leading to patient dissatisfaction [24].

Grafting Procedures

In more advanced deviations >60°, the preferred treatment is plaque incision or partial plaque excision followed by closing of the tunical defect by various grafts, as these procedures can maintain penile length. Penile straightening with this technique is achieved by stretching the concave side of deviation. Grafting procedures are also indicated when patients experience a short penis, to avoid further shortening after plication. This technique is more complex than plication as it requires the complete preparation and lifting of the neurovascular bundle within Buck's fascia. Several autologous and non-autologous grafts can be used for closure of the tunical defect. However, there is a current tendency to use non-autologous "off-the-shelf" grafts like pericardium, small intestinal submucosa, or collagen fleece (Fig. 44.4a–e) [22, 25].

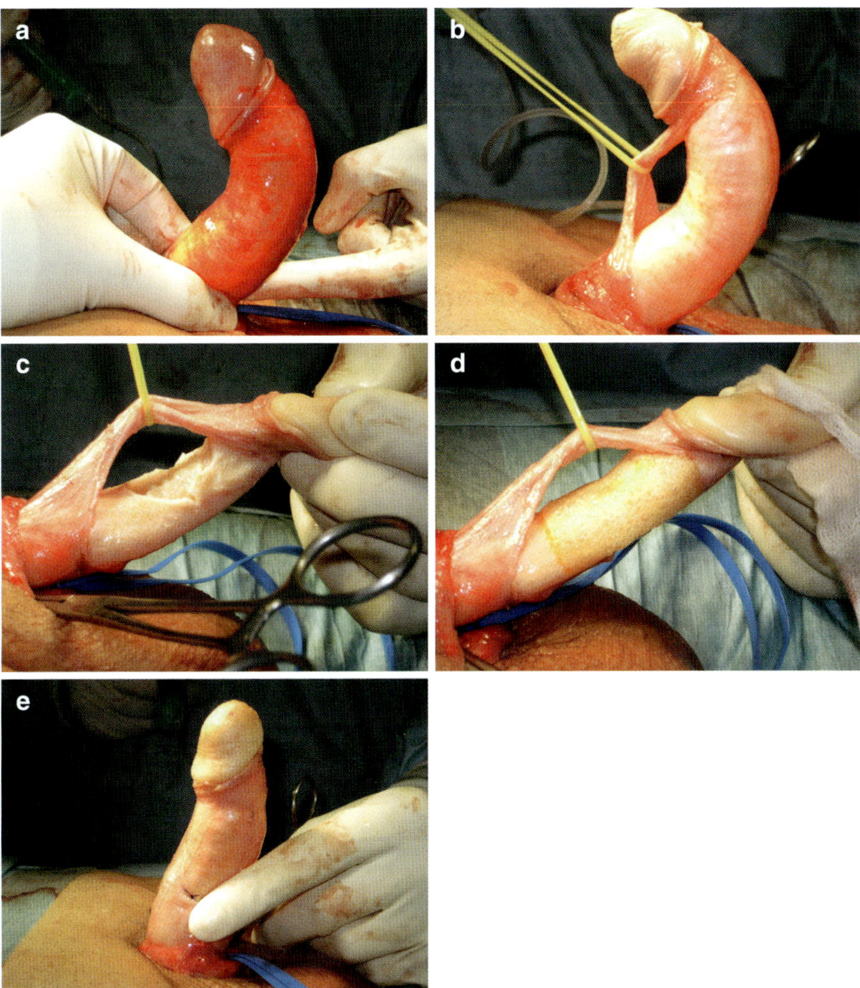

Fig. 44.4 (**a–e**): Surgical therapy of penile deviation by partial plaque excision and grafting with collagen fleece. (**a**): Penile deviation (90° dorsal) after penile degloving (in artificial erection). (**b**): Penile deviation (90° dorsal) after mobilization of neurovascular bundle (in artificial erection). (**c**): Defect of tunica albuginea after partial plaque excision. (**d**): Grafting of tunical defect with collagen fleece. (**e**): Straight penis after reapproximation of neurovascular bundle and closure of Buck's fascia at end of operation (in artificial erection)

The risk of postoperative ED with grafting procedures is higher than with plication; therefore, patients should have strong erectile rigidity preoperatively [21].

Penile Prosthesis Implantation with Simultaneous Correction of Deviation

In PD patients with penile deviation and coexisting ED not responding to medical treatment, e.g., PDE-5 inhibitors or intracavernous injections, penile prosthesis implantation with simultaneous correction of deviation is recommended in order to treat both conditions. This procedure provides the best satisfaction within these patients [21, 26]. When penile deviation is <30°, only prosthesis implantation alone is performed, because this will also correct deviation. However, in patients that show a >30° deviation, additional straightening maneuvers may be necessary. In the first step this is usually done by manual modeling after insertion of the implant cylinders [27]. If deviation persists and exceeds 30°, then further plication or plaque incision/ partial plaque excision and grafting is required to correct penile deviation. Grafting should be performed in these cases to prevent herniation of the cylinders [28].

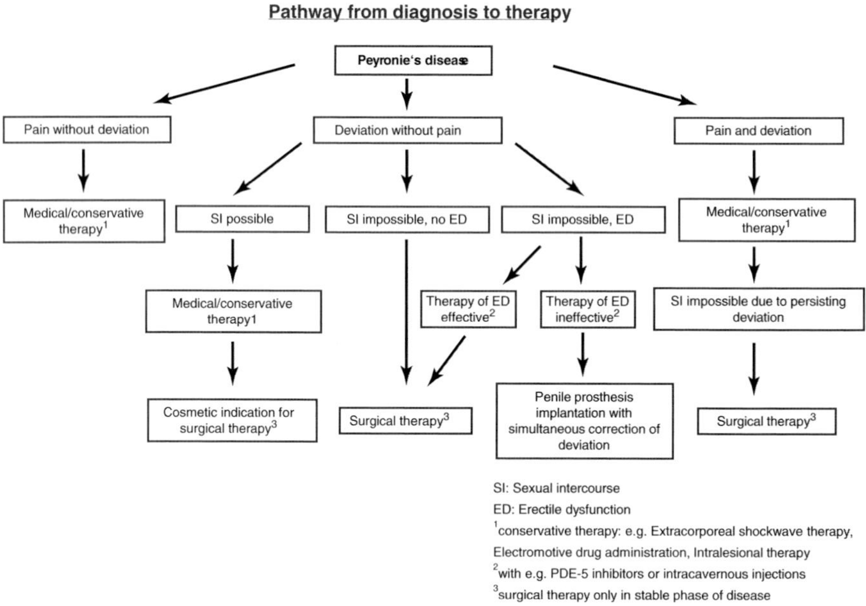

44.2.4 Complications

Preoperative counseling of patients willing to undergo surgical therapy for PD is very important. Several aspects should be discussed with the patient and realistic expectations have to be pointed out. The most important complications/risks associated with surgical therapy are as follows: penile shortening can occur with either plication or grafting procedures. The risk of shortening is obviously less with the later techniques. This is an important aspect as almost all patients already experience penile shortening associated with the disease [1]. Recurrent deviation after successful surgical therapy can occur in about 10 % of cases, when a new episode/inflammation of the disease occurs [2]. In this context, persistent deviation may also be present after surgery. However, when this is <20°, it is considered "functionally straight" with no need for further treatment. The risk of postoperative ED is 30 %. This again is also very important because up to 58 % of PD patients already experience ED concomitantly with the disease [1]. Change or decrease of penile sensation (penile hypoesthesia, glans numbness) is another complication that is found in 8–31 % of cases [22, 29]. However, these changes will resolve spontaneously in nearly all patients with time. As stated above, there is no healing of PD. The patient should be aware of this fact and should therefore know about possible recurrences of symptoms associated with the disease, especially penile deviation.

References

1. Ralph D, Gonzalez-Cadavid N, Mirone V, Perovic S, Sohn M, Usta M, Levine L. The management of Peyronie's disease: evidence-based 2010 guidelines. J Sex Med. 2010;7:2359–74.
2. Levine L, Burnett AL. Standard operating procedures for Peyronie's disease. J Sex Med. 2013;10:230–44.
3. Mulhall J, Schiff J, Guhring P. An analysis of the natural history of Peyronie's disease. J Urol. 2006;175:2115–8.
4. Tal R, Hall MS, Alex B, Choi J, Mulhall JP. Peyronie's disease in teenagers. J Sex Med. 2012;9:302–8.
5. Porst H, Garaffa G, Ralph D. Peyronie's disease (PD) – Morbus de la Peyronie. In: Porst H, Reisman Y, editors. The ESSM syllabus of sexual medicine. Amsterdam: Medix Publishers; 2012. p. 680–731.
6. Bichler K, Lahme S, Mattauch W, Petri E. Untersuchungen zum Kollagenstoffwechsel bei Induration penis plastica. Urologe A. 1998;37:306–11.
7. Hatzichristodoulou G, Dorstewitz A, Gschwend JE, Herkommer K, Zantl N. Surgical management of penile fracture and long-term outcome on erectile function and voiding. J Sex Med. 2013;10:1424–30.
8. Nelson C, Mulhall JP. Psychological impact of Peyronie's disease: a review. J Sex Med. 2013;10:653–60.
9. Hellstrom W, Feldman R, Rosen RC, Smith T, Kaufman G, Tursi J. Bother and distress associated with Peyronie's disease: validation of the Peyronie's disease questionnaire. J Urol. 2013;190:627–34.
10. Cruz N. Congenital penile curvature and penile torsion. In: Porst H, Reisman Y, editors. The ESSM syllabus of sexual medicine. Amsterdam: Medix Publishers; 2012.
11. Conkbayir I, Yanik B, Keyik B, Hekimoglu B. Superficial dorsal penile vein thrombosis (Mondor disease of the penis) involving the superficial external pudendal vein: color doppler sonographic findings. J Ultrasound Med. 2010;29:1243–5.
12. Tunuguntla H. Management of Peyronie's disease-a review. World J Urol. 2001;19:244–50.
13. Pryor J, Farell CR. Controlled clinical trial of vitamin E in Peyronie's disease. Prog Reprod Biol Med. 1983;9:41–5.
14. Paulis G, Brancato T, D'Ascenzo R, De Giorgio G, Nupieri P, Orsolini G, Alvaro R. Efficacy of vitamin E in the conservative treatment of Peyronie's disease: legend or reality? A controlled study of 70 cases. Andrology. 2013;1:120–8.
15. Al-Shaiji T, Brock GB. Peyronie's disease: evolving surgical management and the role of phosphodiesterase 5 inhibitors. Scientific World Journal. 2009;9:822–45.
16. Mehrsai A, Namdari F, Salavati A, Dehghani S, Allameh F, Pourmand G. Comparison of transdermal electromotive administration of verapamil and dexamethason versus intra-lesional injection for Peyronie's disease. Andrology. 2013;1:129–32.
17. Hatzichristodoulou G, Meisner C, Gschwend JE, Stenzl A, Lahme S. Extracorporeal shock wave therapy in Peyronie's disease: results of a placebo-controlled, prospective, randomized, single-blind study. J Sex Med. 2013;10:2815–21.

18. Gelbard M, Lipshultz LI, Tursi J, Smith T, Kaufman G, Levine LA. Phase 2b study of the clinical efficacy and safety of collagenase clostridium histolyticum in patients with Peyronie disease. J Urol. 2012;187:2268–74.
19. Levine L, Newell M, Taylor FL. Penile traction therapy for treatment of Peyronie's disease: a single-center pilot study. J Sex Med. 2008;5:1468–73.
20. Mulhall J, Hall M, Broderick GA, Incrocci L. Radiation therapy in Peyronie's disease. J Sex Med. 2012;9:1435–41.
21. Kadioglu A, Kücükdurmaz F, Sanli O. Current status of the surgical management of Peyronie's disease. Nat Rev Urol. 2011;8:95–106.
22. Hatzichristodoulou G, Gschwend JE, Lahme S. Surgical therapy of Peyronie's disease by partial plaque excision and grafting with collagen fleece: feasibility study of a new technique. Int J Impot Res. 2013;25:183–7.
23. Nesbit R. Congenital curvature of the phallus: report of three cases with description of corrective operation. J Urol. 1965;93:230–2.
24. Gur S, Limin M, Hellstrom WJG. Current status and new developments in Peyronie's disease: medical, minimally invasive and surgical treatment options. Expert Opin Pharmacother. 2011;12(6):931–44.
25. Lahme S, Götz T, Bichler KH. Collagen fleece for defect coverage following plaque excision in patients with Peyronie's disease. Eur Urol. 2001;41:401–5.
26. Garaffa G, Porst H, Ralph D. Peyronie's disease, part II: surgical management. In: Porst H, Reisman Y, editors. The ESSM syllabus of sexual medicine. Amsterdam: Medix Publishers; 2012. p. 715–31.
27. Wilson S, Delk JRII. A new treatment for Peyronie's disease: modeling the penis over an inflatable penile prosthesis. J Urol. 1994;152:1121–3.
28. Levine L, Dimitriou RJ. A surgical algorithm fpr penile prosthesis placement in men with erectile failure and Peyronie's disease. Int J Impot Res. 2000;12:147–51.
29. Taylor F, Levine LA. Surgical correction of Peyronie's disease via tunica albuginea plication or partial plaque excision with pericardial graft: long-term follow up. J Sex Med. 2008;5:2221–8.

Cystitis

45

D. Barski and T. Otto

45.1 General Facts

Cystitis describes a clinical syndrome of dysuria, frequency, urgency, occasional suprapubic pain, usually associated with urinary tract infection (*UTI*), an inflammatory response of the urothelium to bacterial invasion with bacteriuria, and pyuria. UTI affects men and women of all ages. The prevalence in young women is 30 times higher than in men. Almost half of all women experience a UTI during their lifetime [3]. However, with increasing age, the ratio of women to men with bacteriuria progressively decreases.

Bacteria generally ascend into urinary tract from the urethra and rectal reservoir. Most bladder infections are caused by the ascending pathogens: *E. coli* (about 80 % of community-acquired infections), other gram-negative *Enterobacteriaceae* (*Klebsiella*, *Proteus*), gram-positive cocci (*E. faecalis*), and less frequently originating from skin and vaginal flora (*Staphylococcus epidermidis* and *Candida albicans*) [7]. The local bacteriological spectrum varies in different regions.

Nosocomial infection (hospital-acquired UTI, *HAUTI*) occurs in patients who are hospitalized or institutionalized. *HAUTI* is often caused by more antimicrobial-resistant strains (*Pseudomonas*, extended spectrum ß-lactamases, *ESBL*). The prevalence of *HAUTI* varies in different regions between 7 and 21 % [7].

In atypical sequelae or suitable anamnesis infections with mycobacteria and STD (*sexually* transmitted disease) spectrum (*Chlamydia trachomatis*, *Neisseria gonorrhoeae*) should be considered.

An urgent worldwide problem is the increasing resistance of bacterial strains to broad-spectrum antibiotics due to a widespread loose use of the antibiotics (global resistances to F-quinolones up to 84 %, to ß-lactam antibiotica up to 70 %, and to co-trimoxazole up to 76 %) [5]. The development of new antibiotics by the drug industry is lacking.

D. Barski (✉) • T. Otto
Department of Urology, Lukas Hospital, Preußenstraße 84, Neuss 41464, Germany
e-mail: dbarski@lukasneuss.de; thomas_otto@lukasneuss.de

A.S. Merseburger et al. (eds.), *Urology at a Glance*,
DOI 10.1007/978-3-642-54859-8_45, © Springer-Verlag Berlin Heidelberg 2014

45.2 Symptoms and Classification

Clinical manifestations can vary from asymptomatic bacteriuria to irritative symptoms, alguria, and suprapubic pain; sometimes hematuria or foul-smelling urine may develop. The probability of cystitis in a woman with these symptoms alone or in combination is 50–90 %, respectively [1]. Upper tract infections are associated with fever, chills, shivering, and flank pain. In untreated and severe cases, bacteremia can occur; it is associated with severe morbidity, including sepsis and death. The symptoms may also be associated with infection of the urethra or vagina or noninfectious conditions such as interstitial cystitis, bladder carcinoma, or stones.

45.3 Classification

Uncomplicated cystitis describes an infection in a healthy nonpregnant woman without anatomical or functional abnormalities. *A complicated* infection occurs more often in men and is associated with factors that increase a chance of acquiring bacteria and decrease the efficacy of therapy (ORENUC system, Table 45.1). The daily risk for bacteriuria in patients who require a catheter is 5–7 %. Almost all

Table 45.1 Host risk factors in UTI: "ORENUC" [4]

Type	Category of risk factor	Examples of risk factors
O	N*o* known/associated RF	Healthy premenopausal women
R	*R*F of recurrent UTI, but no risk of severe outcome	Sexual behavior and contraceptive devices Hormonal deficiency in post menopause Secretory type of certain blood groups Controlled diabetes mellitus
E	*E*xtra-urogenital RF	Pregnancy Male gender Badly controlled diabetes mellitus Relevant immunosuppression[a] Connective tissue diseases[a] Prematurity, newborn
N	*N*ephropathic disease	Relevant renal insufficiency[a] Polycystic nephropathy
U	*U*rological RF, which can be resolved during therapy	Ureteral obstruction (i.e., stone, stricture) Transient short-term urinary tract catheter Asymptomatic bacteriuria[b] Controlled neurogenic bladder dysfunction Urological surgery
C	Permanent urinary *c*atheter and non-resolvable urological RF	Long-term urinary tract catheter treatment Non-resolvable urinary obstruction Badly controlled neurogenic bladder

RF risk factor
[a]Not well defined
[b]Usually in combination with other RF (i.e., pregnancy, urological intervention)

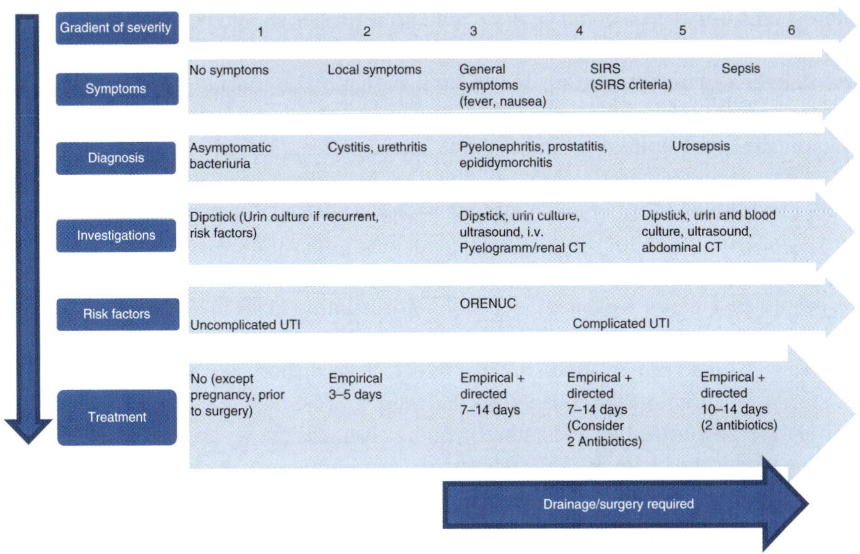

Fig. 45.1 Classification of UTI (Modified from the EAU European Section of Infection in Urology (ESIU) [4]

patients with indwelling catheter show mostly asymptomatic bacteriuria [9]. Special forms of UTI in men are urethritis, prostatitis, epididymitis, and orchitis.

UTI may also be defined by its relationship to other UTI. A *first or isolated* infection is one that occurs in an individual who has never had a UTI or has one remote from a previous UTI. An *unresolved* infection is one that has not responded to antimicrobial therapy. A *recurrent* infection is one that occurs after documented, successful resolution of prior infection (at least two symptomatic episodes per half year or at least three episodes of uncomplicated infection documented by culture in the past 12 months) [10]. The term *reinfection* describes a new event associated with reintroduction of bacteria into the urinary tract from outside. Most reinfections occur after 2 weeks. *Persistent infection is* caused by the same bacteria reemerging from a focus within the urinary tract, such as an infectious stone or the prostate. Because the duration of the infection is not defined, *chronic UTI* is a poor term that should be avoided except for chronic bacterial prostatitis [12] (Fig. 45.1).

45.4 Diagnosis

Midstream urine should be used for dipstick and further laboratory analysis, in order to minimize the contamination with skin flora. Indirect dipstick tests for bacteria (nitrite) or pyuria (leukocyte esterase) may be informative and more convenient but are less sensitive than microscopic examination of the urine. A negative dipstick cannot surely exclude an infection. In uncertain or complicated cases, microscopic urinalysis should be done. The urine probes should be used immediately or stored at 2–8 °C. New molecular diagnostics, like multiplex PCR, are upcoming and deliver fast results within hours with high sensitivity and specificity. Urine culture remains the definitive test by now. The presence of $\geq 10^3$ cfu/mL of bacteria in a midstream sample of urine in symptomatic patients usually indicates infection [8]. After sterile catheterization any count of bacteria is relevant. A urine culture should be obtained for patients with risk factors (ORENUC) or persistent or recurring symptoms after the initial therapy, in order to exclude various or resistant pathogens. However, routine urine cultures are often not necessary, because in uncomplicated cases treatment decisions are usually made and therapy is often completed before culture results are known [4].

Imaging should be performed in order to detect risk factors like residual urine, bladder stone formation, and hydronephrosis that must be corrected immediately. Ultrasound delivers the best available orientating imaging. In recurrent or unclear cases, further invasive diagnostics with VCUG (voiding cystourethrogram), cystoscopy, and urodynamics should be considered. DMSA scan can be used to detect renal scarring.

45.5 Therapy

The aims of cystitis treatment are to relieve the patient's symptoms, eradicate the pathogens, and prevent complications.

Efficacy, local resistance, adverse events, and cost should be considered before the prescription of antibiotics. Early identification and treatment of patients with complicated infections remains a clinical challenge to urologists.

45.5.1 Acute Uncomplicated Cystitis in Nonpregnant Women

Clinical success is significantly more likely in women treated with antibiotics compared with placebo (LE1A). *E. coli* is the causative pathogen in 75–90 % of cases of acute cystitis in young women. According to susceptibility patterns in Europe, oral treatment with fosfomycin (single dose), nitrofurantoin (5 days), and pivmecillinam (3 days) is considered for the first choice (>90 % sensitivity) and F-quinolones or cefpodoxime for the second choice (>80 % sensitivity). Due to high prevalence of resistance of *E. coli* strains (>20 %) in most western countries, trimethoprim, co-trimoxazole, ampicillin, and amoxicillin are not effective for empirical therapy. In regions with high rates of F-quinolone-resistant and *ESBL*-producing *E. coli* (>10 %), urine culture and susceptibility testing should be done before the prescription of oral medication (LE1A) [4, 6]. A three-day therapy is the preferred regimen because a 7-day therapy often causes more adverse affects (i.e., gastrointestinal). In cases of unresolved infection, urine culture should be obtained and the antibiotic therapy should be adjusted. A broader-spectrum antibiotic should be chosen that is also active against *Pseudomonas* (LE1B), i.e., F-quinolone, acyl aminopenicillin (piperacillin) plus a β-lactamase inhibitor, and a group 3b cephalosporin or carbapenem, with or without combination with aminoglycoside (LE1B) [4]. In cases of recurrent cystitis, a proper urological workup should be done during the infection-free interval.

45.5.2 Cystitis During Pregnancy

Asymptomatic bacteriuria ($\geq 10^5$ cfu/ml in two consecutive voidings) detected during pregnancy and acute cystitis or pyelonephritis should be eradicated with antimicrobial therapy (LE1A). Fosfomycin, penicillins, cephalosporins, and nitrofurantoin can be applied; others should be avoided because of fetal toxicity (trimethoprim is toxic in first trimester) [4].

45.5.3 Cystitis in Men

Cystitis in men is almost without exception complicated and associated with prostatitis, epididymitis, and pyelonephritis or indwelling catheter. A minimum treatment duration of 2 weeks is recommended, preferably with a fluoroquinolone since prostatic involvement is frequent (LE 2A) [4]. In epididymitis or prostatitis, an insertion of suprapubic catheter should be considered in order to prevent retrograde irrigation of bacteria. In severe cases patients should be investigated for abscess of the prostate or testicles. In these cases a drainage or surgical removal are urgent.

45.5.4 Cystitis in Children

Pyelonephritis is a common and severe bacterial infection in childhood. In children with fever and UTI, there is a risk of renal scarring, leading to hypertension and chronic renal failure later. Further workup (ultrasound, VCUG, DMSA) should be done early in a specialized center to rule out vesicoureteric reflux (VUR), obstruction (ureteropelvic junction obstruction, ureterocele, posterior urethral valve), or dysfunctional voiding (sphincter dyssynergia) [4]. VUR is a common and important reason for UTI. A longer antibiotic treatment, low-dose antibiotic prophylaxis (LE:2A), and urotherapy seem to be beneficial [2], but only a small percentage of children with VUR needs surgery. Sulfonamides (gastrointestinal symptoms), tetracyclines (tooth staining), F-quinolones (cartilage toxicity), and cetfriaxone (jaundice) should be avoided because of adverse side effects. A circumcision in boys with VUR decreases 10× the risk of UTI.

45.5.5 Complicated Cystitis

Usually predisposing risk factors cause a recurrent or unresolving infection. True cure is only possible if risk factors are eliminated or corrected prior to antibiotic therapy (catheterization, early removal or change of catheter, stone removal, surgery).

The spectrum of uropathogens is larger and more likely to be antibiotic resistant. Antibiotics regimens should be applied in knowledge of local resistance patterns. Urine culture must be obtained before the initiation of therapy. Fungal infections (*Candida*) are common in patients with immunodeficiency and should be treated with antifungals even if asymptomatic. In patients with renal failure, appropriate dose adjustments have to be made (aminoglycoside, nitrofurantoin, and tetracyclines are nephrotoxic). In more severe cases with fever and elevated inflammatory parameters, empiric intravenous application of antibiotics and hospitalization are appropriate. Recurrent UTI in patients with neurogenic bladder may indicate a suboptimal management of the underlying functional problem, e.g., high bladder pressure during storage and voiding or incomplete voiding. Proper urological examination (sonography, urodynamics) and neurourological therapy (clean intermittent catheterization, antimuscarinic medication, etc.) are essential. Asymptomatic bacteriuria in patients with spinal cord injury and generally other neurological disorders should not be treated, even in cases of intermittent catheterization [4].

45.5.6 Nosocomial Cystitis

Local resistance patterns should be taken into account. The crucial preventive measures are monitoring of the infections sequelae and local hygiene protocols, avoid long-term catheters, prudent use of antibiotics, identification of risk patients, avoid infective surgical fields, and tailoring the prophylaxis.

45.5.7 Prophylaxis

Antibiotic prophylaxis is not recommended for most urological operations except for TURP (LE1A), complicated stone endourology (LE2B), prostate biopsy (LE1A), open or laparascopic operation with open urinary tract (LE2B-3) or bowel (LE2A), and implantation of prosthetic device (LE2A). Many antibiotics like second-generation cephalosporins, F-quinolones, or co-trimoxazole are appropriate, but broad-spectrum antibiotics should be reserved for treatment.

Low-dose prophylaxis is recommended if there is a high risk for recurrent pyelonephritis, e.g., children with VUR and female patients with recurrent UTI (continuous or postcoital, if other measures were not successful, LE1A). Immunoprophylaxis (Uro-Vaxom®, StroVac®) and unspecific prophylaxis (urine acidification, cranberry juice) were found to be effective in cases of uncomplicated recurrent UTIs in female (LE1A) [4].

45.6 Complications

Complications of severe cystitis with risk factors or delayed treatment are ascending pyelonephritis (with abscess formation, renal scarring, papillary necrosis), epididymorchitis, or prostatitis (with abscess formation). In severe cases renal failure and bacteremia with urosepsis can develop. A progression to clinical pyelonephritis is more likely in patients with diabetes or other immunodeficiencies.

Acute pyelonephritis is often associated with flank pain, nausea and vomiting, and fever (>38 °C), and it can occur in the absence of symptoms of cystitis. Mild forms can be treated in out-office setting, and patients with severe forms should be hospitalized and need supportive therapy. Abscess formations should be evacuated by percutaneous drainage or surgery (orchidectomy, epididymectomy, abscess splitting). Infected hydronephrosis due to obstruction should immediately be drained by ureteric stent or percutaneous nephrostomy (LE:1A) [4]. In patients with recurrent UTI in the kidney with the end-stage chronic renal failure, a nephrectomy or nephroureterectomy (VUR) should be considered as a last resort.

Urosepsis is defined as systemic inflammatory response syndrome, known as SIRS (fever or hypothermia, hyperleukocytosis or leukopenia, tachycardia, tachypnea) and detection of uropathogens. Severe sepsis is defined by the presence of organ dysfunction and septic shock and is associated with high mortality (20–30 %). Urosepsis treatment needs a special management in collaboration with intense care unit. The treatment of the cause (obstruction of the urinary tract) is mandatory and calls for a combination of adequate life-supporting care and appropriate antibiotic therapy. Clinical algorithms should be followed, and preventive measures (prudent use of antibiotics, short hospital stay, early removal of catheter) are important.

Prostatitis after biopsy is an increasing problem due to growing resistance status (F-quinolones). A symptomatic UTI was found in 5.2 % after prostate biopsy (98 % with antibiotic prophylaxis) and 3.1 % needed a hospitalization [11]. Tailored prophylaxis, alternative antibiotics, and alternative ways of diagnosing prostate cancer are essential and should be a point of current research.

References

1. Bent S, Nallamothu BK, Simel DL, Fihn SD, Saint S. Does this woman have an acute uncomplicated urinary tract infection? JAMA. 2002;287:2701–10.
2. Brandström P, Jodal U, Sillén U, Hansson S. The Swedish reflux trial: review of a randomized, controlled trial in children with dilating vesicoureteral reflux. J Pediatr Urol. 2011;7:594–600.
3. Foxman B, Barlow R, D'Arcy H, Gillespie B, Sobel JD. Urinary tract infection: self-reported incidence and associated costs. Ann Epidemiol. 2000;10:509–15.
4. Grabe M, Bartoletti R, Bjerklund-Johansen TE, et al. EAU Guidelines on Urological Infections Update 2014, published online on www.uroweb.org.
5. Johansen TE, Cek M, Naber KG, et al. Hospital acquired urinary tract infections in urology departments: pathogens, susceptibility and use of antibiotics. Data from the PEP and PEAP-studies. Int J Antimicrob Agents. 2006;28 Suppl 1:S91–107.
6. Naber KG, Schito G, Botto H, Palou J, Mazzei T. Surveillance study in Europe and Brazil on clinical aspects and Antimicrobial Resistance Epidemiology in Females with Cystitis (ARESC): implications for empiric therapy. Eur Urol. 2008;54:1164–75.
7. Ronald A. The etiology of urinary tract infection: traditional and emerging pathogens. Am J Med. 2002;113(Suppl 1A):14S–9.
8. Stamm WE, Counts GW, Wagner KF, et al. Antimicrobial prophylaxis of recurrent urinary tract infections: a double-blind, placebo-controlled trial. Ann Intern Med. 1980;92: 770–5.

9. Tenke P, Kovacs B, Bjerklund Johansen TE, Matsumoto T, Tambyah PA, Naber KG. European and Asian guidelines on management and prevention of catheter-associated urinary tract infections. Int J Antimicrob Agents. 2008;31 Suppl 1:S68–78.
10. Wagenlehner FM, Schmiemann G, Hoyme U, et al. National S3 guideline on uncomplicated urinary tract infection: recommendations for treatment and management of uncomplicated community-acquired bacterial urinary tract infections in adult patients. Urologe A. 2011;50: 153–69.
11. Wagenlehner FM, van Oostrum E, Tenke P, et al. Infective complications after prostate biopsy: outcome of the Global Prevalence Study of Infections in Urology (GPIU) 2010 and 2011, a prospective multinational multicentre prostate biopsy study. Eur Urol. 2013;63:521–7.
12. Wein AJ, Kavoussi LR, et al. Campbell-Walsh urology. 9th ed. 2007, Chapter 8, Saunders Elsevier, Philadelphia, PA 19103-2899, ISBN 10: 0-7216-0798-5

Prostatitis 46

Iason D. Kyriazis, Ioannis Georgiopoulos, and Evangelos N. Liatsikos

46.1 General Facts

Prostatitis is a term used to describe the inflammation of the prostatic gland. Historically, nonspecific disease-associated prostatic pain also referred as chronic pelvic pain syndrome or prostatic pain syndrome had been equated with chronic prostatitis. Nevertheless, in accordance to the 2012 EAU guidelines on chronic pain syndromes, the former syndrome should be regarded as a distinct clinical entity requiring a multimodal and symptom-directed management [1]. For the purposes of this chapter, only prostatitis of infectious origin (bacterial prostatitis) will be discussed.

46.2 Symptoms and Classification

Based on the duration and the severity of symptoms, prostatitis can be classified as acute or chronic [2]. Acute prostatitis is a serious infection that can progress rapidly to urosepsis if remain untreated, especially in immunocompromised patients such as elderly or diabetic. Thus, upon diagnosis prompt treatment with broad-spectrum antibiotics should be initiated. The diagnosis of acute prostatitis is based on clinical symptomatology. Patient is usually febrile demonstrating high fever with shivering. Pain at various locations including perineum, scrotum, lower abdomen, and back in addition to lower urinary tract symptoms such as frequency and dysuria are the predominant symptoms. Although prostatic massage is strongly contraindicated in

I.D. Kyriazis (✉) • I. Georgiopoulos • E.N. Liatsikos
Department of Urology, University of Patras, Rion, Patras 26 504, Greece
e-mail: jkyriazis@gmail.com

A.S. Merseburger et al. (eds.), *Urology at a Glance*,
DOI 10.1007/978-3-642-54859-8_46, © Springer-Verlag Berlin Heidelberg 2014

acute prostatitis, in cases of uncertain diagnosis, a digital rectal examination can be performed revealing a swollen, warm, and tender prostatic gland. Laboratory and radiologic investigation should focus on the assessment of patients' systemic inflammatory response to diagnose urosepsis promptly, the isolation of causative pathogen through midstream urine culture, and the radiologic evaluation of gland if a prostatic abscess is suspected.

Chronic prostatitis is defined as the clinical condition in which prostatitis-like symptoms last more than 3 months following an acute infection. The symptoms of chronic prostatitis are milder than acute infection and fever is usually absent. The isolation of the responsible pathogen is of outmost importance in the laboratory investigation of chronic prostatitis. Midstream urine and Stamey-Meares-expressed prostatic secretion cultures should be available in all cases although the causative agent will be identified only in a minority of cases.

46.3 Therapy

Unless or until a specific pathogen has been isolated, antibiotic treatment of prostatitis should be empirically guided based on the most common causative bacteria. Based on their favorable safety profile, fluoroquinolones are considered the gold standard empirical treatment option for acute and chronic prostatitis. No significant differences in clinical efficacy or adverse effect profile between the different quinolone regimens are apparent. The most commonly recommended treatment options are provided in the following flowchart. In addition, based on the severity of symptoms, patients' septic status, and presence of other comorbidities (e.g., older age, diabetes mellitus, malignancy, immunosuppressive drugs), the clinician should decide whether an initial parenteral antibiotic treatment should be initiated followed by per os substitute of drugs when symptoms have subsided or patient could be safely treated in an outpatient basis [3].

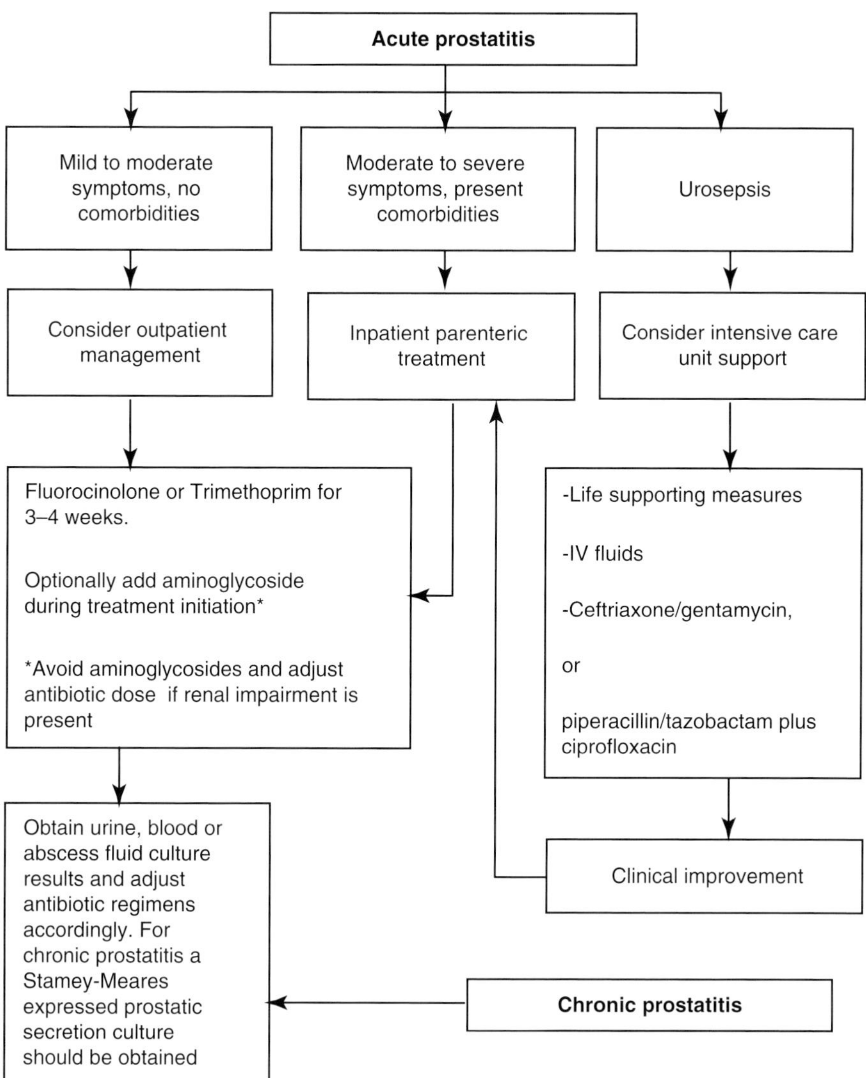

Acute prostatitis
Mild to moderate symptoms, no comorbidities
Moderate to severe symptoms, present comorbidities
Urosepsis
Consider outpatient management
Inpatient parenteric treatment
Consider intensive care unit support
Fluorocinolone or Trimethoprim for 3–4 weeks.
Optionally add aminoglycoside during treatment initiation*
*Avoid aminoglycosides and adjust antibiotic dose if renal impairment is present
-Life supporting measures
-IV fluids
-Ceftriaxone/gentamycin,
or
piperacillin/tazobactam plus ciprofloxacin
Clinical improvement
Obtain urine, blood or abscess fluid culture results and adjust antibiotic regimens accordingly. For chronic prostatitis a Stamey-Meares expressed prostatic secretion culture should be obtained
Chronic prostatitis

46.4 Complications

The most common complications of acute prostatitis are urosepsis, urinary retention, prostatic abscess formation, and progress to chronic disease. In the case of urosepsis, early recognition and treatment initiation without delay including life-supporting measures and broad-spectrum antibiotics in collaboration with intensive care specialists improve prognosis significantly. Urinary retention will complicate the management of acute prostatitis in about 10 % of cases. Both intermittent or indwelling bladder catheterization are reasonable treatment options although suprapubic cystostomy placement is generally recommended to avoid manipulation of the infected gland which might increase the risk of urosepsis or progression to chronic prostatitis. An intraprostatic abscess could be either drained under transrectal ultrasound guidance or managed conservatively with the decision being based mainly on the amount of collection fluid and patient's response to parenteral treatment. Despite prompt antimicrobial treatment, about 10 % of acute prostatitis cases will progress to chronic prostatitis and 10 % of the latter will develop chronic pelvic pain syndrome [4].

References

1. 2013 European Association of Urology guidelines on urological infections. Available on: www.uroweb.org.
2. Engeler DS, Baranowski AP, Dinis-Oliveira P, et al. The 2013 EAU guidelines on chronic pelvic pain: is management of chronic pelvic pain a habit, a philosophy, or a science? 10 years of development. Eur Urol. 2013;64(3):431–9.
3. Perletti G, Marras E, Wagenlehner FM, Magri V. Antimicrobial therapy for chronic bacterial prostatitis. Cochrane Database Syst Rev. 2013;8, CD009071.
4. Wagenlehner FM, Pilatz A, Bschleipfer T, Diemer T, Linn T, Meinhardt A, Schagdarsurengin U, Dansranjavin T, Schuppe HC, Weidner W. Bacterial prostatitis. World J Urol. 2013;31(4):711–6.

Maldescensus Testis

47

Atiqullah Aziz, Wolfgang H. Rösch,
and Maximilian Burger

47.1 Background

Maldescensus testis (MT) represents the most frequent congenital anomaly of the genitourinary tract and is found in roughly 1 % of mature and in up to 30 % of premature male neonates [1]. Maldescensus testis can be subdivided in two forms: retentio testis vs. ectopic testis (Fig. 47.1). Retentio testis describes an incomplete descensus of the testicles positioned within the physiological localizations of the embryological testicular pathway, i.e., abdomen (retentio testis abdominalis, "nonpalpable testis"), inguinal (retentio testis inguinalis), and prescrotal (retentio testis praescrotalis, "gliding testis") regions. The clinical term "cryptorchidism" is a synonym for MT [2]. Maldescensus testis has to be differentiated from retractile testis, a norm variant of descended testicles, predominantly localized in the scrotum and lifted into the inguinal regions by a strong cremasteric reflex upon palpation [2]. Ectopic testis describes a complete descensus of the testicle; however, the testicles are misdirected outside the physiological embryological testicular pathway. While the most frequent localization in ectopic testis is the superficial inguinal region,

A. Aziz (✉)
Department of Urology, Caritas St. Josef Medical Center, University of Regensburg,
Landshuter Str. 65, Regensburg 93053, Germany

Department of Pediatric Urology, St. Hedwig University Medical Center of Regensburg,
Steinmetzstr. 1-3, Regensburg 93049, Germany
e-mail: atiqullah.aziz@gmail.com

W.H. Rösch
Department of Pediatric Urology, St. Hedwig University Medical Center of Regensburg,
Steinmetzstr. 1-3, Regensburg 93049, Germany
e-mail: wolfgang.roesch@barmherzige-regensburg.de

M. Burger
Department of Urology, Caritas St. Josef Medical Center, University of Regensburg,
Landshuter Str. 65, Regensburg 93053, Germany
e-mail: maximilian.burger@ukr.de

A.S. Merseburger et al. (eds.), *Urology at a Glance*,
DOI 10.1007/978-3-642-54859-8_47, © Springer-Verlag Berlin Heidelberg 2014

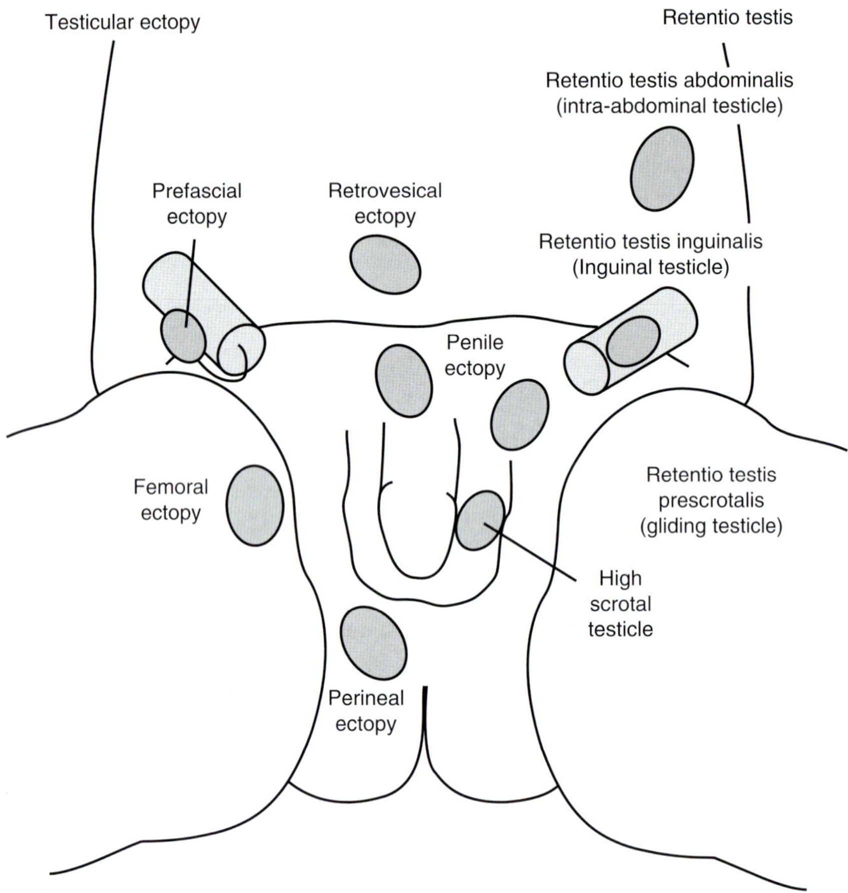

Fig. 47.1 Localizations [7]

it can be positioned in the perineal, femoral, or suprapubic region or in the contralateral hemiscrotum. Table 47.1 gives a brief summary of the several forms of MT.

While the exact pathophysiology of MT remains unclear, intrauterine insufficiency of the hypothalamic-pituitary-gonadal axis is related to a transient, prenatal, and prepubertal hypogonadotropic hypogonadism. Risk factors of MT reported to date include preterm delivery [3], birth weight under 2.5 kg [3], placental insufficiency with reduced secretion of human chorionic gonadotropin (hCG) [3], low maternal estrogen levels [4], maternal smoking [5], and diabetes mellitus [5].

47.2 Symptoms, Classification, and Grading

Physical examination of the child has to be performed in a warm and anxiety-free setting possibly with maternal assistance. Inspection and palpation of the child should be conducted in hanging, lying, supine, or crossed-legged position,

Table 47.1 Definitions [7]

Maldescensus testis	Testicles are localized intra-abdominal or within the inguinal canal, incompletely descended within the physiological embryological testicular pathway and associated with a normal insertion of the gubernaculum
Cryptorchidism	Non-palpable testicles, either located intra-abdominal or completely missing (anorchia)
Ectopic testis	Incomplete descensus of the testicle outlying the physiological embryological testicular pathway. Here, the testicle can be found perineal, femoral, suprapubic, or in the contralateral hemiscrotum with an abnormal insertion of the gubernaculum. The most frequent localization in ectopic testis, however, is the superficial inguinal ring
Inguinal testis (retentio testis inguinalis)	Testicle is palpable within the groin
Gliding testis (retentio testis praescrotalis)	Testicle can be retracted into the scrotum but, however, shifts immediately back to the initial position, which is mostly located prescrotal
Retractile testis	Normally localized in the scrotum and shifted to the groin due to a strong cremasteric reflex

respectively. In order to avoid a missed ectopic testis, inspection of the perineum is mandatory. Palpation should be performed bimanually with one hand striating the inguinal canal and the other hand palpating the scrotum. Differential diagnosis of inguinal MT vs. retractile testis can be obtained: while recoil of the testicle into the groin after release indicates MT, a retractile testicle remains in the scrotum until a subsequent cremasteric reflex.

Imaging, i.e., ultrasound for evaluation of size and parenchyma, can be helpful in some cases, i.e., boys with increased fat tissue [6]. An MRI is not recommended generally due to its low sensitivity and specificity [6]. In bilateral non-palpable testis, testicular function should be assessed by hCG stimulation test and inhibin B proof in serum [7]. Furthermore, the suspicion of a sexual differentiation disorder in case of bilateral non-palpable testis imperatively requires an endocrinological and genetic evaluation.

The most accurate diagnostic method is laparoscopy, which allows discrimination of cryptorchidism vs. monorchidism vs. anorchia and surgical treatment in one procedure [2].

47.3 Therapy

Treatment options in MT involve hormonal therapy, surgery, and a combination of both [2]. Timing of the start of the therapy should be initiated following 6 months and finished after 12 months [2]. Untreated MT conveys fertility disorders and the risk of testicular malignancies [8, 9]. While the aim of MT therapy is preservation of the germinative function of the testicle, the risk of testicular malignancies does not subside following successful treatment; close respective screening during and after puberty is therefore of great importance [2].

Table 47.2 Hormone therapy administration [2]

Drug	Dosage
Luteinizing hormone-releasing hormone (LHRH)	3×400 μg/day (3×daily a spray of 200 μg in each nares) for 4 weeks in the form of a nasal spray
Human chorionic gonadotropin (hCG)	Total dose of 6,000–9,000 U hCG (age and weight dependent) given in four doses over a period of 2–3 weeks in the form of a nasal spray

Within the first 6 months of age, spontaneous descensus should be awaited [2]. Hormone therapy (HT) with luteinizing hormone-releasing hormone (LHRH) and hCG is considered as primary therapy option [10–12]. The aim of the HT is preservation of the germinative function of the testicle and thus fertility rather than to achieve testicular descent [7]. Dependent of age and weight 6,000–9,000 U hCG is applied in four doses over a period of 2–3 weeks together with LHRH for 4 weeks via a nasal spray. A daily total of 1.2 mg is administered divided in three doses (Table 47.2) [2]. Testicular descent is observed in roughly 20 % of the cases under HT and 20 % are reported to fail therapy and to reascend [10]. Accordingly, a close follow-up after successful descent is mandatory. While adjuvant HT following surgery is not generally recommended, a low-dose application of LHRH seems to support fertility [11]. Nevertheless, therapy with hCG remains disputatious due to its potential role in germ cell apoptosis despite contributing to successful testicular descent [7]. Vice versa, LHRH leads to a significant increase of spermatogonia [7]. Conclusively, HT should be initiated as the first therapy option in order to save as many germ cells as possible.

Surgery is primarily indicated in case of an ectopic testis, MT with concomitant persisting processus vaginalis testis, and prior inguinal surgery [2]. The testicle is relocated free of tension to the scrotum following orchidofuniculolysis, and finally orchidopexy is performed at the most distal part of the scrotum to avoid testicular torsion [2]. In the palpable testis, open inguinal approach should be performed [2]. In the non-palpable testis, the laparoscopic approach is the gold standard, since it combines exact diagnostics and therapy (Fig. 47.2) [2]. In case of testicular agenesis or vanishing testis, no further therapy is required during laparoscopy. After laparoscopic verification of the presence of a spermatic cord and of a normal configuration of the inner inguinal ring, a consecutive open inguinal approach is mandatory [2].

In case of insufficient lengths of the spermatic cord preventing tension-free relocation of the testicle, Fowler-Stephens procedure can be conducted [13]. Consisting of clipping and coagulation of the spermatic vessels proximal to the testis and preservation and protection of the spermatic cord vessels [13], the procedure can be performed in one step or in two steps, respectively. The procedure in two steps is indicated in presence of short spermatic vessels and a >3 cm proximal of the inner inguinal ring located testicle [13]. Following development of collateral vessels and thus obtaining sufficient testicular vascularization, the testis is placed into the scrotum in a second step after 6 months [13]. However, a one-step procedure without vascular discontinuation is recommended due to its comparatively

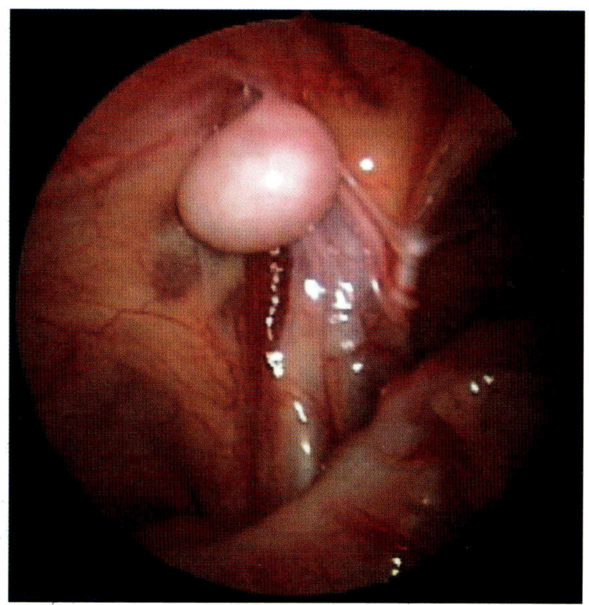

Fig. 47.2 Intraoperative laparoscopic finding of a sinistral intra-abdominal testicle

favorable outcome [13]. Autotransplantation, i.e., microsurgical anastomosis of the spermatic cord vessels with the abdominal wall vessels displays a rarely applied option [14]. In boys aged over 10 years with a unilateral cryptorchidism and normal contralateral testis, removal of the affected testicle should be discussed due to the potentially higher risk of later malignancy [2]. Testicular biopsies are only indicated in case of suspected ovotestis (presence of testicular and ovarian tissue), testicular dysgenesis, or tumor [7]. The flow chart (Fig. 47.3) pictures the pathway from diagnosis to therapy.

47.4 Sequels of MT

Possible sequels of MT are infertility and testicular malignancy. While unilateral MT results in lowered fertility but comparable paternity rates, if respective assistance is sought, compared to bilaterally descended testis, bilateral MT results in lower fertility and paternity rates, respectively [2]. Early treatment of bilateral cryptorchidism improves fertility compared to treatment at older ages (<4 vs. ≥4 years of age; 76 % vs. 26 %) [15].

Cryptorchidism leads to a threefold higher risk of germ cell tumor [16]. Retentio testis abdominalis involves a higher malignancy risk compared to retentio testis inguinalis and bilateral a higher risk than unilateral MT [7]. Orchidopexy under the age of 13 years has been discussed to decrease risk compared to later orchidopexy [8]. A close follow-up including instruction of intermittent self-examination of the testicles is mandatory in boys with MT following therapy.

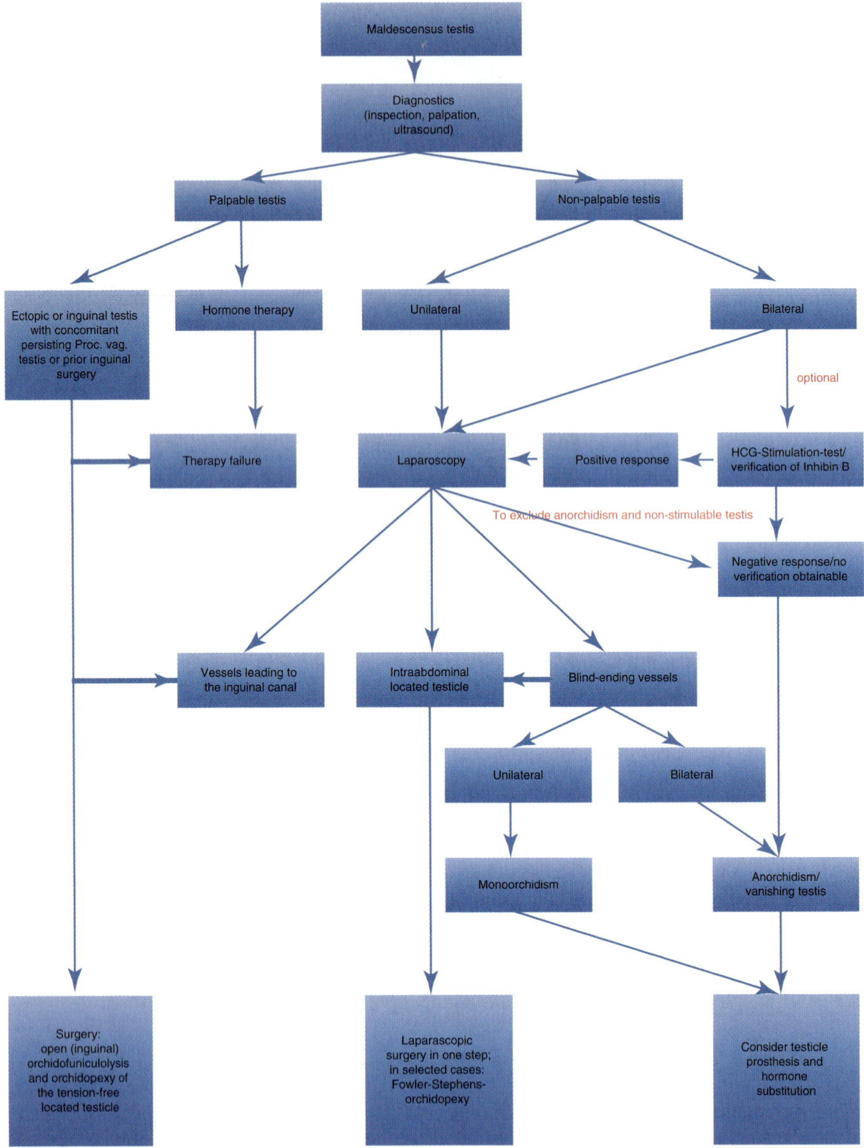

Fig. 47.3 Flow chart demonstrating the pathway from diagnosis to therapy

References

1. Berkowitz GS, Lapinski RH, Dolgin SE, et al. Prevalence and natural history of cryptorchidism. Pediatrics. 1993;92(1):44–9.
2. Tekgül S, Riedmiller H, Dogan HS, et al. Guidelines on paediatric urology. Uroweb 2013. http://www.uroweb.org/gls/pdf/22%20Paediatric%20Urology_LR.pdf.

3. Akre O, Lipworth L, Cnattingius S, et al. Risk factor patterns for cryptorchidism and hypospadias. Epidemiology. 1999;10:364–9.
4. McGlynn KA, Graubard BI, Nam JM, et al. Maternal hormone levels and risk of cryptorchidism among populations at high and low risk of testicular germ cell tumors. Cancer Epidemiol Biomarkers Prev. 2005;14:1732–7.
5. Thorup J, Cortes D, Petersen BL. The incidence of bilateral cryptorchidism is increased and the fertility potential is reduced in sons born to mothers who have smoked during pregnancy. J Urol. 2006;176:734–7.
6. Kanemoto K, Hayashi Y, Kojima Y, et al. Accuracy of ultrasonography and magnetic resonance imaging in the diagnosis of non-palpable testis. Int J Urol. 2005;12:668–72.
7. Mathers MJ, Sperling H, Rübben H, Roth S. The undescended testis: diagnosis, treatment and long-term consequences. Dtsch Arztebl Int. 2009;106(33):527–32.
8. Chilvers C, Dudley NE, Gough MH, et al. Undescended testis: the effect of treatment on subsequent risk of subfertility and malignancy. J Pediatr Surg. 1986;21:691–6.
9. Pettersson A, Richiardi L, Nordenskjold A, et al. Age at surgery for undescended testis and risk of testicular cancer. N Engl J Med. 2007;356(18):1835–41.
10. Pyorala S, Huttunen NP, Uhari M. A review and meta-analysis of hormonal treatment of cryptorchidism. J Clin Endocrinol Metab. 1995;80(9):2795–9.
11. Schwentner C, Oswald J, Kreczy A, et al. Neoadjuvant gonadotropin releasing hormone therapy before surgery may improve the fertility index in undescended testes – a prospective randomized trial. J Urol. 2005;173(3):974–7.
12. Hadziselimovic F, Herzog B. The importance of both an early orchidopexy and germ cell maturation for fertility. Lancet. 2001;358:1156–7.
13. Neissner C, Ebert AK, Rösch WH. Analysis of laparoscopic orchidopexy in intra-abdominal testis. Urologe A. 2011;50(5):573–8.
14. Wacksman J, Billmire DA, Lewis AG, et al. Laparoscopically assisted testicular autotransplantation for management of the intraabdominal undescended testis. J Urol. 1996;156(2 Pt 2): 772–4.
15. Virtanen HE, Bjerknes R, Cortes D, Jørgensen N, Rajpert-De Meyts E, Thorsson AV, Thorup J, Main KM. Cryptorchidism: classification, prevalence and long-term consequences. Acta Paediatr. 2007;96(5):611–6.
16. Lip SZ, Murchison LE, Cullis PS, et al. A meta-analysis of the risk of boys with isolated cryptorchidism developing testicular cancer in later life. Arch Dis Child. 2013;98(1):20–6.

Hypogonadotropic Hypogonadism 48

Jan Adamowicz, Omar M. Aboumarzouk, Piotr L. Chłosta, and Tomasz Drewa

48.1 General

Hypogonadotropic hypogonadism (HH) is a congenital (CHH) or acquired (AHH) clinical condition characterized by low serum testosterone in association with absent or decreased levels of circulating luteinizing hormone (LH) and follicle-stimulating hormone (FSH) concentrations [1]. The FSH and LH secretion and synthesis patterns are impaired in patients with HH. The prevalence of acquired and congenital HH has been estimated in range from 1:4,000 to 1:86,000 in males, and it is reported to be between two and five times less frequent in females [2]. Approximately 60 % cases of CHH are related to Kallmann syndrome. The rest of the causes includes gonadotropin-releasing hormone (GnRH) insensitivity syndrome (20 % of cases) and inactivating mutations in a variety of other genes which regulate GnRH secretion (less than 5–10 %) [3]. Acquired hypogonadotropic hypogonadism in adult males is mainly associated with hyperprolactinemic states,

J. Adamowicz
Department of Tissue Engenering and Urology, Collegium Medicum, University of Nicolaus Copernicus, Toruń, Poland

Katedra i Klinika Urologii Collegium, Medicum Uniwersytetu Jagiellońskiego, ul. Grzegórzecka 18, Kraków, Poland

O.M. Aboumarzouk, MBChB, MSc, PhD, MRCS (Glasg)
College of Medicine, Islamic University of Gaza, Gaza, Occupied Palestine

P.L. Chłosta, MD, PhD, DSci, FEBU
Department of Urology, Jagiellonian University in Krakow, ul. Grzegorzecka 18, Krakow 31-531, Poland

T. Drewa (✉)
Department of Urology, Nicolaus Copernicus Hospital, Batory 17-19 str., Toruń 87-100, Poland

Katedra i Klinika Urologii Collegium, Medicum Uniwersytetu Jagiellońskiego, ul. Grzegórzecka 18, Kraków, Poland
e-mail: tomaszdrewa@wp.pl; sekurol@med.torun.pl

A.S. Merseburger et al. (eds.), *Urology at a Glance*, DOI 10.1007/978-3-642-54859-8_48, © Springer-Verlag Berlin Heidelberg 2014

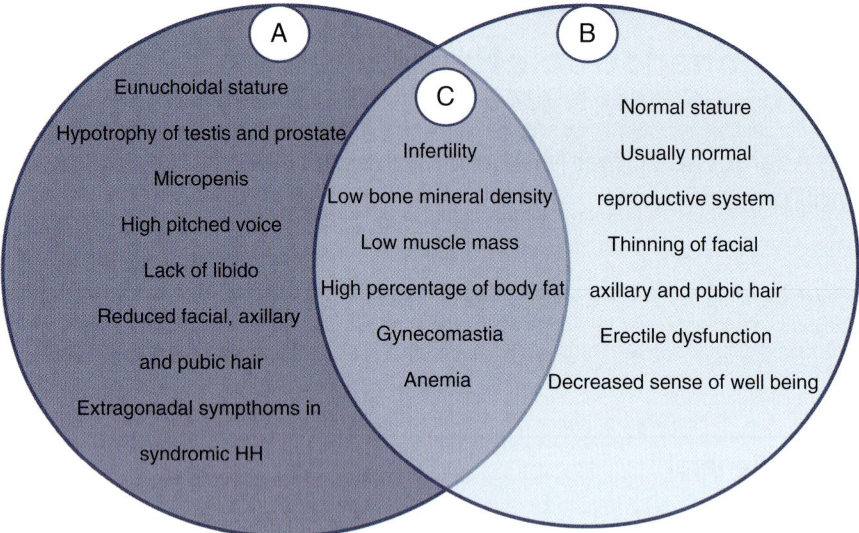

Fig. 48.1 Symptoms of hypogonadotropic hypogonadism depending on time of onset. *A* – Pre-pubertal HH. *B* – Post-pubertal HH. *C* – Common symptoms

obesity, and diabetes type II. The cause of HH is unknown in about 30 % of all cases and these men are diagnosed as having idiopathic isolated HH [4].

48.2 Symptoms, Classification, and Grading

Heterogeneity of clinical manifestation is typical for HH patients because it depends upon the age of onset, the degree of gonadotropin deficiency, and the rapidity of its progression (Fig. 48.1).

The physical examination is usually normal if hypogonadism is of recent onset. Diminished facial and body hair and muscle mass, depression states, gynecomastia, and hypertrophic genitals are observed in long-standing HH. Several months or even a couple of years are needed to develop full-blown HH [5].

Partial or intermediate forms of HH are often difficult to distinguish from constitutional late puberty and need advanced hormonal testing. Typically the diagnosis of HH is made in the second or in the third decade of life, when the patients present delayed pubertal onset or poorly developed secondary sexual characteristics.

CHH is divided in three main classes according to spectrum of clinical disorders combined with insufficient secretion of the pituitary gonadotropins: isolated CHH with normal olfaction, Kallmann syndrome, and complex non-Kallmann syndromes [6] (Fig. 48.2).

48.3 Neonatal Period and Childhood

One of the first signs that can suggest HH is unilateral or bilateral cryptorchidism or micropenis. These symptoms can be diagnosed before the age of 6 months. The

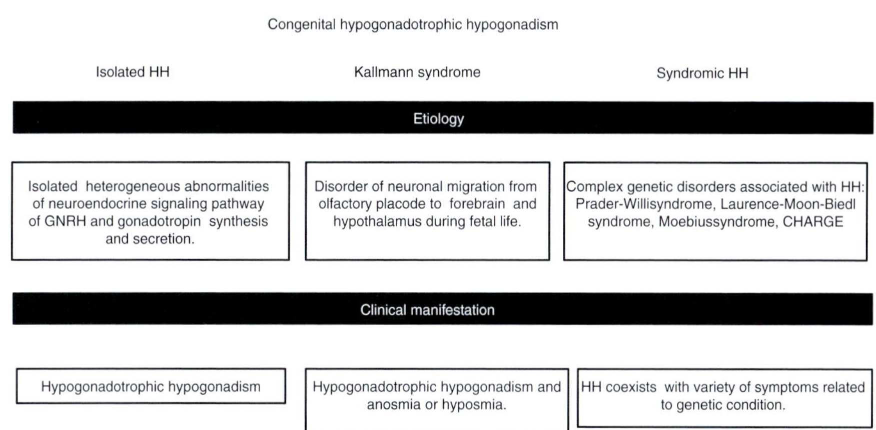

Fig. 48.2 Classification of congenital hypogonadotrophic hypogonadism regarding to causes and clinical manifestation

incidence of micropenis and cryptorchidism is the highest when GnRH deficiency occurs in the late fetal or early neonatal life [7].

The majority of complex syndromic forms of CHH are recognized in early childhood because of predominant extragonadal manifestations such as multiple anterior pituitary hormone insufficiencies, metabolic disorders, adrenal failure, or neurological disorders [8].

48.4 Puberty

The major manifestations of HH in males after the age of 14 are disorders of sexual maturation. The spectrum of symptoms includes delayed, arrested, or absent secondary sexual characteristic development. The altered hormonal milieu determinates lower degree of virilization and infertility. Defective pubertal development represents only less than 30 % of HH diagnosed in male adolescent because of the low specificity of its symptoms [9].

The abnormalities in skeletal proportion become also noticeable during puberty. Especially eunuchoid stature (arm span exceeds height by 5 cm, pubic to floor length exceeds crown to pubic length by >5 cm) and tallness due to absence of long bone epiphyseal closure are most expressed. Abnormalities attributed to altered hormonal milieu adversely affect skeletal system and initiate retarded bone maturation, osteopenia, and osteoporosis that are then discovered in adulthood [10].

Anosmia or hyposmia, always associated with Kallmann syndrome, may be discovered in prepubertal or postpubertal males. However, in most of the cases, quantitative disabilities of sense of smell are not spontaneously reported by young patients. Only 20 % of all Kallmann syndrome cases are diagnosed due to olfactory disorders [11].

48.5 Adulthood

HH diagnosed in adulthood is usually an acquired disorder due to pituitary tumors, Cushing's disease, Cushing's syndrome, and obesity. Congenital forms of HH are less frequently diagnosed in adulthood and mainly account for isolated CHH. Symptoms of acquired HH are more subtle than congenital ones due to extragonadal testosterone production.

Infertility is one of the most frequent complaints among patients at the age of 20–35 years. Men with HH may also present less stamina, diminished libido, erectile dysfunction, and considerable weight gain. In about 10 % of HH cases, only worsened sense of well-being led to further hormonal diagnostic [12].

48.6 Treatment

The major goals of therapy for HH depend upon age and needs of each patient. Treatment of hypogonadotropic hypogonadism may be initiated for two purposes, androgenization and fertility. In cases where the onset of hypogonadism occurred before puberty, the most important is to induce and to maintain normal puberty. In adults with HH the treatment objective is to improve the symptoms and signs of hypogonadism.

48.7 Testosterone Replacement Therapy

Testosterone replacement therapy based on long- or short-acting testosterone esters is a classic treatment in all groups of patients. It aims at restoring hormone levels in the normal range. Testosterone esters have been used for decades as first-line treatment, given their low cost, convenience of use, and reliable effectiveness. Agents are available as oral preparations, intramuscular injections, and transdermal gel or patches. Androgen replacement therapy is used to initiate complex virilization in males with impaired maturation due to HH. In adolescents and young men, testosterone supplementation is recommended to improve sexual function (increase penis size and libido) and sense of well-being and increase muscle mass and bone mineralization [13]. Successful management of testosterone replacement therapy requires optimizing based on the age of the patient and the extent of hormonal changes associated with HH. The initial treatment should be particularly carefully planned due to risk of adverse events after abrupt increase of testosterone level. In this phase gradually increased low doses of testosterone esters and short-acting preparations are preferred so that any probable side effects can be observed and mitigated.

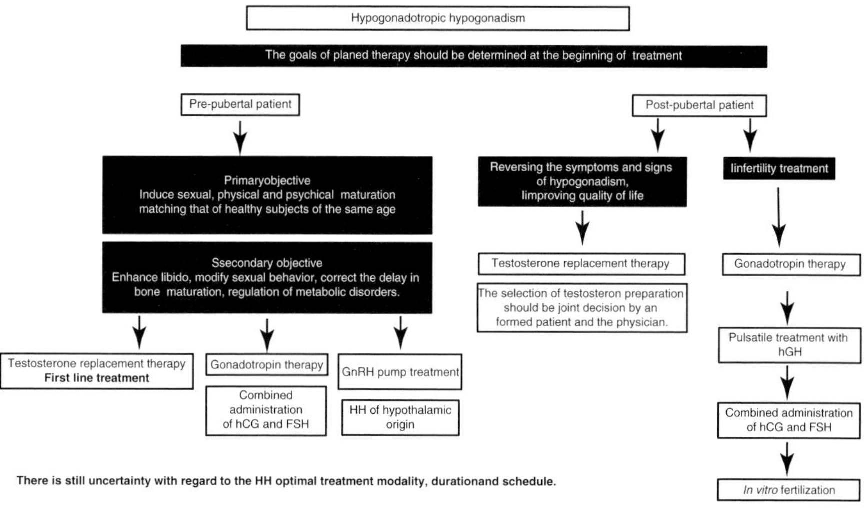

48.8 Gonadotropin Treatment

Testosterone replacement treatment does not increase testicular volume or induce spermatogenesis. Patient-desired fertility can be offered with human chorionic gonadotropin (hCG) treatment which stimulates testosterone production of Leydig cells. This approach is recommended for patients with HH and fertility issues. Human chorionic gonadotropin is used alone or combined with FSH. This second scheme increases effectiveness of spermatogenesis induction. The administration of hCG with FSH results in testicular growth and enhanced spermatogenesis in up to 90 % of patients [14]. Natural conception can be achieved within 4–24 months after the beginning of gonadotropin treatment. The hormonally induced fertility is achieved later in men with complete CHH than in men with HH of postpubertal onset. Intracytoplasmic sperm injection can be considered, in addition to gonadotropins to enhance the fertility of men with HH [15].

Gonadotropin treatment could be also an alternative therapy to ART for the induction of puberty in selected patients with HH. In comparison with ART gonadotropin-based therapies demand rigid discipline and are very expensive. This in turn limits their application in clinical practice.

48.9 Complications

The risks of testosterone replacement therapy depend upon age, life circumstances, and other medical conditions. There is a risk for prostate cancer and worsening symptoms of benign prostatic hypertrophy, liver toxicity, sleep apnea, congestive heart failure, gynecomastia, infertility, and skin diseases. The important part of HH hormonal treatment is monitoring of laboratory parameters that should be checked before and during treatment which include PSA, hemoglobin, hematocrit, lipid profiles, and liver function tests [16].

References

1. Hayes FJ, Seminara SB, Crowley Jr WF. Hypogonadotropic hypogonadism. Endocrinol Metab Clin North Am. 1998;27:739–63.
2. Seminara SB, Hayes FJ, Crowley Jr WF. Gonadotropin-releasing hormone deficiency in the human (idiopathic hypogonadotropic hypogonadism and Kallmann's syndrome): pathophysiological and genetic considerations. Endocr Rev. 1998;19:521–39.
3. Dode C, Teixeira L, Levilliers J, Fouveaut C, Bouchard P, Kottler ML, Lespinasse J, Lienhardt-Roussie A, Mathieu M, Moerman A, Morgan G, Murat A, Toublanc JE, Wolczynski S. Isolated hypogonadotropic hypogonadism. Eur Endocrynol. 2010;162:847856.
4. Coll GS, Jacobs HS, Conway GS, Besser M, Stanhope RG, Bouloux PM. Idiopathic gonadotrophin deficiency: genetic questions addressed through phenotypic characterization. Clin Endocrinol (Oxf). 2001;55:163–74.
5. Young J. Approach to the male patient with congenital hypogonadotropic hypogonadism. J Clin Endocrinol Metab. 2012;97:707–18.
6. Brioude F, Bouligand J, Trabado S, Francou B, Salenave S, Kamenicky P, Brailly-Tabard S, Chanson P, Guiochon-Mantel A, Young J. Non-syndromic congenital hypogonadotropic hypogonadism: clinical presentation and genotype-phenotype relationships. Eur J Endocrinol. 2010;162:835–51.
7. Versiani BR, Trarbach E, Koenigkam-Santos M, Dos Santos AC, Elias LL, Moreira AC, Latronico AC, de Castro M. Clinical assessment and molecular analysis of GnRHR and KAL1 genes in males with idiopathic hypogonadotrophic hypogonadism. Clin Endocrinol (Oxf). 2007;66:173–9.
8. Pinto G, Abadie V, Mesnage R, Blustajn J, Cabrol S, Amiel J, Hertz- Pannier L, Bertrand AM, Lyonnet S, Rappaport R, Netchine I. CHARGE syndrome includes hypogonadotropic hypogonadism and abnormal olfactory bulb development. J Clin Endocrinol Metabol. 2005;90:5621–6.
9. Martin MM, Martin AL. Constitutional delayed puberty in males and hypogonadotropic hypogonadism: a reliable and cost-effective approach to differential diagnosis. J Pediatr Endocrinol Metab. 2005;18:909–16.
10. Placzkiewicz E, Baldys-Waligorska A. Kallmann's syndrome: skeletal and psychological aspects of late diagnosis. Ann Endocrinol (Paris). 2003;64:277–80.
11. Nishio H, Mizuno K, Moritoki Y, Kamisawa H, Kojima Y, Mizuno H, Kohri K, Hayashi Y. Clinical features and testicular morphology in patients with Kallmann syndrome. Urology. 2012;79:684–6.
12. Seftel A. Male hypogonadism. Part II: etiology, pathophysiology, and diagnosis. Int J Impot Res. 2006;18:223–8.
13. Corona G, Rastrelli G, Forti G, Maggi M. Update in testosterone therapy for men. J Sex Med. 2011;8:639–54.
14. Akarsu C, Caglar G, Vicdan K, Isik AZ, Tuncay G. Pregnancies achieved by testicular sperm recovery in male hypogonadotrophic hypogonadism with persistent azoospermia. Reprod Biomed Online. 2009;18:455–9.
15. Zorn B, Pfeifer M, Virant-Klun I, Meden-Vrtovec H. Intracytoplasmic sperm injection as a complement to gonadotrophin treatment in infertile men with hypogonadotrophic hypogonadism. Int J Androl. 2005;28:202–7.
16. Bassil N, Alkaade S, Morley JE. The benefits and risks of testosterone replacement therapy: a review. Ther Clin Risk Manag. 2009;5:427–48.

49 Erectile Dysfunction

Rebecca Bongers and George Kedia

49.1 General Facts

Erectile dysfunction (ED) is defined as the persistent inability to attain and maintain an erection sufficient to permit satisfactory sexual performance [1]. Referring to bigger epidemiological studies, the incidence of ED which requires medical treatment is reported to be 20 % in the mean. It is age-related and increases up to 70 % in 70-year-old patients. But also younger patients suffer from ED: 5 % of 40-year-old patients have a complete and 17 % a moderate ED [2, 3]. Risk factors are lack of exercise, obesity, smoking, hypercholesterolemia, and metabolic syndrome [4]. Psychological, vascular, neurogenic, endocrine, or myogenic disorders as well as drugs can be the cause of ED. Patients with ED have to be screened for diabetes, hypertension, and dyslipidemia since ED can be an early manifestation of cardiovascular disease [5, 6].

49.2 Symptoms, Classification, and Grading

ED is not a disease, but a symptom itself. The causes for ED can be classified to psychological, vascular, neurogenic, or endocrine disorders and drug-related factors.

Psychological reasons for ED include loss of libido, often times partner-related because of different sexual interests in the relationship. Other reasons can be fear of failure, former traumatic events, parenting style, or religious education.

R. Bongers • G. Kedia (✉)
Department of Urology and Urological Oncology, Hannover University Medical School, Carl-Neuberg-Str. 1, Hannover 30625, Germany
e-mail: bongers.rebecca@mh-hannover.de; kedia.george@mh-hannover.de

A.S. Merseburger et al. (eds.), *Urology at a Glance*,
DOI 10.1007/978-3-642-54859-8_49, © Springer-Verlag Berlin Heidelberg 2014

A vascular cause for ED is arteriosclerosis due to lack of exercise, obesity, smoking, hypercholesterolemia, and metabolic syndrome. These risk factors are the same as for cardiovascular disease, and therefore ED can be an early manifestation of coronary artery and peripheral vascular disease [4]. Other vascular reasons for ED can be pelvic injury or pelvic surgery. After radical prostatectomy 25–75 % of men show a postoperative ED [7]. Radiotherapy for prostate cancer is also a risk factor for ED. The mechanisms contributing to ED after prostate irradiation involve injury to the neurovascular bundles, penile vasculature, and cavernosal structural tissue [8, 9]. Morphological changes such as Peyronie's disease or penile fracture can also disturb the blood flow and cause ED.

Parkinson's disease, traumatic paraplegia, peripheral neuropathy (diabetes), or alcohol abuse can be neurogenic reasons for ED.

Endocrine causes for ED can be hormonal disorders, e.g., testosterone deficiency due to primary testicular failure or secondary to pituitary or hypothalamic causes, including pituitary tumors resulting in hyperprolactinemia.

Drug-related ED can be due to antihypertensive medication (non-cardioselective beta-blockers), tranquilizers, antidepressants, and antihistamines.

49.3 Therapy

Before treating the symptom reversible risk factors for ED must be identified and changed including lifestyle changes; treating cardiovascular or metabolic disorders, e.g., diabetes or hypertension [4]; and changing drug-related factors (e.g., beta-blocker treatment).

If low serum testosterone is found to be the reason for ED, an intramuscular, oral, or transdermal replacement therapy can be offered to the patient if there is no contraindication (untreated prostate cancer or unstable cardiac disease). Before initiating testosterone substitution endocrine causes for testicular failure must be excluded [10], and digital rectal examination, serum PSA, hematocrit, liver function tests as well as lipid profile should be performed [11].

Psychosexual counseling and therapy can be offered to patients with psychosomatic causes for ED.

If there is no curable cause for ED, first-line therapy includes oral pharmacotherapy. Three selective PDE5 inhibitors are available for the treatment of ED (sildenafil, tadalafil, and vardenafil). PDE5 hydrolyses cGMP in the cavernosal tissue. The inhibition of PDE5 results in smooth muscle relaxation with increased arterial blood flow, leading to compression of the subtunical venous plexus and penile erection [12]. Sexual stimulation is required to facilitate an erection. The choice of drug will depend on the frequency of intercourse. PDE5 inhibitors can be taken on-demand or daily.

If oral drug treatment fails, patients can be offered intracavernous injection therapy, intraurethral alprostadil, or the use of a vacuum erection device.

Alprostadil (Caverject®) was the first and only drug approved for intracavernous treatment of ED [13] with a high success rate of 85 % [14].

Intraurethral pharmacotherapy can be offered as an alternative to intracavernous injections to patients who prefer a less-invasive treatment. Alprostadil (500–1,000 μg) in a medicated pellet (MUSE®) is reabsorbed by a vascular interaction between the urethra and the corpora cavernosa [15]. Efficacy rates are significantly lower than intracavernous pharmacotherapy [16].

A drug-free method is a vacuum erection device (VED). It can be offered to patients with infrequent sexual intercourse and comorbidity requiring noninvasive drug-free treatment of ED [17]. The vacuum provides a passive engorgement of the corpora cavernosa. A constrictor ring placed at the base of the penis retains the blood within the corpora.

If all conservative treatment options have failed, the implantation of a penile prosthesis may be considered. Inflatable and malleable devices are available [18] and show high satisfaction rates of 92–100 % in patients and 91–95 % in partners [19].

49.4 Complications

Patients under testosterone treatment should be monitored for elevated hematocrit and development of hepatic or prostatic disease. Untreated prostate cancer is a contraindication for testosterone therapy.

Common adverse events of PDE5 inhibitors are headache, flushing, dyspepsia, nasal congestion, dizziness, and abnormal vision. Nitrates are contraindicated with PDE5 inhibitors. They result in cGMP accumulation and an unpredictable hypotension.

Complications of intracavernous alprostadil include penile pain, prolonged erections (5 %), priapism (1 %), and fibrosis (2 %) [20]. It should not be used by men at risk of priapism and men with bleeding disorders.

Adverse events of intraurethral alprostadil are local pain (29–41 %) and dizziness with possible hypotension (1.9–14 %). Urethral bleeding (5 %) and urinary tract infections (0.2 %) are related to the mode of administration.

Risks in using vacuum erection devices (VEDs) are pain, inability to ejaculate, petechiae, bruising, and numbness which occur in <30 % of patients [21]. Skin necrosis can be avoided if patients remove the constriction ring within 30 min. VEDs are contraindicated in patients with bleeding disorders or on anticoagulant therapy.

The two main complications of penile prosthesis implantation are mechanical failure and infection (Fig. 49.1).

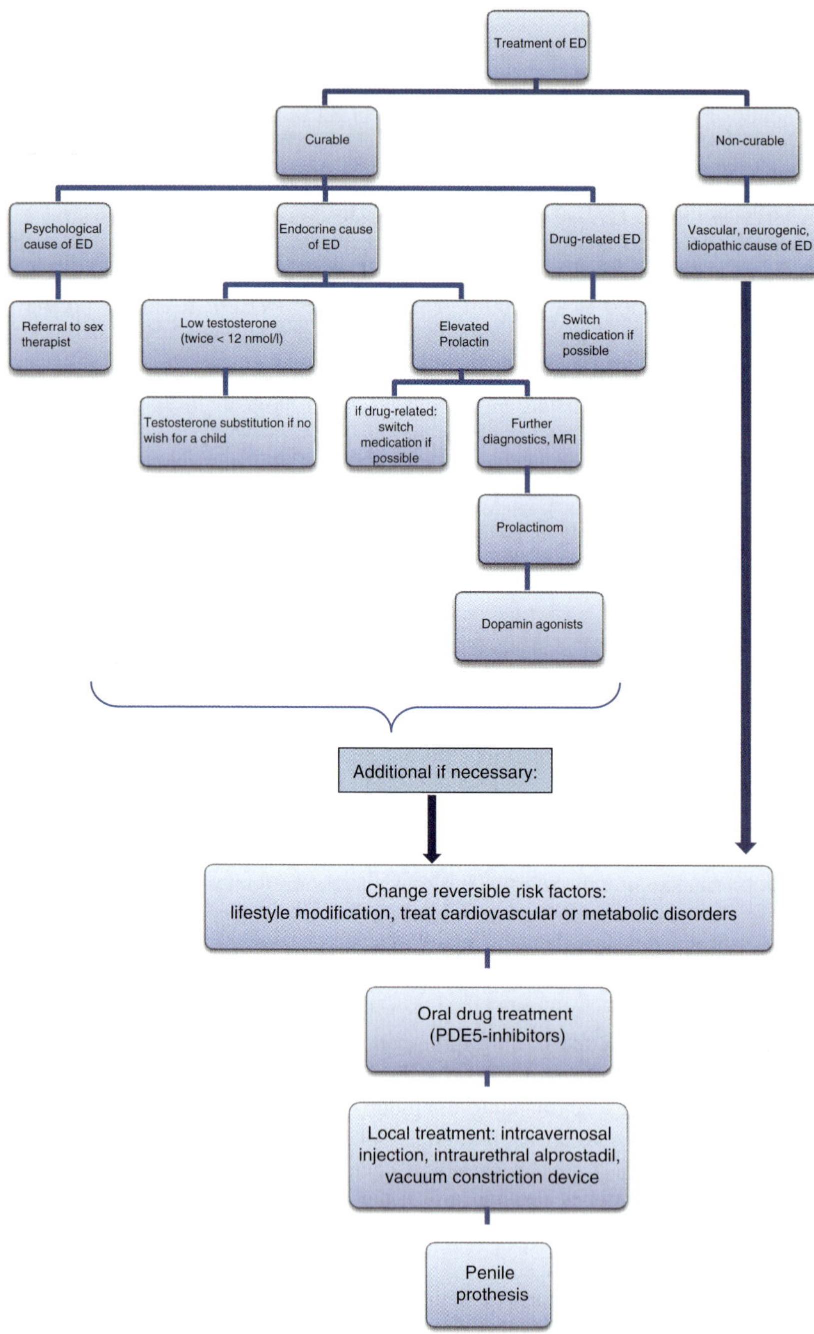

Fig. 49.1 Flow chart demonstrating the pathway from diagnosis to therapy

References

1. Lue TF, Giuliano F, Montorsi F, et al. Summary of the recommendations on sexual dysfunctions in men. J Sex Med. 2004;1:6–23.
2. Feldman HA, Goldstein I, Hatzichristou DG, et al. Impotence and its medical and psychosocial correlates: results of the Massachusetts Male Aging Study. J Urol. 1994;151(1):54–61.
3. Braun M, Wassmer G, Klotz T, et al. Epidemiology of erectile dysfunction: results of the 'Cologne Male Survey'. Int J Impot Res. 2000;12(6):305–11.
4. Gupta BP, Murad MH, Clifton MM, et al. The effect of lifestyle modification and cardiovascular risk factor reduction on erectile dysfunction: a systematic review and meta-analysis. Arch Intern Med. 2011;171(20):1797–803.
5. Kostis JB, Jackson G, Rosen R, et al. Sexual dysfunction and cardiac risk (the Second Princeton Consensus Conference). Am J Cardiol. 2005;96:313–21.
6. Guo W, Liao C, Zou Y, Li F, Li T, Zhou Q, Cao Y, Mao X. Erectile dysfunction and risk of clinical cardiovascular events: a meta-analysis of seven cohort studies. J Sex Med. 2010;7(8):2805–16.
7. Sanda MG, Dunn RL, Michalski J, et al. Quality of life and satisfaction with outcome among prostate cancer survivors. N Engl J Med. 2008;358(12):1250–61.
8. van der Wielen GJ, Mulhall JP, Incrocci L. Erectile dysfunction after radiotherapy for prostate cancer and radiation dose to the penile structures: a critical review. Radiother Oncol. 2007;84(2):107–13.
9. Stember DS, Mulhall JP. The concept of erectile function preservation (penile rehabilitation) in the patient after brachytherapy for prostate cancer. Brachytherapy. 2012;11(2):87–96.
10. Greenstein A, Mabjeesh NJ, Sofer M, et al. Does sildenafil combined with testosterone gel improve erectile dysfunction in hypogonadal men in whom testosterone supplement therapy alone failed? J Urol. 2005;173(2):530–2.
11. Morales A, Heaton JP. Hormonal erectile dysfunction. Evaluation and management. Urol Clin North Am. 2001;28(2):279–88.
12. Lue TF. Erectile dysfunction. N Engl J Med. 2000;342(24):1802–13.
13. Leungwattanakij S, Flynn Jr V, Hellstrom WJ. Intracavernosal injection and intraurethral therapy for erectile dysfunction. Urol Clin North Am. 2001;28(2):343–54.
14. Coombs PG, Heck M, Guhring P, Narus J, Mulhall JP. A review of outcomes of an intracavernosal injection therapy programme. BJU Int. 2012;110(11):1787–91.
15. Padma-Nathan H, Hellstrom WJ, Kaiser FE, et al. Treatment of men with erectile dysfunction with transurethral alprostadil. Medicated Urethral System for Erection (MUSE) Study Group. N Engl J Med. 1997;336(1):1–7.
16. Shabsigh R, Padma-Nathan H, Gittleman M, et al. Intracavernous alprostadil alfadex is more efficacious, better tolerated, and preferred over intraurethral alprostadil plus optional actis: a comparative, randomized, crossover, multicentre study. Urology. 2000;55(4):109–13.
17. Levine LA, Dimitriou RJ. Vacuum constriction and external erection devices in erectile dysfunction. Urol Clin North Am. 2001;28(2):335–41, ix–x.
18. Martinez-Salamanca JI, Mueller A, Moncada I, et al. Penile prosthesis surgery in patients with corporal fibrosis: a state of the art review. J Sex Med. 2011;8(7):1880–9.
19. Bernal RM, Henry GD. Contemporary patient satisfaction rates for three-piece inflatable penile prostheses. Adv Urol. 2012;2012:707321.
20. Lakin MM, Montague DK, Vander Brug Medendorp S, et al. Intracavernous injection therapy: analysis of results and complications. J Urol. 1990;143(6):1138–41.
21. Lewis RW, Witherington R. External vacuum therapy for erectile dysfunction: use and results. World J Urol. 1997;15(1):78–82.

Hypospadias

50

Christian Niedworok and Iris Rübben

50.1 Definition

Hypospadias is a defect in the development of the male genital resulting in an abnormal localized position of the external urethral orifice, curvature of the penis, and failed closure of the foreskin in the ventral part of the penis (Fig. 50.1). The urethral orifice, usually localized at the glanular tip, occurs ectopic on the ventral side of the glans in so-called distal hypospadias, on the penile shaft in midshaft or penile hypospadias, and in the scrotal or perineal area in so-called proximal hypospadias. Hypospadias is a common birth defect with an incidence of one in 150–300 male births [1, 2]. Multiple factors were shown to influence male genital development disorders: several target genes have been identified to be associated with hypospadias [3], advanced maternal age was seen to increase severity of hypospadias [4], placental insufficiency [5] and preterm newborns as well as newborns with low birth weight [6] were shown to have a higher risk to develop a hypospadias, and finally endocrine disruptors are currently discussed to play an important role in the occurrence of genital malformations [7–10]. Hypospadias is often related with other genitourinary malformations like undescended testicles and development disorders like the testicular dysgenesis syndrome [11].

C. Niedworok, FEBU (✉)
Department of Urology, Essen Medical School, University Duisburg-Essen,
Hufelandstrasse 55, Essen 45122, Germany
e-mail: christian.niedworok@uk-essen.de

I. Rübben, FEAPU
Pediatric Urology Division of Department of Urology, Essen Medical School,
University Duisburg-Essen, Hufelandstrasse 55, Essen 45122, Germany
e-mail: iris.ruebben@uk-essen.de

A.S. Merseburger et al. (eds.), *Urology at a Glance*,
DOI 10.1007/978-3-642-54859-8_50, © Springer-Verlag Berlin Heidelberg 2014

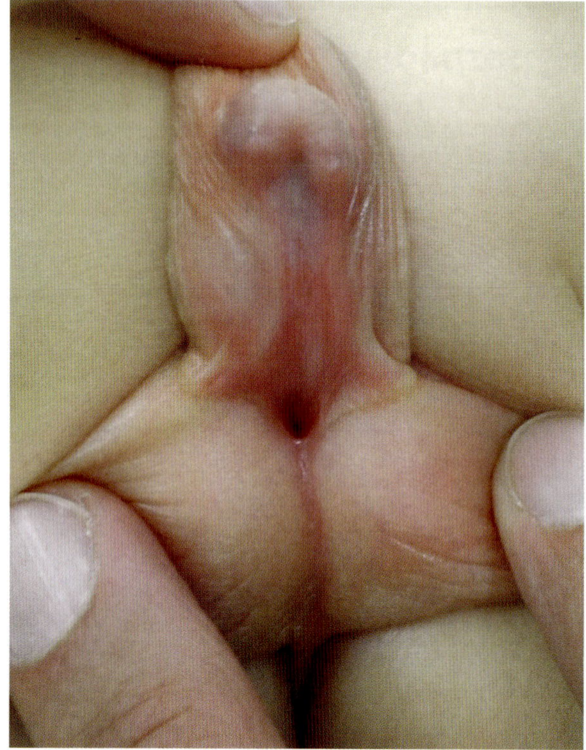

Fig. 50.1 Appearance of a hypospadiac genital in a 1-year-old boy suffering from a penoscrotal hypospadias. The external urethral orifice is dislocated to the root of the penis; the urethral plate is exposed on the whole penile distance. Closure of the foreskin on the ventral side has failed resulting in a wrinkled aspect with the impression of redundant foreskin tissue on the dorsal side of the penis

50.2 Symptoms and Diagnosis

The diagnosis is confirmed immediately after birth in most of the cases. The inspection of the penis usually enables a visual diagnosis, especially in severe cases. Very distal hypospadias, hypospadias with only marginal dislocation of the urethral meatus, and hypospadias without hypospadias, a seldom subform of hypospadias with a short urethra ending at the tip of the glans resulting in a distinct penile curvature but missing of foreskin disorders, can lead to a deferred time of diagnosis. Sometimes the leading symptom is not the dislocated urethral meatus but a severe penile curvature. Further symptoms are rare in childhood. In adolescence, with the beginning of sexual activity and in adult age, some patients consult the urologist due to impotence, pain during sexual intercourse, or disturbing cosmetic appearance of the penis.

50.3 Therapy

The therapy for hypospadias is surgery. Regardless of the particular type of repair, the surgical procedure has to include a correction of penile chordee and a urethroplasty to create a normal cosmetic appearance. A good cosmetic appearance and

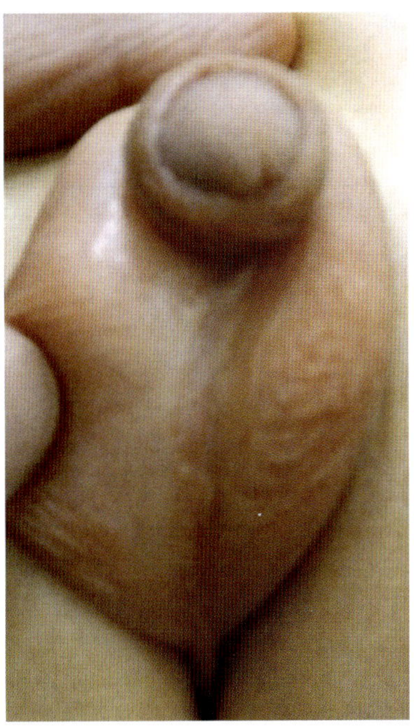

Fig. 50.2 Same patient 6 months after hypospadias repair. The external urethral orifice is located at the tip of the glans penis; the penis is straightened. Redundant foreskin is removed and the urethra closed on the ventral side, so that the penis has a normal cosmetic appearance

functional result is important to avoid severe physical and psychic problems in adolescence and adult age like impotence, relationship problems, or lack of confidence (Fig. 50.2). Suggested age to perform surgery is the age between 6 and 18 months. The incidence of postoperative complications is higher when hypospadias is repaired in older patients [12]. Preoperatively the local androgen treatment of the penis is an optional stimulation for penile growth in order to decrease complication rates although only few clinical trials have shown encouraging results [13, 14].

Numerous surgical procedures are described for hypospadias repair. The appropriate choice of the technique depends on the appearance of the hypospadias, location of the meatus, appearance of the shaft, presence and extent of penile curvature and rotation of the shaft, configuration and proportion of the foreskin, extent of the urethral plate, and residuum of the urethra.

For distal and midshaft hypospadias, either local perimeatal tissue is used to perform hypospadias repair, or pedicled tissue has to be dislocated from a more distant part of the penis. The Thiersch-Duplay procedure, modified by Snodgrass as TIP technique (tubularized incised-plate urethroplasty), is the standard technique [15]. The urethral plate is preserved and incised when necessary, and the adjacent glanular and inner foreskin tissue is used to form a tubularized replacement of missing urethral structure. Further techniques were described by Mathieu (incision at the glandular tip and lateral of the estimated urethral line, preparation of the inner foreskin at a length suitable to the distance to span and closing the ventral defect with the prepared tissue) [16] and Duckett (MAGPI and preputial onlay island flap) [17, 18].

The repair of severe proximal hypospadias is a challenging surgical approach. Due to the fact that severe proximal hypospadias are rare compared to the distal

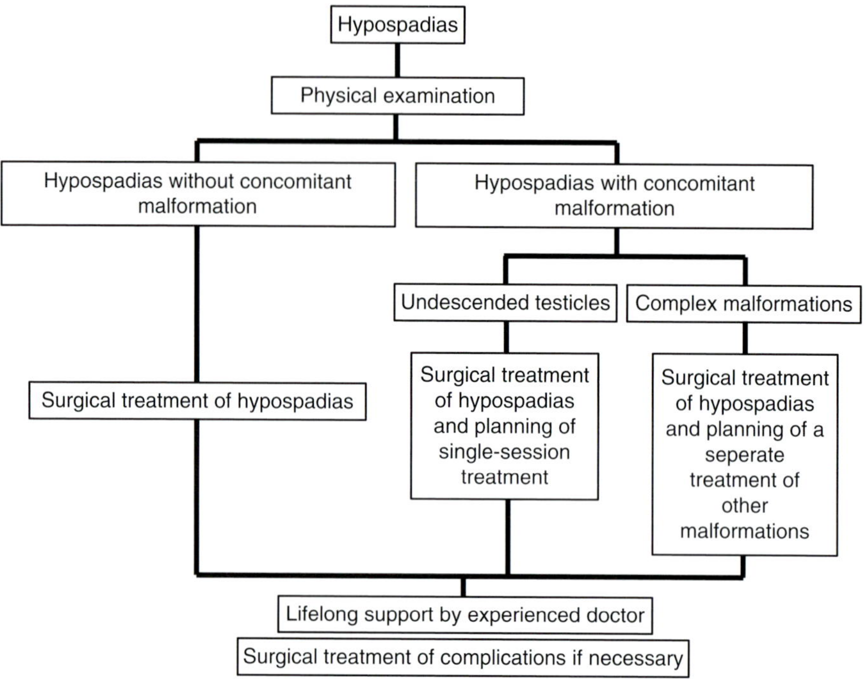

Fig. 50.3 Flow chart of therapy and support of hypospadias

forms, surgical experience is limited and the literature is lacking clinical trials comparing different techniques. There are approaches to perform one-stage or two-stage repair. Long defects of the urethral plate and chordee removal with the destruction of remnants of the urethral plate require the use of pedicled skin flaps or free-autologous buccal mucosa grafts (Fig. 50.3).

50.4 Complications

Hypospadias surgery should only be performed in experienced centers. Complication rates for fistula forming differ between 2 and 30 %, depending on severity of hypospadias and experience of the surgeon [19]. Other complications are wound healing disorders, unsatisfying cosmetic results, and urethral strictures with consecutive obstructive voiding disorders [20]. Special attention should be taken to the fact that the rate of patients with sexual function disorders and psychosocial worries is higher in patients with hypospadias [21, 22]. Sexual and social problems should be addressed in follow-up examinations by the doctor as the treatment of a patient with hypospadias should not be considered to be finished with the end of the surgical treatment. There should be a lifelong support of hypospadias patients with a target-orientated treatment of emerging problems by experienced doctors.

References

1. Paulozzi LJ. International trends in rates of hypospadias and cryptorchidism. Environ Health Perspect. 1999;107(4):297–302.
2. Toppari J, Kaleva M, Virtanen HE. Trends in the incidence of cryptorchidism and hypospadias, and methodological limitations of registry-based data. Hum Reprod Update. 2001;7(3):282–6.
3. Kojima Y, Kohri K, Hayashi Y. Genetic pathway of external genitalia formation and molecular etiology of hypospadias. J Pediatr Urol. 2010;6(4):346–54.
4. Carlson WH, Kisely SR, MacLellan DL. Maternal and fetal risk factors associated with severity of hypospadias: a comparison of mild and severe cases. J Pediatr Urol. 2009;5(4):283–6.
5. Fujimoto T, Suwa T, Kabe K, Adachi T, Nakabayashi M, Amamiya T. Placental insufficiency in early gestation is associated with hypospadias. J Pediatr Surg. 2008;43(2):358–61.
6. Sun G, Tang D, Liang J, Wu M. Increasing prevalence of hypospadias associated with various perinatal risk factors in chinese newborns. Urology. 2009;73(6):1241–5.
7. Wang MH, Baskin LS. Endocrine disruptors, genital development, and hypospadias. J Androl. 2008;29(5):499–505.
8. Wang Z, Liu BC, Lin GT, Lin CS, Lue TF, Willingham E, Baskin LS. Up-regulation of estrogen responsive genes in hypospadias: microarray analysis. J Urol. 2007;177(5):1939–46.
9. Liu B, Agras K, Willingham E, Vilela ML, Baskin LS. Activating transcription factor 3 is estrogen-responsive in utero and upregulated during sexual differentiation. Horm Res. 2006;65(5):217–22. Epub 2006 Mar 28.
10. Liu B, Lin G, Willingham E, Ning H, Lin CS, Lue TF, Baskin LS. Estradiol upregulates activating transcription factor 3, a candidate gene in the etiology of hypospadias. Pediatr Dev Pathol. 2007;10(6):446–54.
11. Skakkebaek NE, Rajpert-De Meyts E, Main KM. Testicular dysgenesis syndrome: an increasingly common developmental disorder with environmental aspects. Hum Reprod. 2001;16(5):972–8.
12. Ziada A, Hamza A, Abdel-Rassoul M, Habib E, Mohamed A, Daw M. Outcomes of hypospadias repair in older children: a prospective study. J Urol. 2011;185(6 Suppl):2483–5.
13. Bastos AN, Oliveira LR, Ferrarez CE, de Figueiredo AA, Favorito LA, Bastos Netto JM. Structural study of prepuce in hypospadias–does topical treatment with testosterone produce alterations in prepuce vascularization? J Urol. 2011;185(6 Suppl):2474–8.
14. Gorduza DB, Gay CL, de Mattos E, Silva E, Demède D, Hameury F, Berthiller J, Mure PY, Mouriquand PD. Does androgen stimulation prior to hypospadias surgery increase the rate of healing complications? – A preliminary report. J Pediatr Urol. 2011;7(2):158–61.
15. Snodgrass WT, Bush N, Cost N. Tubularized incised plate hypospadias repair for distal hypospadias. J Pediatr Urol. 2010;6(4):408–13.
16. Mathieu P. Traitement en un temps de l'hypospadias balanique ou juxta balanique. J Chir. 1932;39:481–7.
17. Duckett J. MAGPI (Meatal advancement and glanuloplasty) a procedure for subcoronal hypospadias. Urol Clin North Am. 1981;8(3):513–9.
18. Duckett Jr JW. Transverse preputial island flap technique for repair of severe hypospadias. J Urol. 1980;167(2 Pt 2):1179–82.
19. Wood HM, Kay R, Angermeier KW, Ross JH. Timing of the presentation of urethrocutaneous fistulas after hypospadias repair in pediatric patients. J Urol. 2008;180(4 Suppl):1753–6.
20. Niedworok C, Jürgensen K, Vom Dorp F, Rossi R, Füllhase C, Rübben I, Rübben H. Pedicled prepuce flap plasty: results in patients with hypospadias or urethral stricture. Urologe A. 2013; 52(5):672–6. doi:10.1007/s00120-013-3124-6.
21. Mureau MA, Slijper FM, Slob AK, Verhulst FC. Psychosocial functioning of children, adolescents, and adults following hypospadias surgery: a comparative study. J Pediatr Psychol. 1997;22(3):371–87.
22. Bubanj TB, Perovic SV, Milicevic RM, Jovcic SB, Marjanovic ZO, Djordjevic MM. Sexual behavior and sexual function of adults after hypospadias surgery: a comparative study. J Urol. 2004;171(5):1876–9.

Varicocele

51

Annika Simon

51.1 General Facts

Varicocele can be defined as dilatation of veins in the pampiniform plexus of the spermatic cord. Approximately 15 % of all men are affected. Furthermore, varicocele is found in around about 30 % of males with primary infertility and 45–85 % with secondary infertility. It can occur unilaterally or bilaterally; the left side is the most commonly affected [1–5].

In regard to aetiology, in most cases, incompetent valves in the spermatic veins lead to retrograde blood flow and vessel dilatation of the pampiniform plexus. Because it plays an important role for certain heat-exchange mechanisms cooling the arterial blood of the testicles, varicocele may cause symptoms of pain and discomfort, growth disturbance and at least infertility [1].

51.2 Symptoms, Classification and Grading

Generally, the majority of varicoceles are asymptomatic; the incidence of pain and discomfort is 2–10 % [1]. The most common classification distinguishes four stages which are summarized in Table 51.1. Another common grading system respects size and distinguishes the three grades: small, moderate and large. Their definition corresponds to the description of grades 1–3 listed in Table 51.1 [2–5].

The diagnosis is generally made by clinical examination (inspection, palpation, Valsalva manoeuvre), scrotal Doppler sonography, vasography and even X-ray. In regard to infertility, semen analysis is advisable [1–4].

A. Simon
Department of Urology and Urological Oncology, Hannover University Medical School, Carl-Neuberg-Str. 1, Hannover 30625, Germany
e-mail: psychosomatik.simon@googlemail.com

A.S. Merseburger et al. (eds.), *Urology at a Glance*,
DOI 10.1007/978-3-642-54859-8_51, © Springer-Verlag Berlin Heidelberg 2014

Table 51.1 Classification and grading of varicocele [2–5]

Subclinical stage	Not visible or palpable; demonstrated in diagnostic tests (e.g. ultrasound)	
Grade 1	Not visible, only palpable during Valsalva manoeuvre	Small
Grade 2	Not visible, palpable at rest	Medium
Grade 3	Visible and palpable	Large

51.3 Therapy

Because the majority demonstrates no symptoms, the necessity of special treatment depends on the individual situation and symptoms of the patient [1–5]. Up to today, the treatment is object of discussion and there are many therapy approaches available. The most common strategies of treatment are embolization with coils or other sclerosing agents and surgical ligation of spermatic veins [3–4]. However, the selection of intervention depends on the surgeon's experience. The flow chart demonstrates the pathway from diagnosis to therapy and its complications.

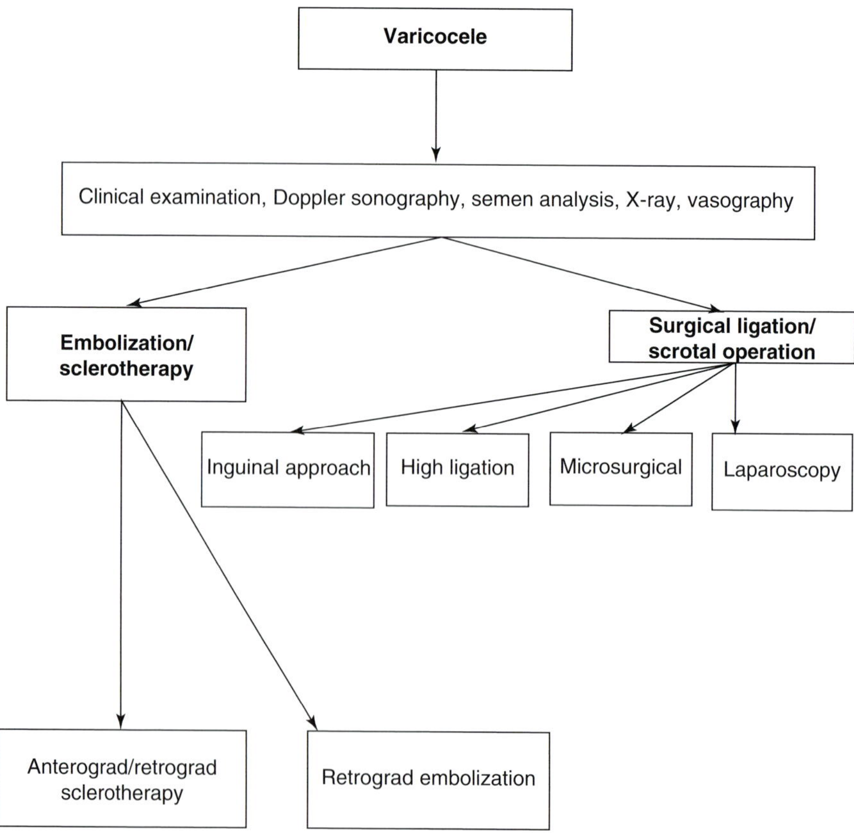

51.4 Complications

Varicocele may lead to infertility; most surgical complications are recurrence, hydrocele formation atrophy of testicles and nerve damage of the ilioinguinal cord [6–7].

References

1. Diamond DA, Gargollo PC, Caldamone AA. Current management principles for adolescent varicocele. Fertil Steril. 2011;96(6):1294–8.
2. EAU. EAU Guidelines, edition presented at the 25th EAU Annual Congress, Barcelona 2010. ISBN 978-90-79754-70-0.
3. Kroese AC, de Lange NM, Collins J, Evers JL. Surgery or embolization for varicoceles in subfertile men. Cochrane Database Syst Rev. 2012;10, CD000479.
4. Iaccarino V, Venetucci P. Interventional radiology of male varicocele: current status. Cardiovasc Intervent Radiol. 2012;35(6):1263–80.
5. Reynard J, Brewster S, Biers S. Oxford handbook of urology. New York: Oxford University Press; 2009.
6. Serefoglu EC, Saitz TR, La Nasa JA, Hellstrom Jr WJ. Adolescent varicocoele management controversies. Andrology. 2013;1(1):109–15.
7. Will MA, Swain J, Fode M, Sonksen J, Christman GM, Ohl D. The great debate: varicocele treatment and impact on fertility. Fertil Steril. 2011;95(3):841–52.

Hydrocele

52

Hendrik Borgmann

52.1 General Facts

Hydrocele is an abnormal fluid collection in the scrotum between the visceral and the parietal layers of the tunica vaginalis [1]. Pathogenesis of hydrocele is due to an imbalance between secretion and reabsorption of this fluid. On the contrary, inguinal hernia occurs after protrusion of a portion of organs or tissues through the abdominal wall. The incidence of hydrocele is 1–5 % [2] in neonates and 1 % in older boys and men. In most cases, the hydrocele is noncommunicating and fluid disappears by 1 year of age. In older boys and men, it results secondary to testicular torsion, epididymitis, trauma, tumor, and varicocele operation or as a recurrence after primary repair of a communicating hydrocele. Hydrocele is almost exclusively seen in males, but newborn girls can have hydroceles of the canal of Nuck or meconium hydrocele of the labia [3].

52.2 Symptoms and Classification

The main symptom of a hydrocele is a testicular swelling. In the case of a communicating hydrocele, the swelling vacillates in size, usually related to activity. The hydrocele then is small in the morning and becomes progressively larger during the day. On the other hand, a noncommunicating hydrocele does not vacillate in size. A large hydrocele can cause pain and a sensation of heaviness. If the hydrocele occurs secondary or as a reactive process, it may also have preceding symptoms associated with the primary pathology.

H. Borgmann
Department of Urology, University Hospital Frankfurt,
Theodor-Stern-Kai 7, Frankfurt 60590, Germany
e-mail: hendrik.borgmann@kgu.de

A.S. Merseburger et al. (eds.), *Urology at a Glance*,
DOI 10.1007/978-3-642-54859-8_52, © Springer-Verlag Berlin Heidelberg 2014

Hydrocele can be categorized as communicating and noncommunicating. A communicating hydrocele occurs due to an open processus vaginalis that leads to varying amounts of serous fluid in the cavum vaginalis testis. The long-term risk of a communicating hydrocele is the development of an inguinal hernia. In most cases, the hydrocele is noncommunicating because the processus vaginalis obliterates during development. A noncommunicating hydrocele can be categorized according to its location into hydrocele of the testis, hydrocele of the cord, and abdominoscrotal hydrocele. The latter is a rare variant, in which there is a large, tense hydrocele that extends into the lower abdominal cavity [4].

52.3 Therapy

Since hydroceles have a tendency for spontaneous resolution, surgical treatment is not indicated within the first 12–24 months in the majority of infants. Surgery in the early months should be done if there is suspicion of an underlying testicular pathology or of a concomitant inguinal hernia. If a scrotal hydrocele persists beyond 2 years of age, this may be an indication for inguinal surgical correction because the hydrocele is then often accompanied by inguinal hernia. Synchronous contralateral exploration should be considered in case of a past or present history of contralateral inguinal or scrotal pathology [5]. Furthermore, contralateral exploration should be performed in children with increased peritoneal fluid due to a ventriculoperitoneal shunt or due to peritoneal dialysis.

Indications for surgery of a noncommunicating hydrocele are pain, disturbing size, and sensation of heaviness [6]. For hydrocelectomy of the cord, inguinal approach is used. For hydrocelectomy of the testis, two surgical techniques are available. Using Winkelman's or Jaboulay's technique hydrocelectomy is performed with excision of the hydrocele sac. This technique is used for large or thick-walled hydroceles and multilocular hydroceles. Using Lord's technique, the hydrocele sac is reduced by placation sutures. This placation technique is suitable for medium-sized and thin-walled hydroceles.

The flow chart (Fig. 52.1) demonstrates the pathway from diagnosis to therapy.

52.4 Complications

General surgical complications include bleeding and infection [7]. There is a low risk for recurrence of the hydrocele or damage to the epididymitis or vas deferens with infertility. The incidence of testicular damage during hydrocele or inguinal hernia repair is very low.

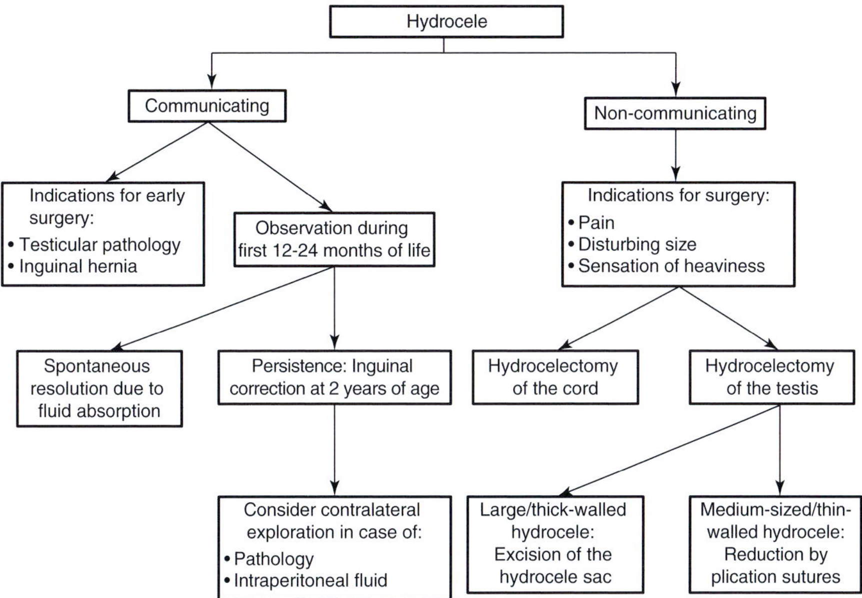

Fig. 52.1 Flow chart demonstrating the pathway from diagnosis of a hydrocele to its therapy

References

1. Kapur P, Caty MG, Glick PL. Pediatric hernias and hydroceles. Pediatr Clin North Am. 1998;45(4):773–89.
2. Ben-Ari J, Merlob P, Mimouni F, Rosen O, Reisner SH. The prevalence of high insertion of scrotum, hydrocele and mobile testis in the newborn infant (36–42 weeks gestation). Eur J Pediatr. 1989;148(6):563–4.
3. Block RE. Hydrocele of the canal of nuck. A report of five cases. Obstet Gynecol. 1975;45(4):464–6.
4. Saharia PC, Bronsther B, Abrams MW. Abdominoscrotal hydrocele. Case presentation and review of the literature. J Pediatr Surg. 1979;14(6):713–4.
5. Antonoff MB, Kreykes NS, Saltzman DA, Acton RD. American Academy of Pediatrics Section on Surgery hernia survey revisited. J Pediatr Surg. 2005;40(6):1009–14.
6. Cimador M, Castagnetti M, De Grazia E. Management of hydrocele in adolescent patients. Nat Rev Urol. 2010;7(7):379–85.
7. Swartz MA, Morgan TM, Krieger JN. Complications of scrotal surgery for benign conditions. Urology. 2007;69(4):616–9.

Enuresis

53

Katrin Harrer and Thomas Knoll

53.1 Definition

Enuresis is a very prevalent condition within children. Five to ten percent of 7-year-olds are affected, and in 7 % of them symptoms continue until adulthood. Enuresis is defined as nocturnal wetting (continuous or intermittent) after completion of the 5th year of age, differentiated into primary and secondary enuresis. The latter describes new-onset nocturnal incontinence in a child with a previous dry period of at least 6 months. Simple nocturnal incontinence is described as monosymptomatic enuresis. If the child shows additional urinary tract symptoms (LUTS), e.g., daytime incontinence, urgency, holding maneuvers, incomplete bladder emptying, increased voiding frequency, etc., one speaks of non-monosymptomatic enuresis. Reasons for enuresis can be increased nighttime urine output, arousal problems, low bladder capacity, or elevated detrusor activity. Furthermore, enuresis can be based on genetical disorders but also might be due to psychological issues.

53.2 Medical History

Doctors should ask about the frequency of wetting, if there has ever been a dry period before, if wetting only occurs at night or also during the day, and whether incontinence episodes correlate to special conditions (psychological aspects). Parents should also be asked about the incidence of urinary tract infections. Questions about the social background of the child and problems within the family or at school are important, just like other illnesses, for example, attention deficit disorder (ADD). It is also interesting to know if other family members were affected

K. Harrer (✉) • T. Knoll
Department of Urology, Klinikum Sindelfingen-Böblingen,
Arthur-Gruber-Str. 70, Sindelfingen 71065, Germany
e-mail: k.harrer@klinikverbund-suedwest.de; t.knoll@klinikverbund-suedwest.de

A.S. Merseburger et al. (eds.), *Urology at a Glance*,
DOI 10.1007/978-3-642-54859-8_53, © Springer-Verlag Berlin Heidelberg 2014

by the condition in their younger years. The parents should be asked about any daytime symptoms of the child, like urgency, holding maneuvers, etc., and about the bowel function which means frequency of defecation and consistency of the stool. This can be important because preexisting urgency due to low bladder capacity or increased detrusor activity might be triggered by constipation.

53.3 Diagnostics

The intake-and-voiding diary is a pivotal basis for evaluating enuresis. Besides the assessment of time, amount, and type of fluid intake, parents are supposed to help the child with the measurement of each voided portion day and night. The regular fluid intake should be 30 ml/kg body weight per day, and the normal bladder capacity in ml can be calculated by age × 30 + 30. For the measurement of nighttime urine production, the weighing of diapers might be necessary. A nocturnal urine output higher than 130 % of age-related bladder capacity is considered as nocturnal polyuria. Another basic diagnostic means is a urine sample (dipstick) to detect urinary tract infections or diabetes. For monosymptomatic enuresis, these basic instruments are sufficient to start treatment. In the case of non-monosymptomatic enuresis, further examinations are to be carried out like physical examination (anatomical anomalies, spina bifida, etc.) and ultrasound of the kidneys and bladder. The normal value for a children's bladder wall is up to 3 mm for a full bladder and up to 5 mm for an empty bladder. Residual volume is also to be measured. In addition it is useful to induce a uroflowmetry, preferably in combination with pelvic floor EMG, to detect dysfunctional voiding. Invasive diagnostic means like cystoscopy or urodynamic testing is reserved for complicated therapy-resistant cases or when neurologic diseases are known or suspected (Fig. 53.1).

53.4 Differential Diagnosis

Differential diagnosis	Diagnostics
Monosymptomatic enuresis	
Increased nighttime urine output	Bladder diary
Low bladder capacity	Bladder diary
Arousal problems	Anamnesis (parents)
Non-monosymptomatic enuresis	
Low bladder capacity/elevated detrusor activity	Bladder diary, anamnesis (urgency, daytime incontinence)
Dysfunctional voiding	Flow-EMG, ultrasound (residual volume)
"Lazy voider"	Bladder diary, ultrasound (resid. volume)
Urinary tract infection	Dipstick
Obstruction (e.g., urethral valves, strictures)	Medical history (former surgery)
	Ultrasound (bladder wall, hydronephrosis)
	Cystoscopy

Differential diagnosis	Diagnostics
Neurogenic bladder disturbance	Physical examination (e.g., spina bifida), urodynamic, MRI of the spine
Ectopic ureter	Anamnesis (constant incontinence), physical examination, MRI urography
Psychological issues (stress, trauma, etc.)	Psychological assessment
Hormonal disorders (e.g., diabetes)	Dipstick, intake-voiding diary (increased intake)

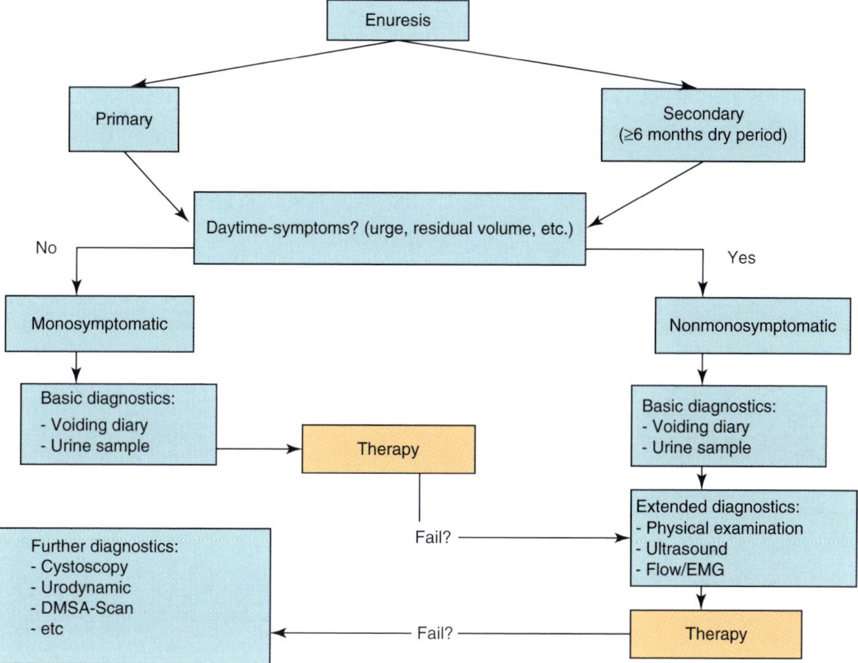

Fig. 53.1 Flow chart for the diagnosis of enuresis

Neurogenic Bladder Dysfunction (NBD) 54

Burkhard Karl-Heinz Domurath
and Johannes Friedrich Kutzenberger

54.1 Definition

Neurogenic bladder dysfunction is a general term for any type of bladder dysfunction due to a defined neurological disorder. It comprises all facets of neurogenic dysfunction of the urinary bladder – the sensitivity, the storage function, and the voiding function. The term is not a diagnosis by exclusion. The location and the extent of the nerve cell injury determine the kind and the degree of the bladder dysfunction (see Table 54.1). Different types of neurogenic bladder dysfunction are understandable in the model of lower and upper motor neuron injury in patients after spinal cord injury (SCI). Neurogenic overactivity after upper motor neuron lesion usually causes a detrusor-sphincter dyssynergia.

Disorders of the brain may also lead to bladder dysfunction. The focus is on the change in bladder sensitivity and impaired inhibition of areas situated below the damage. The pontine coordination center (PMC, PSC) is seldom affected. Therefore, there is no detrusor-sphincter dyssynergia in diseases of the brain.

54.2 Medical History

Starting point for the diagnosis of suspected NBD is the detailed knowledge of the neurological history. Occasionally symptoms of NBD are the first of a hitherto undiagnosed neurological illness. The physician has to ask within the urological part about the sensitivity of the bladder (normal, hyposensitive, hypersensitive), the way of emptying the bladder (normally, triggered, straining, Crédé maneuver, catheterizing, urinary diversion – transurethral, suprapubic, etc.), the frequency of

B.K.-H. Domurath, MD, PhD (✉) • J.F. Kutzenberger, MD, PhD
Department of Neuro-Urology, Werner Wicker Clinic,
Im Kreuzfeld 4, Bad Wildungen 34537, Germany
e-mail: bdo@werner-wicker-klinik.de;
jkutzenberger@werner-wicker-klinik.de

A.S. Merseburger et al. (eds.), *Urology at a Glance*,
DOI 10.1007/978-3-642-54859-8_54, © Springer-Verlag Berlin Heidelberg 2014

Table 54.1 What causes NBD

Brain diseases	Demyelinating disorders Cerebrovasculary disorders Craniocerebral trauma Craniocerebral tumor Basal nuclei disorders (f. e. M. Parkinson) Dementia
Spinal cord pathologies	Spinal cord injury Spine or spinal cord tumor Spinal vascular disorders Neural tube defects Inflammatory disorders Demyelinating disorders
Lumbosacral neuropathologies	Trauma Congenital malformations, tethered cord inclusively Tumor of cauda equina Herpes zoster Demyelinating disorders Disc herniation
Disorders of peripheral nerval structures	Radical pelvical surgery Pelvic fractures

micturition, and the nocturnal micturition. Mandatory is a drinking and voiding diary in which has to be notified incontinence episodes and methods of management of urinary incontinence, too. Questions about defecation and sexual dysfunction should be raised specifically.

54.3 Diagnostics

NBD can never be classified solely on the basis of symptoms. A thorough clinical examination using neurological examination techniques forms the basis for assessing the results of further investigation procedures. Special attention has to be paid to sacral reflex arcs and the sacral dermatomes.

Only by means of video-urodynamics it is possible to recognize every functional state within one examination, including the extent of morphological damage during reservoir function and the coordinated or discoordinated emptying phase in order to identify and formulate a diagnosis of NBD. Ultrasound examinations of the urinary tract, urine tests, and the determination of endogenous creatinine clearance are used to estimate secondary damage caused by the NBD. Only in case of minor muscular failure the determination of renal function may be done by estimation formulas (e.g., after surgery in the pelvis, after pelvic fractures, or after unisegmental disorders because of disc herniation).

A urodynamic examination in spinal anesthesia (or if not possible under general anesthesia) will be helpful in case of doubtful low-compliance bladder. An organically fixed low-compliance bladder will not improve appreciably under spinal anesthesia; a low compliance as a result of neurogenic overactivity will normalize.

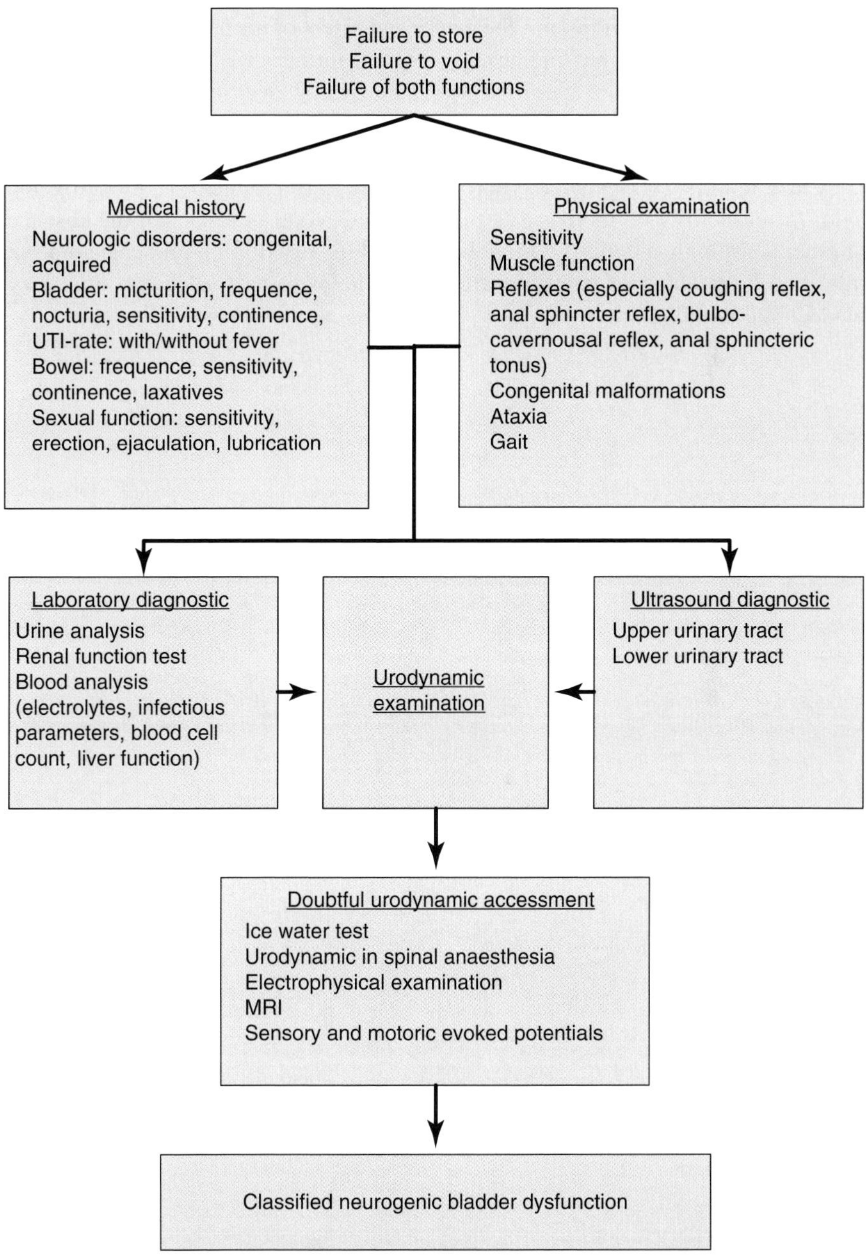

54.4 Differential Diagnosis

NBD can be distinguished from the non-neurogenic bladder disorders by the absence of neurological symptoms. There are more difficulties to demarcate NBD from psychosomatic disorders of any kind. Here the key point is the discrepancy between the described symptoms, the nature and extent of the neurological manifestations, and the urodynamic findings. To confirm, further investigations are helpful such as urodynamics under anesthesia with a transrectal electrical stimulation of the ventral sacral roots. A normal-shaped detrusor contraction argues against a damage to the lower motor neuron.

A lazy bladder (lazy voider syndrome) can be differentiated from neurogenic hypo-/acontractility on the basis of the sustained sacral reflexes and the absence of other neurological deficits. Often the medical history (high liquid consumption rates and a rare bladder emptying frequency) helps to cast suspicion on a lazy bladder syndrome.

Urethritis

55

Katrin Harrer and Thomas Knoll

55.1 Definition

Urethritis describes an inflammation of the urethra, which can be either infectious or noninfectious. The most common symptoms are dysuria, urethral discharge and urethral pruritus. Infectious urethritis is divided into gonococcal and nongonococcal urethritis (NGU). NGU can be caused by *Chlamydia trachomatis (*most common), *Mycoplasma genitalium*, *Candida*, herpes, *Trichomonas* or common bacteria, for example, *E. coli.* Infectious urethritis is most likely spread by sexual contact. Reasons for noninfectious urethritis can be, for example, allergic or mechanical. Risk factors are young age (≤25 years), promiscuity and unprotected sexual contact.

55.2 Medical History

Concerning the ongoing symptoms, doctors are supposed to ask about the presence of urethral discharge including colour and viscosity. Mucoid or clear discharge can be a hint for NGU while purulent discharge indicates infection with *N. gonorrhoeae*. Questions about problems with urination, like higher frequency, urgency, pain or difficulty to start to urinate, should also be asked. Furthermore, the patient should be asked about recent sexual contacts (changing partners, unprotected sex) and about possible symptoms of the sexual partner. Incubation time ranges from 2 to 6 days after exposure of *N. gonorrhoeae* and around 2 weeks for NGU. Information about previous urinary tract infections, previous surgery or other illnesses might also be helpful.

K. Harrer (✉) • T. Knoll
Department of Urology, Klinikum Sindelfingen-Böblingen,
Arthur-Gruber-Str. 70, Sindelfingen 71065, Germany
e-mail: k.harrer@klinikverbund-suedwest.de; t.knoll@klinikverbund-suedwest.de

A.S. Merseburger et al. (eds.), *Urology at a Glance*,
DOI 10.1007/978-3-642-54859-8_55, © Springer-Verlag Berlin Heidelberg 2014

55.3 Diagnostics

Besides the assessment of medical history, physical examination of the penis and testes is the basic diagnostic means. Special attention should be turned on possible urethral secretion; sometimes discharge can be provoked by "milking" the urethra. Furthermore, urine sample of first-void urine (at least 2 h after last urination) is to be analysed. A finding of >10 leucocytes per field of view (400-times magnified) in the urine sample indicates an infectious urethritis. If existent, an examination of urethral discharge with >5 leucocytes per high-power field (1,000-times magnified Gram-stain microscopy) is proof for infectious urethritis. With the help of the Gram-stain test, it is even possible to determine gonococcal infection by detecting leucocytes containing gram-negative intracellular diplococci. If these rapid tests are negative but infectious urethritis is suspected, further examination is necessary. Even if the rapid tests give proof for infectious urethritis but no diplococci are present, microbiological tests are useful to determine the specific pathogen. Although treatment for the different types of bacterial infections is very similar, it is proven that the patients' compliance is higher in case of determination of a specific pathogen, and it also might be of importance for the treatment of the patient's sexual partner as, for example, some pathogens might lead to infertility or even cancer in women. By using nucleic acid amplification testing (NAAT), distinction between, for example, *N. gonorrhoeae*, *Chlamydia trachomatis* and herpes is possible.

55.4 Differential Diagnosis

Differential Diagnosis	Diagnostics
Infectious	
N. gonorrhoeae	Microscopy of urethral discharge (UD): Gram-negative diplococci (Fig. 55.1)
Chlamydia trachomatis	PCR/NAAT of first-catch morning urine or UD
Mycoplasma	PCR/NAAT of first-catch morning urine or UD
Candida	Mycological culture of urine or UD
Herpes	PCR of urethral swab
Trichomonas	Microscopy (native preparation) of urethral swab
Gram-negative bacteria (e.g. *E. coli*)	Microbiological culture of urine, UD or urethral swab
Noninfectious	
Diabetes	Dipstick, blood analysis (HbA1c)
Typhus abdominalis	Anamnesis, blood analysis (eosinopenia), blood culture
Reiter's disease	Anamnesis/symptoms (conjunctivitis, arthritis)
Mechanical	Anamnesis (trauma, self-manipulation), physical examination
Allergic	Anamnesis, dermatological examination (allergy test)
Anomalies of the lower urinary tract	Physical examination, urethrography, micturition urethrocystography (Fig. 55.2)

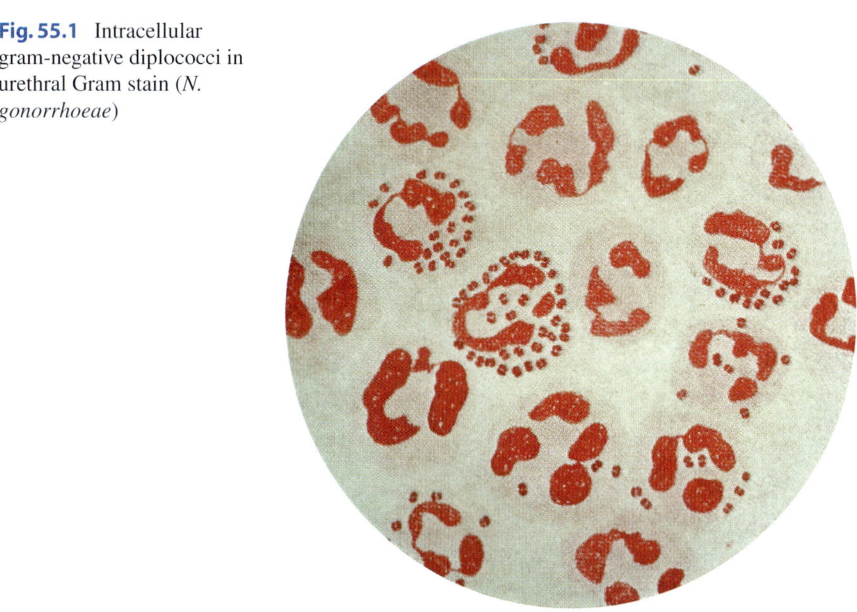

Fig. 55.1 Intracellular gram-negative diplococci in urethral Gram stain (*N. gonorrhoeae*)

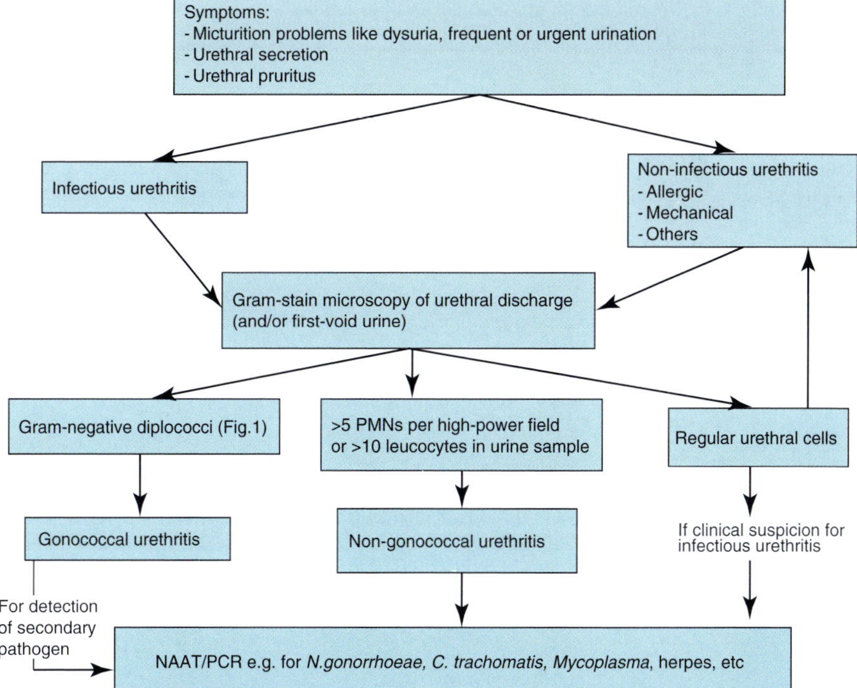

Fig. 55.2 Flow chart for the diagnosis of urethritis

Upper Urinary Tract Cancer

56

Marie C. Hupe, Thomas R. Herrmann, and Axel S. Merseburger

56.1 General Facts

Urothelial cancers are the fourth most common cancer of which more than 95 % originate from the urothelium. The majority of these tumors arise within the bladder (90–95 %) while only 5–10 % occur in the upper urinary tract, i.e., renal pelvis and ureter (upper urinary tract urothelial cell carcinomas (UUTUCCs)). Tumors of the pyelocaliceal system are more common than ureteral tumors. Two thirds (60 %) of the UUTUCCs are invasive when diagnosed and 8–13 % of all patients present with concomitant bladder cancer. UUTUCC more commonly affects patients at approximately 80 years of age with a male to female ratio of 3:1 [1]. Patients with an invasive tumor (T2-4) have a significantly lower 5-year disease-specific survival rate than patients with a superficial tumor (Ta and T1), 16.8 and 70.8 %, respectively [2]. Risk factors for UUTUCC include smoking, analgesics, chronic urinary tract infection, stone disease, and chemotherapeutic agents such as cyclophosphamide. There is also an increased risk for UUTUCC with patients who have been diagnosed with primary bladder cancer (10 %). Prognostic factors include stage, grade, lymph node invasion, lymphovascular invasion, tumor necrosis, and tumor architecture (infiltrative) [3].

56.2 Symptoms, Classification, and Grading

Patients with UUTUCC may present with hematuria, flank pain, or a lumbar mass. Symptoms such as massive weight loss, night sweats, and/or fever may indicate a more advanced stage of disease. UUTUCCs can be grouped into noninvasive papillary tumors, flat lesions (carcinoma in situ), or invasive carcinomas. The 2004 World

M.C. Hupe • T.R. Herrmann • A.S. Merseburger (✉)
Department of Urology and Urological Oncology, Hannover University Medical School, Carl-Neuberg-Str. 1, Hannover 30625, Germany
e-mail: hupe.marie@mh-hannover.de; herrmann.thomas@mh-hannover.de; merseburger.axel@mh-hannover.de

A.S. Merseburger et al. (eds.), *Urology at a Glance*,
DOI 10.1007/978-3-642-54859-8_56, © Springer-Verlag Berlin Heidelberg 2014

Table 56.1 TNM classification of UUTUCCs [1]

T – primary tumor	
TX	Primary tumor cannot be assessed
T0	No evidence of primary tumor
Ta	Noninvasive papillary tumor
Tis	Carcinoma in situ
T1	Tumor invades subepithelial connective tissue
T2	Tumor invades muscularis
T3	(Renal pelvis) tumor invades beyond muscularis into peripelvic fat or renal parenchyma
	(Ureter) tumor invades beyond muscularis into periureteric fat
T4	Tumor invades adjacent organs or through the kidney into perinephric fat
N – regional lymph nodes	
NX	Regional lymph nodes cannot be assessed
N0	No regional lymph node metastasis
N1	Metastasis in a single lymph node ≤2 cm in the greatest dimension
N2	Metastasis in a single lymph node >2 cm but no more than 5 cm in the greatest dimension or multiple lymph nodes, none >5 cm in greatest dimension
N3	Metastasis in a lymph node >5 cm in greatest dimension
M – distant metastasis	
M0	No distant metastasis
M1	Distant metastasis

Health Organization (WHO) grading system subclassifies the noninvasive papillary tumors into papillary neoplasms of low malignant potential, low-grade carcinomas, and high-grade carcinomas. Prior to this, UUTUCC was classified into Grades 1–3 according to the 1973 WHO grading system. Tumor staging is most commonly characterized according to the current tumor node metastasis (TNM 2009) staging system (Table 56.1) [1, 3].

56.3 Therapy

Computed tomographic urography (CTU) and urine cytology should be performed for diagnosis. However, a positive urine cytology result can only be linked to UUTUCC when a malignant transformation of the bladder and prostatic urethra can be ruled out by cystoscopy. Additionally, it can be decided individually whether a ureteroscopy should be performed in order to provide a specimen or a selective ureteral cytology (Fig. 56.1) [1].

The gold standard for treatment of UUTUCC is open nephroureterectomy (ONU) including resection of the bladder cuff surrounding the ureteral orifice. Figure 56.1 shows the current recommendations for treatment. Laparoscopic nephroureterectomy (LNU) is becoming more common. Advantages of LNU include decreased perioperative pain, decreased blood loss, and a shortened hospital stay, while the oncological outcome including cancer-specific and recurrence-free survival is comparable to ONU. LNU should not be performed in T3/T4 and/or N+/M+ tumors or multifocal tumors. Besides radical NU, there is also the possibility of conservative management/surgery for selected patients. Especially when applying oncological

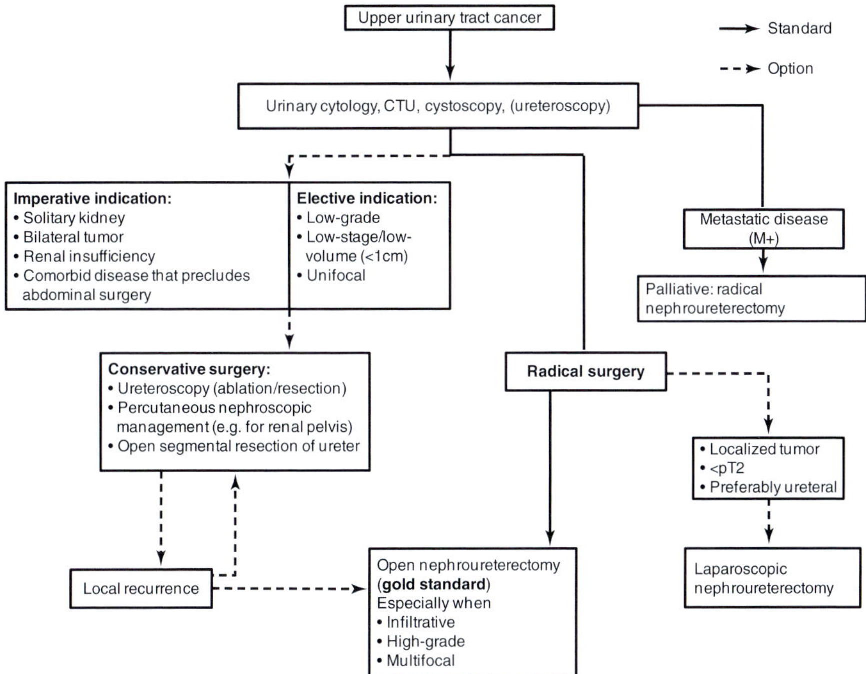

Fig. 56.1 Flow chart demonstrating the pathway from diagnosis to therapy

surgery to a growing number of patients in an ageing cohort with a considerably high prevalence of preoperative latent or apparent chronic renal insufficiency, postoperative renal function has to be taken into account when considering radical vs. organ-preserving approaches. Thus, imperative indications for organ-preserving management include renal insufficiency, as well as, a solitary kidney, a bilateral tumor, or comorbidities precluding abdominal surgery. Elective indications for organ-preserving management include a low grade, low stage/low volume (<1cm), and unifocal tumor (Fig. 56.1). Patients who underwent organ-preserving management need to comply with a strict follow-up plan over at least 5 years, including cystoscopy, ureteroscopy, urinary cytology, and CTU due to the high risk for recurrence. Patients who underwent radical NU also need to comply with a follow-up plan (cytology, cystoscopy, CTU) in order to be able to detect a contralateral cancer, bladder cancer, or metastases. Muscle-invasive UUTUCCs have a high risk for lymph node metastases (30 %). Some studies have shown a staging and therapeutic benefit of lymphadenectomy, e.g., it may be an independent factor for cancer-specific survival. Nevertheless, whether or not a lymphadenectomy should be performed remains controversial due to the lack of a standard lymphadenectomy template and thus comparable studies. In cases of advanced disease (M+), nephroureterectomy is performed for palliative measures. The role of instillation of BCG or mitomycin (e.g., as adjuvant therapy after endoscopic treatment), or chemotherapy, is not clearly defined yet and requires further evaluation. Radiation has not proven to be of significant benefit in the treatment for UUTUCC [1, 3–9].

56.4 Complications

Complications associated with UUTUCC can include renal obstruction with subsequent renal failure, hematuria, and/or pain at an advanced stage.

Additionally, there is a high risk of recurrence in the bladder or the contralateral urinary tract (30–51 %) [6].

References

1. Roupret M, Zigeuner R, Palou J, Boehle A, Kaasinen E, Sylvester R, Babjuk M, Oosterlinck W. European guidelines for the diagnosis and management of upper urinary tract urothelial cell carcinomas: 2011 update. Eur Urol. 2011;59(4):584–94.
2. Simsir A, Sarsik B, Cureklibatir I, Sen S, Gunaydin G, Cal C. Prognostic factors for upper urinary tract urothelial carcinomas: stage, grade, and smoking status. Int Urol Nephrol. 2011;43(4):1039–45.
3. Verhoest G, Shariat SF, Chromecki TF, Raman JD, Margulis V, Novara G, Seitz C, Remzi M, Roupret M, Scherr DS, et al. Predictive factors of recurrence and survival of upper tract urothelial carcinomas. World J Urol. 2011;29(4):495–501.
4. Ristau BT, Tomaszewski JJ, Ost MC. Upper tract urothelial carcinoma: current treatment and outcomes. Urology. 2012;79(4):749–56.
5. Kondo T, Tanabe K. Role of lymphadenectomy in the management of urothelial carcinoma of the bladder and the upper urinary tract. Int J Urol. 2012;19(8):710–21.
6. Roupret M, Smyth G, Irani J, Guy L, Davin JL, Saint F, Pfister C, Wallerand H, Rozet F. Oncological risk of laparoscopic surgery in urothelial carcinomas. World J Urol. 2009; 27(1):81–8.
7. Rai BP, Shelley M, Coles B, Somani B, Nabi G. Surgical management for upper urinary tract transitional cell carcinoma (UUT-TCC): a systematic review. BJU Int. 2012;110(10):1426–35.
8. Hollingsworth JM, Miller DC, Daignault S, Hollenbeck BK. Rising incidence of small renal masses: a need to reassess treatment effect. J Natl Cancer Inst 2006;98(18):1331–34.
9. Herrmann TR, Kruck S, Nagele U. Transperitoneal in situ intraarterial cooling in laparoscopic partial nephrectomy. World J Urol 2011;29(3):337–42.

Testicular Cancer

57

Kathleen F. McGinley and Edward N. Rampersaud Jr.

57.1 General Facts

Though testicular cancer (TC) is the most common malignancy in 15–35-year-old men [1], it accounts for only 1–2 % of all neoplasms in men [2]. Worldwide, the incidence of TC has doubled in 40 years [3]. Risk factors for TC include cryptorchidism, a personal or family history of TC, and intratubular germ cell neoplasia. Over 95 % of testicular cancers are germ cell tumors, including seminomas and nonseminomatous tumors; non-germ cell tumors, including Leydig and Sertoli cell tumors, account for <5 % of all testicular cancers [4]. Men generally present with localized disease (69 %). Five-year relative survival, inclusive of all stages, is 95.3 % [5].

57.2 Symptoms, Classification, and Grading

A painless mass or swelling of the testicle is the presenting symptom in approximately 50 % of patients with TC. A painful scrotum, with or without swelling, is reported in 25–50 % of TC patients [6]. Less commonly, back pain, gynecomastia, flank pain, and weight loss are reported [1]. Scrotal ultrasonography is the imaging modality of choice [4]. If a hypoechoic area within the tunica albuginea, or a testicular mass with irregular borders or calcifications, is identified, serum tumor markers, including AFP, LDH, and beta-hCG, should be obtained preoperatively [3].

TC is classified histologically (Fig. 57.1) and by the TMN system (Fig. 57.2). Following a diagnosis of TC, a CT of the abdomen and pelvis, chest x-ray, and repeat serum markers are obtained to enable stage grouping (Fig. 57.3).

K.F. McGinley • E.N. Rampersaud Jr. (✉)
Division of Urology, Department of Surgery, Duke University Medical Center,
DUMC 2812, Durham, NC 27710, USA
e-mail: edward.rampersaud@duke.edu

A.S. Merseburger et al. (eds.), *Urology at a Glance*,
DOI 10.1007/978-3-642-54859-8_57, © Springer-Verlag Berlin Heidelberg 2014

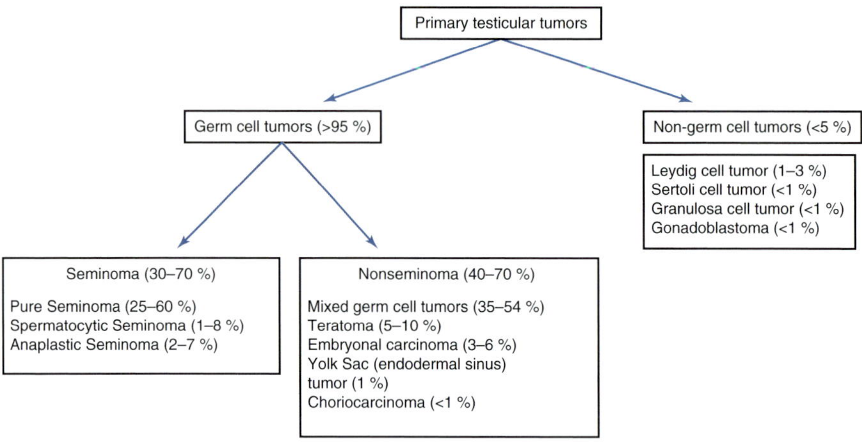

Fig. 57.1 Data derived from Reuter [9], Stephenson and Gilligan [4]

TNM Staging			
Definition of TNM			
Primary Tumor (T)			
PTX	Primary tumor cannot be assessed		
PT0	No evidence of primary tumor		
PTis	Intratubular germ cell neoplasia (carcinoma *in situ*)		
PT1	Tumor limited to the testis and epididymis and no vascular/lymphatic invasion		
PT2	Tumor limited to the testis and epididymis with vascular/lymphatic invasion or tumor extending through the tunica albuginea with involvement of tunica vaginalis		
PT3	Tumor invades the spermatic cord with or without vascular/lymphatic invasion		
PT4	Tumor invades the scrotum with or without vascular/lymphatic invasion		
Regional Lymph Nodes (N)			
Clinical			
Nx	Regional lymph nodes cannot be assessed		
N0	No regional lymph node metastasis		
N1	Lymph node mass ≤2 cm in greatest dimension or multiple lymph nodes masses, none >2 cm in greatest dimension		
N2	Lymph node mass >2 cm but <5 cm in greatest dimension, or multiple lymph node masses >2 cm but < 5 cm in greatest dimension		
N3	Lymph node mass >5 cm in greatest dimension		
Pathologic			
PN0	No evidence of tumor in lymph nodes		
PN1	Lymph mass ≤2 cm in greatest dimension and ≤5 nodes positive, none >2 cm in greatest dimension		
PN2	Lymph node mass >2 cm but <5 cm in greatest dimension; >5 nodes positive, none >5 cm; evidence of extranodal extension of tumor		
PN3	Lymph node mass >5 cm in greatest dimension		
Distant Metastases (M)			
M0	No evidence of distant metastases		
M1	Non-regional nodal or pulmonary metastases		
M2	Non -pulmonary visceral metastases		
Serum Tumor Markers (S)			
	LDH	HCG	AFP
S0	≤ Upper Limit of Normal (ULN)	≤ULN	≤ULN
S1	<1.5 x ULN	< 5,000	< 1,000
S2	1.5 –10 x ULN	5,000 – 50,000	1,000 –10,000
S3	> 10 x ULN	> 50,000	> 10,000

Fig. 57.2 Testicular cancer staging system of the American Joint Committee of Cancer (Data from Carver and Feldman [10])

Testicular cancer staging				
Stage Grouping	T	N	M	S
Stage 0	PTis	N0	M0	S0
Stage IA	T1	N0	M0	S0
Stage IB	≥T2	N0	M0	S0
Stage IS	Any T	N0	M0	S1-S3
Stage IIA	Any T	N1	M0	S0, S1
Stage IIB	Any T	N2	M0	S0, S1
Stage IIC	Any T	N3	M0	S0, S1
Stage IIIA	Any T	Any N	M1	S0, S1
Stage IIIB	Any T	Any N	M0, M1	S2
Stage IIIC	Any T	Any N	M0, M1	S3

Fig. 57.3 Testicular cancer staging system of the American Joint Committee of Cancer (Data from Carver and Feldman [10])

57.3 Therapy

Discuss sperm banking prior to surgical intervention [3]. Initial therapy for suspected TC is a radical inguinal orchiectomy. Serum tumor markers should be followed postoperatively to assess for response to therapy, persistence of disease, and recurrence of disease in follow-up [3]. Nonseminomatous germ cell tumors are associated with a higher stage at diagnosis, a higher incidence of occult metastasis, and a higher incidence of systemic relapse following treatment of the retroperitoneum. In comparison, seminomas have a relatively favorable natural history and are exquisitely sensitive to radiotherapy and platinum-based chemotherapy [4]. Following radical orchiectomy, treatment is dictated by tumor histology, stage, and the presence of residual disease (Figs. 57.4 and 57.5).

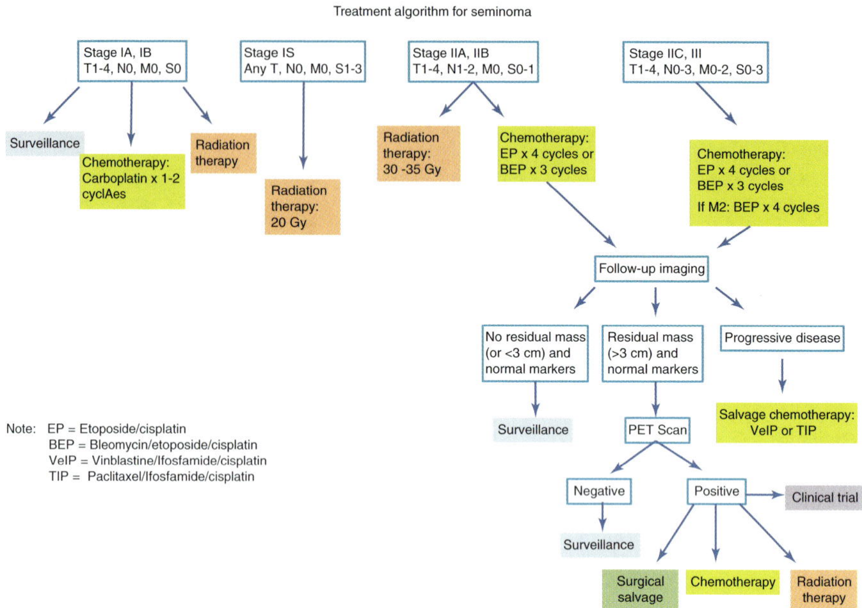

Fig. 57.4 Algorithm modified from the National Comprehensive Cancer Network [3]

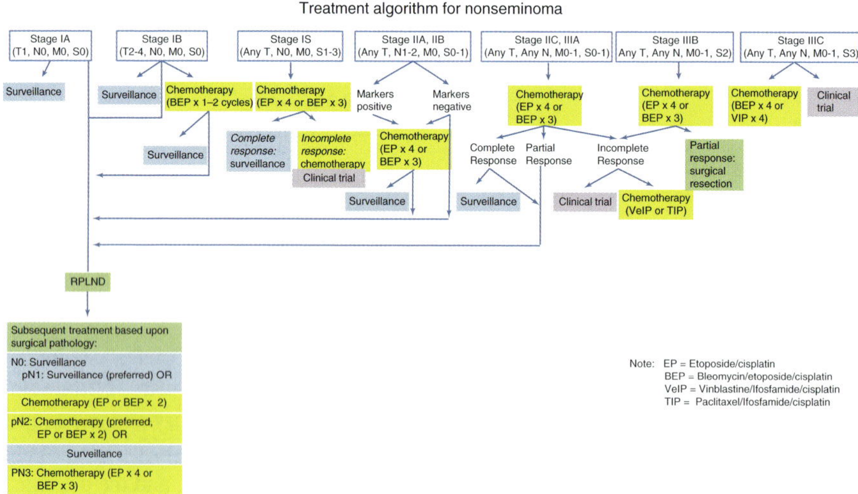

Fig. 57.5 Algorithm modified from the National Comprehensive Cancer Network [3]

57.4 Complications

Morbidity associated with inguinal orchiectomy is limited. Possible complications of a retroperitoneal lymph node dissection include adjacent organ injury, ejaculatory dysfunction, infertility, thromboembolic events, and chylous ascites. Adverse effects of chemotherapy for TC include sensory neuropathy, ototoxicity, pulmonary toxicity, neurotoxicity, cardiotoxicity, nephrotoxicity, infertility, and secondary malignancies. Complications of radiotherapy include cutaneous changes, secondary malignancies, cardiotoxicity, and infertility. On surveillance, disease relapse occurs in 25–35 % of patients [7]. Anxiety [7] and a possible increased risk of secondary malignancies due to the volume of ionizing radiation [8] associated with surveillance imaging are cited.

References

1. Masterson TA, Beck SDW. Testicular cancer: clinical signs and symptoms. In: Scardino PT, Linehan WM, Zelefsky MJ, Vogelzang NJ, editors. Comprehensive textbook of genitourinary oncology. Philadelphia: Wolters Kluwer; 2011. p. 505–8.
2. Huyghe E, Matsuda T, Thonneau P. Increasing incidence of testicular cancer worldwide: a review. J Urol. 2003;170(1):5–11.
3. National Comprehensive Cancer Network. Testicular cancer (Version 1.2013). http://www.nccn.org/professionals/physician_gls/pdf/testicular.pdf. Accessed 15 Sept 2013.
4. Stephenson AJ, Gilligan TD. Neoplasms of the testis. In: Wein AJ, Kavoussi LR, Novick AC, Partin AW, Peters CA, editors. Campbell-Walsh urology. 10th ed. Philadelphia: Elsevier; 2011. p. 837–70.
5. National Cancer Institute SEER Stat Fact Sheets: Testis. http://seer.cancer.gov/statfacts/html/testis.html. Accessed 15 Sept 2013.
6. Moul JW. Timely diagnosis of testicular cancer. Urol Clin North Am. 2007;34(2):109–17.
7. Kaufman MR, Chang SS. Short and long-term complications of therapy for testicular cancer. Urol Clin North Am. 2007;34(2):259–68.
8. Tarin TV, Sonn G, Shinghal R. Estimating the risk of cancer associated with imaging related radiation during surveillance for stage I testicular cancer using computed tomography. J Urol. 2009;181(2):627–33.
9. Reuter VE. Anatomy and pathology of testis cancer. In: Scardino PT, Linehan WM, Zelefsky MJ, Vogelzang NJ, editors. Comprehensive textbook of genitourinary oncology. 4th ed. Philadelphia: Wolters Kluwer; 2011. p. 531–41.
10. Carver BS, Feldman DR. Staging of testicular cancer. In: Scardino PT, Linehan WM, Zelefsky MJ, Vogelzang NJ, editors. Comprehensive textbook of genitourinary oncology. 4th ed. Philadelphia: Wolters Kluwer; 2011. p. 544–7.

Penile Cancer

58

Chris Protzel, Brant A. Inman, and Oliver W. Hakenberg

58.1 General Facts

Penile cancer is a rare tumor entity in Europe and North America, e.g., the estimated incidence in Germany is 1.4 cases per 100,000 men [1, 2]. Due to poor economic and hygienic conditions, the incidence in countries of South America and Southeast Asia is tenfold higher [1]. Penile cancer is most frequently found in men between 60 and 80 years. Younger patients often suffer from more aggressive subtypes. This fact has to be taken into consideration for treatment.

Penile cancer represents a group of different histological subtypes of squamous cell carcinomas which show great differences in pathogenesis, biological behavior and prognosis. The conventional squamous cell carcinoma, the most frequent subtype, is associated with high-risk human papillomavirus (HPV) in only 30–50 % of the cases, while the more aggressive warty and basaloid subtypes show an HPV association in 80–100 % [3]. Verrucous and papillary subtypes are characterized by a low tendency of metastatic spread and good prognosis [3, 4].

Besides the histological subtype, the presence of lymph node metastasis is the most important prognostic factor for survival in penile cancer. Patients without lymph node metastasis show a 5-year survival rate of over 90 %, while the 5-year survival rate for patients with lymph node metastasis is around 80 % for pN1, 10–60 % in pN2, and below 10 % for pN3 patients [5, 6].

The most important risk factors for penile cancer are chronic inflammation and phimosis. The role of HPV infection for pathogenesis of conventional squamous

C. Protzel (✉) • O.W. Hakenberg
Department of Urology, University of Rostock,
Ernst-Heydemann-Straße 6, Rostock 18055, Germany
e-mail: chris.protzel@med.uni-rostock.de

B.A. Inman, MD, MS, FRCSC
Division of Urology, Department of Surgery, Duke University
Medical Center, DUMC 2812, Durham, NC 27710, USA
e-mail: brant.inman@duke.edu

A.S. Merseburger et al. (eds.), *Urology at a Glance*,
DOI 10.1007/978-3-642-54859-8_58, © Springer-Verlag Berlin Heidelberg 2014

cell carcinomas remains under discussion. Tobacco smoking, alcohol abuse, and promiscuity are other risk factors [7].

58.2 Symptoms, Classification, Grading

Persistent penile efflorescences lead to a consultation and diagnosis in early stages of carcinoma in situ or invasive tumors in most cases. Diagnosis is frequently delayed due to phimosis in older patients. Carcinoma in situ is characterized by red efflorescences at the glans or prepuce. Penile carcinomas appear as exophytic tumors or ulcerous lesions. In advanced stages, the penis can be completely destroyed by the tumor. In a number of cases, enlarged metastatic inguinal lymph nodes are the reason for the first consultation.

Diagnosis of the primary tumor includes clinical examination (number of lesions, size, morphology, involved sites). Infiltration of the corpora cavernosa can be examined by ultrasonography. MRI was shown as a diagnostic tool in case of planned organ-sparing surgery [2].

Clinical examination of the inguinal lymph nodes is not a reliable predictor for lymph node metastases. Metastases are found in 50 % of palpable lymph nodes, while up to 20 % of patients with non-palpable lymph node may suffer from micrometastases [8]. Common imaging techniques like ultrasonography and computed tomography (CT) are not able to distinguish between reactive lesions and metastases. Although PET CT shows a sensitivity of 80 % for enlarged inguinal lymph nodes, it is not suitable for the diagnosis of micrometastases [9]. Since the presence of lymph node metastases is the most important prognostic factor for patients with penile cancer, an invasive lymph node staging (modified inguinal lymphadenectomy or dynamic sentinel node biopsy) has to be recommended for every patient with invasive penile cancer [8].

In order to improve the indication for lymphadenectomy, the current TNM classification of the UICC subdivided early invasive stages into pT1a (no vascular invasion, G1 or G2 grading) and pT1b (vascular invasion or G3 or G4 grading). Since recent studies have shown great interobserver differences in grading, the new classification of pT1 tumors remains under discussion [10]. A new grading system has to be established for penile cancer in the next years. Due to the poor prognosis of patients with fixed inguinal lymph nodes, the clinical N3 stage now includes palpable fixed inguinal lymph nodes and pelvic lymph node metastases. Extranodal extension of lymph node metastases is now also classified as pN3 due to the poor prognosis. The complete TNM classification is shown in Table 58.1 [10].

58.3 Therapy

Since chemotherapy is not able to cure patients with advanced penile cancer, an early and complete resection of the primary tumor and lymph node metastases has to be the aim in all patients. Therefore, therapy has to include the first step of

Table 58.1 TNM classification by the UICC

T – primary tumor
TX Primary tumor cannot be assessed
T0 No evidence of primary tumor
Tis Carcinoma in situ
Ta Noninvasive verrucous carcinoma, not associated with destructive invasion
T1 Tumor invades subepithelial connective tissue
T1a
Tumor invades subepithelial connective tissue without lymphovascular invasion and is not poorly differentiated or undifferentiated (T1G1-2)
T1b
Tumor invades subepithelial connective tissue without with lymphovascular invasion or is poorly differentiated or undifferentiated (T1G3-4)
T2 Tumor invades corpus spongiosum/corpora cavernosa
T3 Tumor invades urethra
T4 Tumor invades other adjacent structures
N – regional lymph nodes (clinical)
NX Regional lymph nodes cannot be assessed
N0 No palpable or visibly enlarged inguinal lymph node
N1 Palpable mobile unilateral inguinal lymph node
N2 Palpable mobile multiple or bilateral inguinal lymph nodes
N3 Fixed inguinal nodal mass or pelvic lymphadenopathy, unilateral or bilateral
pN – regional lymph nodes (pathologic)
pNX Regional lymph nodes cannot be assessed
pN0 No regional lymph node metastasis
pN1 Intranodal metastasis in a single inguinal lymph node
pN2 Metastasis in multiple or bilateral inguinal lymph nodes
pN3 Metastasis in pelvic lymph node(s), unilateral or bilateral or extranodal extension of regional lymph node metastasis
M – distant metastases
M0 No distant metastasis
M1 Distant metastasis

resection of the primary tumor and the second step of a sufficient lymph node management.

The resection of the primary tumor has to be adapted to the size and site of the tumor as well as to the depth of infiltration. In early stages, organ-preserving surgery is an option but has to include an intraoperative pathologic assessment of tumor-free margins. Carcinoma in situ can be treated with excision or circumcision in case of involvement of the prepuce. Local chemotherapy shows control rates of 50 % and can be recommended for patients with good compliance [11]. Laser therapy is also a first-line option. In case of local recurrence, a complete excision and glans resurfacing has to be discussed as a therapeutic option. All pTa and small pT1 (pT1a) tumors can be treated by excision or circumcision followed by plastic reconstructions. Skin grafts can be used in case of larger lesions. For pT1b tumors and pT2 tumors without infiltration of the corpora cavernosa, a glansectomy with skin graft reconstruction can be offered to the patient. All pT2 tumors with infiltration of the corpora cavernosa and pT3 and pT4 tumors need to be treated with partial penectomy or complete penectomy with perineal urethrostomy. An intraoperative pathologic assessment of tumor-free margins of at least 10 mm is recommended in these cases [2].

The lymph node management depends on the clinical appearance of inguinal lymph nodes. For patients with palpable fixed inguinal lymph node metastases, a neoadjuvant chemotherapy followed by a salvage inguinal and pelvic lymphadenectomy is recommended. All patients with enlarged palpable inguinal lymph nodes have to undergo radical inguinal lymphadenectomy after histological confirmation of metastases [8]. In case of negative excision biopsy, at least a modified inguinal lymphadenectomy is necessary.

Since a relevant number of patients without palpable inguinal lymph nodes have micrometastases, an invasive lymph node staging is recommended by the EAU guidelines [2]. Therefore, all patients with pT1G2 tumors or higher should undergo a modified inguinal lymphadenectomy or a dynamic sentinel lymph node biopsy in experienced centers. For patients undergoing dynamic sentinel node biopsy, a relevant number of false-negative examinations has to be taken into consideration (5–12 %). In case of positive lymph nodes, a radical inguinal lymphadenectomy has to be performed.

For all patients with two or more inguinal lymph node metastases or extranodal tumor growth, a pelvic lymphadenectomy of the iprilateral side is recommended. Since a survival benefit for patients after adjuvant chemotherapy in comparison to a historical control group was shown, all patients with pN2 and pN3 status may benefit from an adjuvant chemotherapy [12].

The regimen of chemotherapy remains under discussion. Due to the data of recent studies, a paclitaxel-/cisplatin-based regimen seems useful in a neoadjuvant and adjuvant setting. The results of chemotherapy for advanced tumors with distant metastases are very poor (Fig. 58.1).

58.4 Complications

Psychological problems of the treatment of the primary tumor can be reduced by an early diagnosis and an organ-preserving surgery. The risk of local recurrence has to be taken into consideration and has to be discussed with the patient.

Inguinal lymphadenectomy may cause lymphorrhea, lymphocele, and lymph edema in a relevant number of patients. Wound-healing problems and skin necrosis can be avoided or reduced by subtle intraoperative handling and postoperative vacuum treatment.

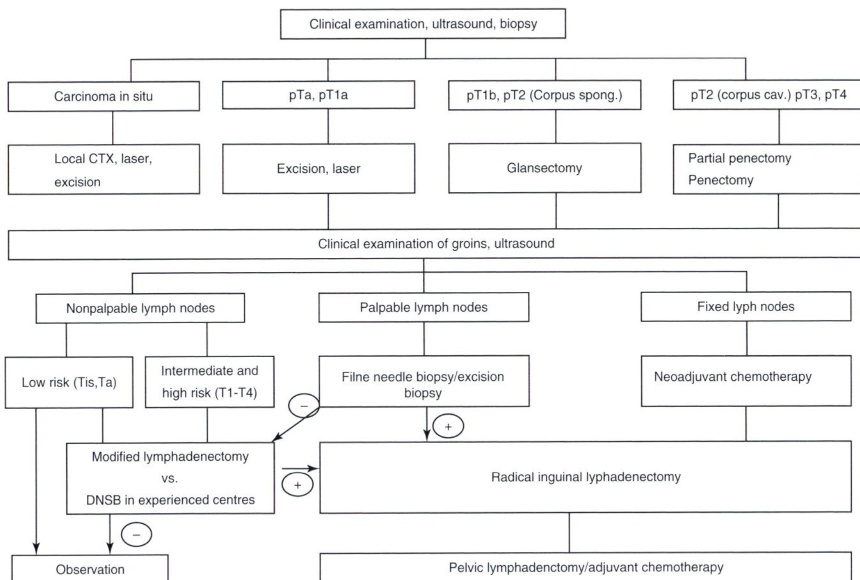

Fig. 58.1 Flow chart for treatment of penile cancer

References

1. Parkin DM, WS, Ferlay J, Teppo L, Thomas DB, editors. Cancer incidence in five continents. IARC scientific publications no 155. Lyon: IARC; 2002.
2. Pizzocaro G, Algaba F, Horenblas S, et al. EAU penile cancer guidelines 2009. Eur Urol. 2010;57:1002–12.
3. Rubin MA, Kleter B, Zhou M, et al. Detection and typing of human papillomavirus DNA in penile carcinoma: evidence for multiple independent pathways of penile carcinogenesis. Am J Pathol. 2001;159:1211–8.
4. Chaux A, Lezcano C, Cubilla AL, Tamboli P, Ro J, Ayala A. Comparison of subtypes of penile squamous cell carcinoma from high and low incidence geographical regions. Int J Surg Pathol. 2010;18:268–77.
5. Ficarra V, Zattoni F, Cunico SC, et al. Lymphatic and vascular embolizations are independent predictive variables of inguinal lymph node involvement in patients with squamous cell carcinoma of the penis: Gruppo Uro-Oncologico del Nord Est (Northeast Uro-Oncological Group) Penile Cancer data base data. Cancer. 2005;103:2507–16.
6. Leijte JA, Kirrander P, Antonini N, Windahl T, Horenblas S. Recurrence patterns of squamous cell carcinoma of the penis: recommendations for follow-up based on a two-centre analysis of 700 patients. Eur Urol. 2008;54:161–8.
7. Dillner J, von Krogh G, Horenblas S, Meijer CJ. Etiology of squamous cell carcinoma of the penis. Scand J Urol Nephrol Suppl. 2000;205:189–93.

8. Protzel C, Alcaraz A, Horenblas S, Pizzocaro G, Zlotta A, Hakenberg OW. Lymphadenectomy in the surgical management of penile cancer. Eur Urol. 2009;55:1075–88.
9. Scher B, Seitz M, Albinger W, et al. Value of PET and PET/CT in the diagnostics of prostate and penile cancer. Recent Results Cancer Res. 2008;170:159–79.
10. Sobin LH, Gospodariwicz M, Wittekind C, editors. TNM classification of malignant tumours. UICC International Union Against Cancer. 7th ed. New York: Wiley-Blackwell; 2009.
11. Alnajjar HM, Lam W, Bolgeri M, Rees RW, Perry MJ, Watkin NA. Treatment of carcinoma in situ of the glans penis with topical chemotherapy agents. Eur Urol. 2012;62:923–8.
12. Pizzocaro G, Piva L, Bandieramonte G, Tana S. Up-to-date management of carcinoma of the penis. Eur Urol. 1997;32:5–15.

Urogenital Trauma

59

Christian Zeckey, Marcel Winkelmann, Christian Macke, Philipp Mommsen, Hossein Tezval, Andrew C. Peterson, and Danielle A. Stackhouse

59.1 Kidney, Ureter, and Bladder Trauma

Marcel Winkelmann, Christian Macke, Philipp Mommsen, and Christian Zeckey

59.1.1 General Facts

The two main reasons of kidney, ureter, and bladder injuries are blunt abdominal trauma and pelvic ring fractures (high energy trauma) [5, 22]. With an incidence of 3–8 % of all fractures, pelvic fractures are relatively rare [3, 26], but within polytrauma, the percentage ascends to 25 % [1, 24, 36]. The incidence of uronephrologic injuries is low. One to five percent of all polytraumatized patients have a renal injury, 90–95 % of it due to blunt trauma [22]. Blunt abdominal trauma occurs in 2–4 % of all accidental injured patients [69, 70]. Penetrating trauma, e.g., stab and bullet wounds, in Europe is seldom, but is accompanied with an increased rate of nephrectomy. Two percent of all operatively treated abdominal injuries concerning the bladder, 67–86 % due to blunt trauma associated to pelvic ring fractures in 70–97 % [6, 8, 22]. The incidence of ureteral injuries is very

C. Zeckey (✉) • M. Winkelmann • C. Macke • P. Mommsen
Trauma Department, Hannover Medical School, Carl-Neuberg-Str. 1, Hannover 30625, Germany
e-mail: zeckey.christian@mh-hannover.de

H. Tezval
Department of Urology and Urological Oncology, Hannover Medical School, Carl-Neuberg-Str. 1, Hannover 30625, Germany
e-mail: tezval.hossein@mh-hannover.de

A.C. Peterson • D.A. Stackhouse
Division of Urology, Department of Surgery, Duke University Medical Center, DUMC 2812, Durham, NC 27710, USA

A.S. Merseburger et al. (eds.), *Urology at a Glance*,
DOI 10.1007/978-3-642-54859-8_59, © Springer-Verlag Berlin Heidelberg 2014

Table 59.1 Kidney

Grade	Type of injury	Description of injury	AIS
1	Contusion	Microscopic or gross hematuria, urologic studies normal	2
	Hematoma	Subcapsular, nonexpanding without parenchymal laceration	2
2	Hematoma	Nonexpanding perirenal hematoma confirmed to renal retroperitoneum	2
	Laceration	<1.0 cm parenchymal depth of renal cortex without urinary extravagation	2
3	Laceration	<1.0 cm parenchymal depth of renal cortex without collecting system rupture or urinary extravagation	3
4	Laceration	Parenchymal laceration extending through the renal cortex, medulla, and collecting system	4
	Vascular	Main renal artery or vein injury with contained hemorrhage	4
5	Laceration	Completely shattered kidney	5
	Vascular	Avulsion of renal hilum which devascularizes the kidney	5

Table 59.2 Ureter

Grade	Type of injury	Description of injury	AIS
1	Hematoma	Contusion or hematoma without devascularization	2
2	Laceration	<50 % transection	2
3	Laceration	≥50 % transection	3
4	Laceration	Complete transection with <2 cm devascularization	3
5	Laceration	Avulsion with >2 cm of devascularization	3

low, concerning only 1 % of all urogenital injuries. 75 % of it are iatrogenic and only 18 % due to blunt and 7 % due to penetrating trauma [29]. But one should be aware of a concomitant urologic injury in case of polytraumatized patients with suspicion of pelvic and/or abdominal trauma, especially motor vehicle accidents and falls from great height [5, 22].

59.1.2 Symptoms and Diagnostic

Because there are no typical clinical signs, medical history is of special importance. The mechanism of injury is helpful for suspicion of urologic injury. One should be aware in case of every pelvic ring fracture and/or blunt abdominal trauma. For optimal treatment, knowledge of preexisting renal diseases and renal dysfunction is necessary [5, 12, 22].

Clinical signs are various and rarely specific. They reach from external signs like bruises, hematoma (e.g., suprapubic in case of bladder lesion), and swelling of the perineum, scrotum, or abdominal wall to abdominal pain and distention, urinary retention/voiding disorder, or suprapubic discomfort. The most suggestive sign is (gross) hematuria, which occurs in 80 % of all bladder lesions, but is not correlated with injury severity [4, 12]. Injury severity can be classified into five grades

Table 59.3 Bladder

Grade	Type of injury	Description of injury	AIS
1	Hematoma	Contusion, intramural hematoma	2
	Laceration	Partial thickness	3
2	Laceration	Extraperitoneal bladder wall laceration <2 cm	4
3	Laceration	Extraperitoneal (>2 cm) or intraperitoneal (<2 cm) bladder wall laceration	4
4	Laceration	Intraperitoneal bladder wall laceration >2 cm	4
5	Laceration	Intraperitoneal or extraperitoneal bladder wall laceration extending into the bladder neck or ureteral orifice (trigone)	4

according to the American Association for the Surgery of Trauma (AAST) (Tables 59.1, 59.2, and 59.3).

Focusing on trauma, isolated kidney, ureter, or bladder lesions are rare. Usually, it is a concomitant injury in multiple injured patients. Therefore, diagnostic depends on the leading symptoms or lesions and hemodynamic stability of the patient. A thorough whole-body examination including palpation of the abdomen and testing pelvic stability is practically obligatory. If blunt thoracic/abdominal trauma or pelvic fracture is suspected, urine should be collected and screened for hematuria in the early phase of diagnostic. Gross hematuria, and microscopic hematuria in combination with other conditions, is a strong indicator for renal and bladder injury, although missing hematuria does not exclude a relevant injury. The diagnostic imaging depends on the hemodynamic stability of the patient. In case of insufficient hemodynamic stabilization with suspected intra-/retroabdominal or pelvic bleeding source, a laparotomy is indicated. Focused assessment with sonography in trauma (FAST) can help to make a decision. If it shows free peritoneal fluid, it is a clear indication for diagnostic laparotomy (and/or early stabilization of pelvic ring in case of fracture) [15, 19, 21, 27]. However, one must acknowledge that a negative FAST does not exclude free peritoneal fluid [13, 39]. Within laparotomy, one-shot intravenous pyelogram (IVP) is best suitable to evaluate the extent of kidney injury [7, 28]. In case of hemodynamic stability, one should aspire to a diagnosis as precise as possible. Contrast-enhanced CT scan with 10–20 min delayed cuts (time until the contrast agent has been excreted into the collecting system) is a diagnostic gold standard in kidney and ureteral injury [22, 34, 35, 38]. Diagnostic peritoneal lavage (DPL) is a safe and sensitive diagnostic approach to identify free peritoneal fluid and reduce the use of CT in blunt abdominal trauma, but is meanwhile not used routinely [15, 37]. The standard diagnostic tool for detecting bladder injuries is a retrograde cystogram that is almost 100 % sensitive and can be performed by conventional radiology or by CT scan but might not be feasible in a notable number of trauma patients due to overall injury severity and other diagnostic and therapeutic needs [9, 18, 20, 31, 33]. When combined upper and lower tract urologic injuries are suspected, the upper tract contrast study should be performed prior to the cystogram, as retained contrast in the abdomen or retroperitoneum can obscure upper tract pathology [12].

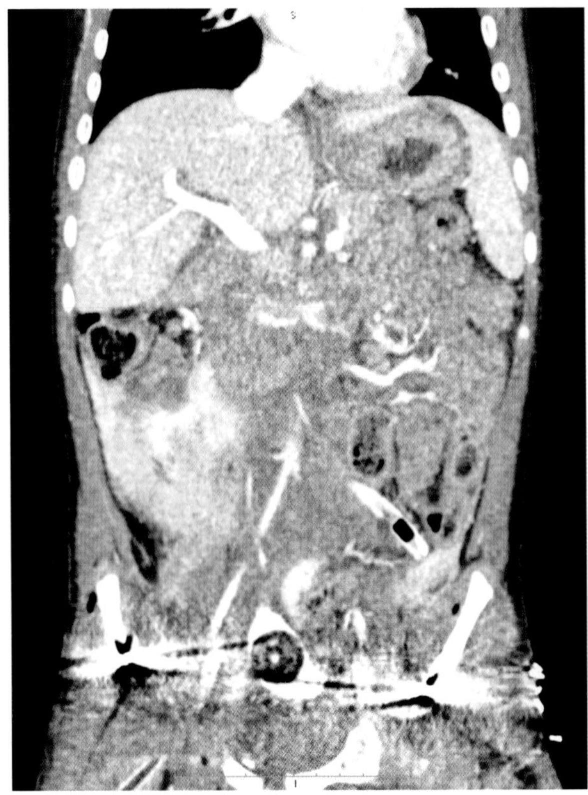

Rupture of right ureter near crossing over the iliac artery

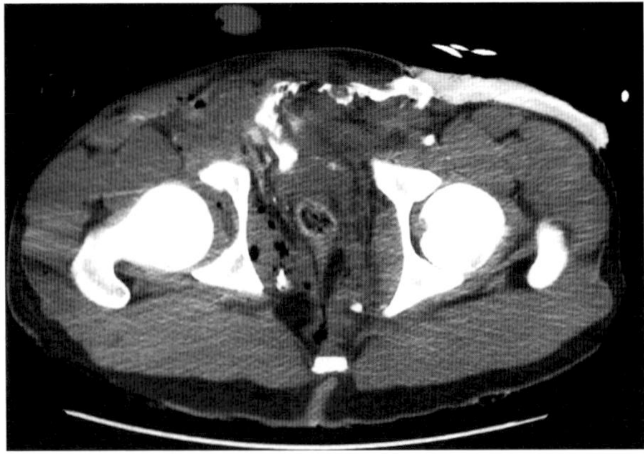

Accompanying rupture of the bladder within a complex pelvic ring fracture

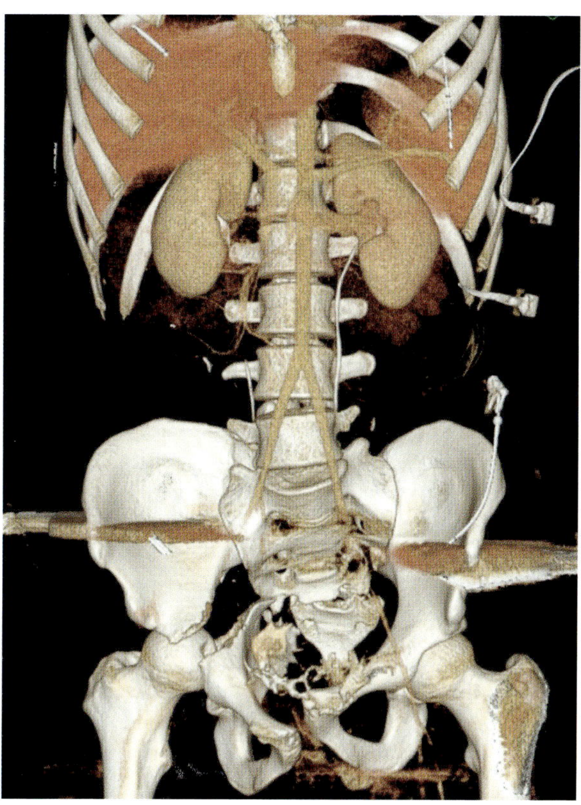

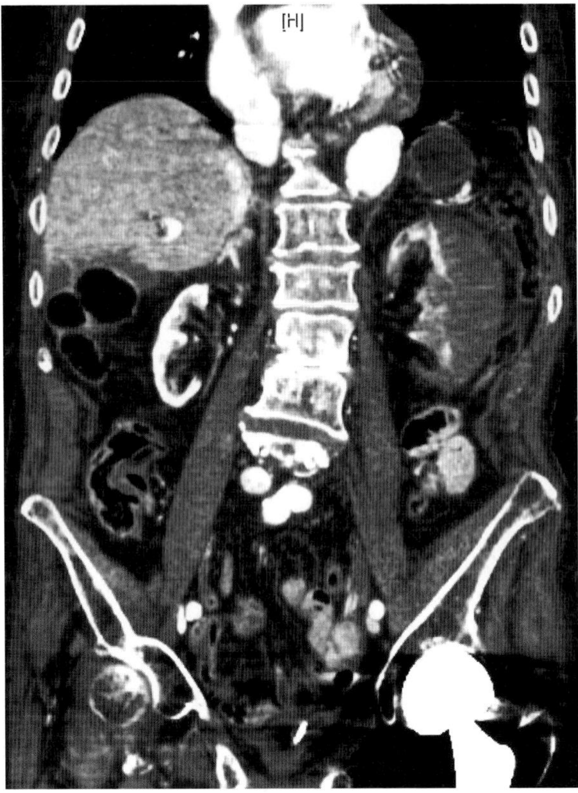

Rupture of the left kidney with capsule hematoma

59.1.3 Therapy

Specific therapy depends on the hemodynamic stability of the patient and the injury severity.

Kidney injuries Grades I–III (and even IV–V under special conditions) could be treated nonoperatively that comprises appropriate imaging, close follow-up of vital signs, red blood count laboratory results, volume therapy, antibiotics, and bed rest [40]. Indications for operative treatment are hemorrhagic shock without response to volume therapy or suspected increasing perirenal hematoma or brisk bleeding [11, 17]. Prolonged bleeding, suspicion of associated injury of renal pelvis or ureteral lesions, and renal artery thrombosis are relative indications. Renovascular injuries or occlusion requires an instant nephrectomy (Grade V) or delayed nephrectomy (Grade IV). Renorrhaphy and partial nephrectomy can be performed to salvage the renal function [5, 40]. Selective or superselective embolization or stenting (in case of intima lesion) eventually in combination with ureteral catheterization or percutaneous nephrostomy is reserved for special indications [16].

Ureteral injuries Grades I and II should be treated with retrograde ureteropyelography and implantation of double-J catheter. Grades 3–5 injuries usually require a surgical treatment. Specific surgical technique required depends on the localization of the impairment. Injuries of the proximal third should be treated with ureteroureterostomy, calico-ureteral anastomosis (ureterocalicostomy), or ipsilateral renal autotransplantation; injuries of the mid-third with ureteroureterostomy (possible, if <3 cm loss of ureteral length) or transureteroureterostomy (contralateral ureter); and injuries of the distal third with ureterovesical reimplantation into the vesical dome (ureteroneocystostomy with psoas hitch of the bladder). Intestinal replacement plastics (ureteroilioplasty, ureterocoloplasty, appendiculoplasty) remain reserved for complex injuries [2, 5, 40].

Treatment of bladder lesions primarily is nonoperative. This can be performed in most extraperitoneal injuries with transurethral catheterization. In about 90 %, healing occurs within 10 days [18]. Operative approach is necessary in case of intraperitoneal lesion, penetrating bladder injury, involved vesical neck, bone fragments in the vesical wall, or bony incarceration of the bladder [25]. The preferred standard of care is a formal surgical repair with absorbable suture [23].

59.1.4 Complications

The most important complications after kidney injury are urinoma, perinephric abscess, secondary hemorrhage, arteriovenous fistula, hypertension, and renal failure [34]. Persistent urinary extravasation can result in urinoma, perinephric infection, and late renal loss and therefore warrants a percutaneous drainage. Delayed bleeding (up to 30 days after trauma) can occur in 13–25 % of higher-grade renal injuries that could be treated best with selective or superselective angiographic embolization. Late stenosis or thrombosis of renal arteries can lead to devitalizing of renal fragments or late-onset hypertension (long-term follow-up of blood pressure) [5, 30, 32, 34].

Urinoma, periureteral abscess, fistula, and stricture are the most frequent complications. Stenting the ureter can surely prevent most of these complications [10, 41].

There is a variety of complications after bladder injury. An unnoticed urinary extravasation can result in uroascites, ileus, abdominal distension, sepsis, peritonitis, and localized abscesses that require a surgical treatment. Other complications like incontinence, fistula, or stricture may necessitate complex reconstruction procedures if repair of bladder neck or vaginal and rectal involvement has not or poorly been performed at once. Distinct plexus or nerve lesions within pelvic ring fractures can lead to denervation of the bladder and consecutive voiding disturbances [14, 40].

59.2 Penile, Urethral, and Scrotal Trauma

Andrew C. Peterson, Hossein Tezval, and Danielle A. Stackhouse

During the evaluation for genitourinary trauma, the mechanism of injury is an important factor to consider. Genitourinary trauma can be broadly classified as blunt or penetrating. The treatment principles are the same for the entire perineum, scrotum, and penis.

While the obvious injuries in these cases are at the skin level with maceration, burns, and traumatic avulsion of the skin, it is imperative to appreciate the possible involvement of surrounding structures. The urethra, bladder, and corporal bodies always must be completely evaluated. When not detected, injuries to these organs may result in prolonged bleeding and possible future erectile dysfunction. Likewise, untreated urethral and bladder injuries may result in prolonged urinary leak with extravasation and resultant urinoma, abscess, and sloughing along with infection of the perineum, penis, and scrotum. In addition, urethral injuries may result in significant stricture disease or fistula down the road thus complicating matters even more when an acute injury is missed.

Initial evaluation for trauma to the lower genitourinary tract depends upon both the presence or absence of hematuria (gross or microscopic) and the mechanism and location of the injury [42].

In all cases, a careful genitourinary examination must be performed including diligent palpation of the penis, scrotum, abdomen, and perineum with a digital rectal examination in order to evaluate for the involvement of the prostate. Complete radiographic evaluation is necessary when there is blood at the meatus, gross hematuria, and penetrating trauma to the lower abdomen or perineum and in almost all pediatric patients. Patients with microscopic hematuria who have accompanying shock with any mechanism of injury should also be imaged. And those without microscopic or gross hematuria should be imaged when the mechanism of injury is concerning for a genitourinary involvement (pelvic fractures or blunt trauma to the lower abdomen, penis, or scrotum and perineum) [43]. Cystourethroscopy, retrograde urethrogram, and cystogram should be used liberally in patients with injury to the penis, scrotum, and perineum and should be used in any patient with blood at the meatus or difficulty urinating after experiencing blunt or penetrating injuries in the vicinity of the genitalia and lower abdomen [44].

59.2.1 Penile Trauma

59.2.1.1 General Facts

Penile trauma can be classified into blunt, penetrating, avulsions, and burns. External injuries to the penis may include damage to the corporal bodies and the urethra in up to 50 % of the cases despite the absence of blood at the meatus on presentation [45]. In cases of penetrating trauma to the penis, early surgical exploration is indicated and gives a significantly better long-term outcome with respect to erectile dysfunction and voiding [46]. Blunt trauma however often responds better to stabilization and delayed repair especially when involving the urethra. The use of cystoscopy and the retrograde urethrogram is imperative prior to exploration in order to plan the surgical approach and repair.

59.2.1.2 Symptoms, Classification, and Grading

Penetrating injuries are rare in the civilian setting, however, relatively common in wartime situations. The algorithm for penetrating injuries involves a common theme of immediate exploration, copious irrigation, and excision of all foreign matter, antibiotic prophylaxis, and surgical closure [42]. When urethral injury is suspected or if blood is present at the meatus, always perform a retrograde urethrogram or cystoscopy.

Penile "fracture" occurs due to rupture of the tunica albuginea when an excessive bending force is applied to the erect penis [47]. This most commonly occurs due to vigorous intercourse. The patient will report that this happens when the penis slips out of the introitus and thrusts against the perineum or pubic bone. This also is reported to occur during excessive angulation with masturbation. In the Middle East, the most common etiology of fracture is the practice of "taghaandan" in which the penis is forcibly pushed downward in order to achieve rapid detumescence [48, 49]. In all cases, the patient often gives a history of hearing a "popping" sound and pain, followed by rapid detumescence. Often, the physical exam will demonstrate the classic eggplant deformity and the defect may be palpable in the corpora cavernosa (Fig. 59.1a, b). This injury can be associated with concomitant urethral injury, and, therefore, a retrograde urethrogram or cystoscopy must be performed to rule out urethral involvement. Cavernosography has fallen out of favor because many urologists and radiologists are not familiar with this imaging technique and the diagnosis can almost always be made by history and physical exam alone.

Though most patients present with a classic history and physical exam that points to a diagnosis of penile fracture, sometimes this is not the case. MRI is a noninvasive method and sensitive method to evaluate for disruption of the tunica albuginea in patients who present with an atypical history or equivocal physical exam [50]. In these cases, the tunica albuginea will show a low signal intensity relative to the high signal intensity of the corpora cavernosa and corpus spongiosum. T1-weighted plane images can demonstrate discontinuity of the tunica albuginea, therefore making the diagnosis.

Bites to the penis can also occur from animals or humans and can cause significant injury to deep tissues. Animal bites should be copiously irrigated and tissues debrided. They may be closed primarily and broad-spectrum antibiotics should be administered. In the case of a dog bite, penicillin V should be administered to cover for *Pasteurella* which is present in ~25 % of dog bites. Human bites often present in a delayed fashion and these wounds have the potential for significant infection. They should also be thoroughly irrigated and debrided, but primary closure should be avoided. Patients should be given broad-spectrum antibiotics to cover for polymicrobial infection [51].

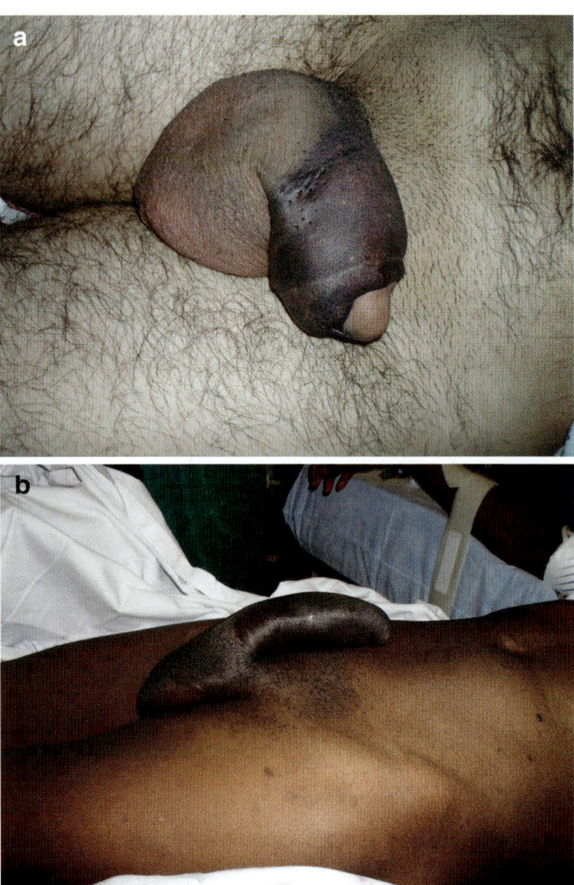

Fig. 59.1 Common physical examination finding of the eggplant deformity seen in penile fracture (**a**, **b**)

Traumatic amputation of the penis is rare but may result from industrial accidents and explosion injuries. In fact, the most common cause of penile amputation is genital self-mutilation, a situation most often accompanied by patients with active psychotic and urgent psychiatric issues. Therefore, appropriate mental health consultation should always be sought [52].

59.2.1.3 Therapy

Early reports in the literature advocated conservative management of penile fracture to include compressive dressings, anti-inflammatory medications, and pharmacologic suppression of erection. However, nonoperative management has been shown to result in an increased incidence of penile curvature, fibrosis, and erectile dysfunction, and now early surgical intervention is recommended [47, 49, 53].

Observation is not appropriate for penetrating trauma (GSW or stab injury) and penile fractures and again, early surgical intervention is recommended for gunshot wounds to the penis.

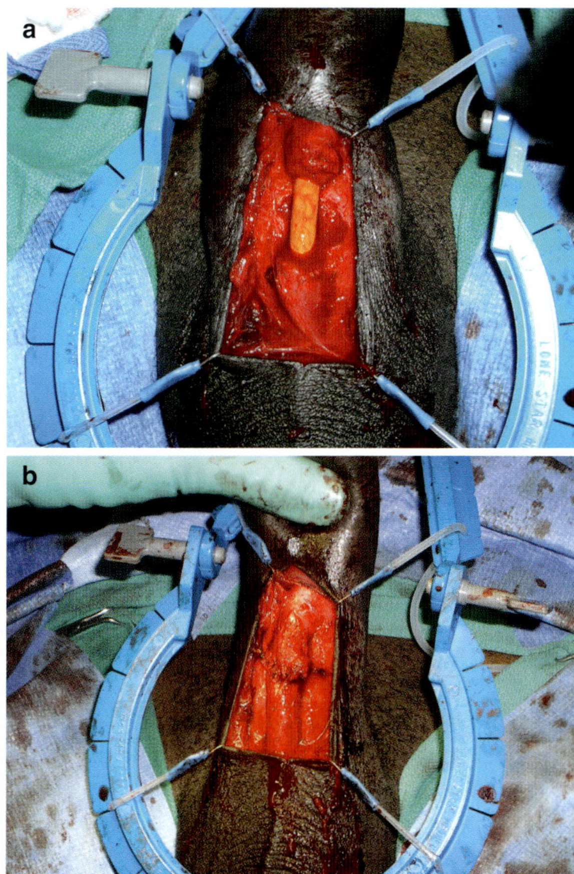

Fig. 59.2 Penile fracture may involve the tunica corporal bodies as well as the urethra (**a**). (**b**) shows the repaired urethra and tunical defects after debridement

The best way to expose the penis for penetrating or blunt injuries is through a circumcising incision via a subcoronal approach. Placing a catheter prior to surgery can help minimize the risk of injury to the urethra during dissection, especially if extensive hematoma is present. The shaft skin may be degloved from the penis and the corporal bodies and urethra directly inspected. On exploration, significant hemorrhage can be controlled initially with direct compression and gauze sponges. If bleeding is extremely brisk, control can be easily obtained through the use of a tourniquet at the base of the penis consisting of a Penrose drain held in place with a Kelley clamp. Any lacerations or injuries to the corporal bodies should be minimally debrided and closed with interrupted 2-0 Vicryl for a watertight closure. In the uncircumcised patient, a completion circumcision may be required to avoid phimosis and paraphimosis from the postoperative edema. Injecting saline into the corporal body with a tourniquet in place at the base of the penis can help assess integrity of the repair. If a urethral injury is found at exploration, devitalized tissue should be debrided. The urethra should be spatulated and reapproximated in a watertight fashion with interrupted 5-0 Vicryl (Fig. 59.2a, b).

An amputated penis should be wrapped in sterile gauze that is moistened with saline and placed into a sterile bag that is placed into a second container of ice. Successful reimplantation has been reported after 16 h of cold ischemia and after 6 h of warm ischemia [54]. A step-by-step approach for the reattachment of the amputated penis should be performed in the following order: urethra, cavernosal artery, tunica albuginea, dorsal artery, dorsal vein, and dorsal nerve [54]. Microscopic repair of the dorsal vessels and nerves should be performed whenever possible. The urethra should be stented with a small Foley catheter and a suprapubic cystotomy tube should be placed [52]. When the penis is not available for reimplantation, reconstruction should be performed in a similar manner to a partial penectomy. The corporal bodies must be closed in a watertight fashion to prevent bleeding. The urethra should be spatulated ventrally into a neo-meatus and the remaining skin should be closed.

59.2.1.4 Complications

Complications of repair of traumatic penile injuries include urethral stricture, fistula, skin loss, decreased sensation, chordee, and impotence. Excessive edema after reimplantation may be controlled with the use of medical leeches [55].

59.2.2 Urethral Trauma

59.2.2.1 General Facts

Any penetrating or blunt traumatic injury to the penis, perineum, scrotum, or pelvis may cause injury to the urethra. It is imperative to promptly diagnose urethral injury, accurately assess the extent of the injury, perform appropriate treatment, and minimize possible complications. One should have a high index of suspicion based on the mechanism of injury prior to insertion of a Foley catheter in a trauma situation.

Urethral injuries may present with blood at the meatus, difficulty or inability to void, a distended and palpable bladder, characteristic bruising patterns (butterfly or sleeve hematoma), and, in cases with associated pelvic fracture, a high-riding prostate on physical exam [56].

59.2.2.2 Symptoms, Classification, and Grading

It is best to classify urethral injuries based on location, as well as the mechanism of injury. Urethral injuries in the male should be classified into posterior urethral injuries, those involving the urethra from the bladder neck to the membranous urethra, and anterior urethral injuries, those in the area between the membranous urethra and the meatus.

The retrograde urethrogram is key to the accurate classification of urethral injuries and imperative in order to assess the extent of injury.

A correct understanding of how to conduct a retrograde urethrogram is imperative to the proper diagnosis of urethral injuries [57]. This should be performed in a semi-oblique position, rotated ~30°. A scout film should be performed in this position to allow visualization of the entire urethra and to inspect for any foreign bodies. Many injuries in the posterior urethra and proximal bulbar urethra can be missed on an anterior-posterior film. To verify appropriate amount of oblique, the obturator fossa should be obliterated on the scout film. We recommend using a mix 40 cc of Cysto-Conray in 10 cc of lidocaine jelly and place this into the Toomey syringe with sterile technique. The penis is then prepped with Betadine swabs at the tip. Sterile gloves are used and a 4×4 sterile gauze is placed under the tip of the penis. The penis is then grasped and the contrast solution is instilled into the penis in a retrograde fashion. Place the tip of the Toomey syringe inside the meatus of the penis and grasp the glans of the penis with the nondominant hand. Then under fluoroscopy, the penis is bent downward in order to view the location of the suspensory ligament of the penis. Under fluoroscopy, retrograde infusion of the contrast is placed into the penis until it can be seen to fill the entire urethra and a small amount can be seen to infuse into the bladder. The patient then is allowed to void in the same position showing complete emptying of the contrast from the system thus providing a voiding phase of the retrograde urethrogram. If fluoroscopy is not available, a series of plain X-rays can be used.

The posterior urethra includes the bladder neck, prostatic urethra, and membranous urethra. Ten percent of men who sustain a pelvic fracture may also present with a concomitant urethral injury, so a high index of suspicion is required. In the posterior urethra, the injury is most commonly from blunt trauma which causes a distraction injury where the membranous urethra is pulled off of the prostate at the apex, resulting in a pelvic fracture urethral distraction defect or "PFUDD" [58]. This results in a high-riding prostate on physical exam or a "pie in the sky" bladder on cystogram. Other causes of posterior urethral injury may include gunshot wounds, stab wounds, and other penetrating injuries, but pelvic fractures (motor vehicle collisions, industrial accidents) and iatrogenic injuries (prostatectomy or TURP) remain the most common [56] (Fig. 59.3).

Anterior urethral injuries can be subdivided into pendulous and bulbar location. Bulbar urethral injuries are typically caused by blunt trauma caused by a straddle injury or direct blow to the perineum where the urethra is crushed against the pubic bone. These injuries may present with a butterfly hematoma on the perineum and can also have an associated scrotal hematoma or blood at the meatus. The pendulous urethra may also be injured in this way and typically present with sleeve hematomas of the penis in which the blood is confined to Buck's fascia.

59.2.2.3 Therapy

For the anterior urethra, there are three valid management options for urethral trauma regardless of the location or mechanism of injury:

- Immediate suprapubic tube placement with delayed urethral repair
- Immediate realignment by placing a catheter across the urethral injury with delayed repair if needed
- Immediate repair with debridement of injured urethra and surgical anastomosis

When an anterior urethral injury is suspected, aggressive attempt at catheterization is discouraged because this may convert a partial laceration into a complete

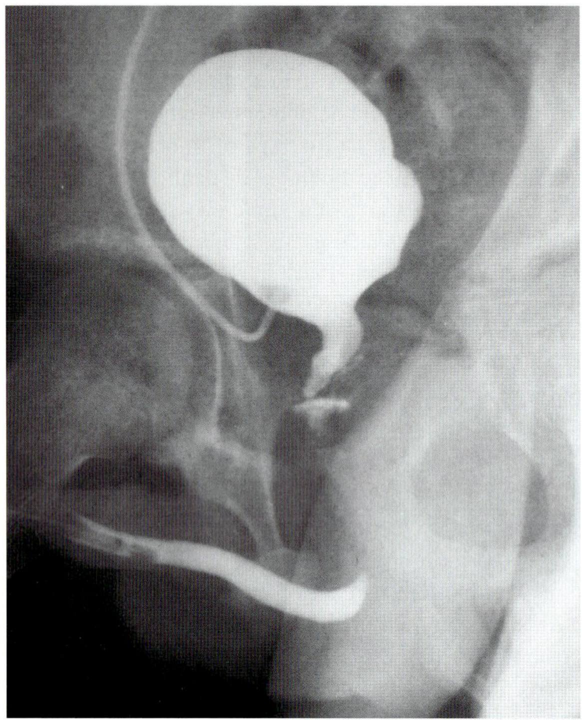

Fig. 59.3 Retrograde urethrogram showing the posterior defect resulting from a pelvic fracture

urethral injury though the chance of this is scarce [59]. A single, gentle attempt to place a Foley catheter by an experienced member of the urology team in the case of a partial disruption is reasonable [60].

Penetrating wounds can cause injuries at any location in the urethra. Treatment has classically consisted of simple suprapubic tube or Foley catheter urinary diversion to allow the injury to heal. Recent reports however indicate that when injuries include the anterior urethra, exploration with primary closure of the injury to the urethra results in a better long-term outcome with decreased scar and stricture formation [61]. When urethral injury is found on surgical exploration, the edges need to be carefully debrided and the penetration or laceration to the urethra closed with interrupted fine absorbable sutures such as 4-0 or 5-0 Vicryl. At this point, a small Foley catheter (12–14 French) should be left in place for 3 weeks. A pericatheter retrograde urethrogram should be performed to show no extravasation of contrast prior to removal of the catheter. If the urethral injury is too significant for an acute repair, or there is too much tissue loss for adequate debridement and closure, then placement of a suprapubic tube is recommended in order to stabilize the patient for transport and a definitive repair at a later date.

Injuries to the posterior urethral from high velocity gunshot wounds should be managed with suprapubic drainage and a Foley catheter if possible. If there are concomitant injuries to the distal gastrointestinal tract, a diverting colostomy may be required. Early attempt at repair is not indicated since it may cause a significant amount of bleeding, incontinence, and possible erectile dysfunction.

Management of a posterior urethral distraction defect caused by blunt trauma is a topic of debate within the urologic community. Some authors recommend primary realignment using endoscopic techniques, while others recommend early suprapubic drainage with delayed repair in 3–6 months. Our preference is the latter. This approach allows acute decompression of the urinary system, convalescence of the patient, and definitive reconstruction later in a controlled setting. Primary repair of posterior urethral injury is not recommended due to high rates of postoperative impotence and incontinence [59].

A suprapubic tube can be placed either percutaneously (when the bladder is distended) or by an open technique (if the bladder has been recently emptied or in the case of concomitant bladder neck injury).

59.2.2.4 Open Suprapubic Tube

When placing an open suprapubic tube, care should be taken not to disrupt the pelvic hematoma. A vertical midline skin incision is made from the symphysis pubis to two to three fingerbreadths below the umbilicus. The external oblique fascia is incised and the rectus muscles split in the midline. It is not necessary to separate them from their insertion on the pubic bone. One should stay extraperitoneal and the bladder can be identified in the midline as it likely will be full of urine at this point. Place 2 silk stay sutures on each side of the dome of the bladder and make a vertical incision in the dome of the bladder with the Bovie electrocautery or knife. Once urine is obtained, the cystotomy may be extended in order to provide inspection of the inside of the bladder should there be concomitant bladder injuries. A 20–24 French Foley catheter is placed through the cystotomy and the opening is closed with a purse string suture of absorbable 2-0 or 3-0 Vicryl suture for watertight closure. The balloon on the suprapubic tube is inflated with 10 cc of sterile water. The suprapubic tube may then be brought out through the inferior portion of the abdominal wound or through a separate stab incision only 2–3 cm lateral to the wound. Tension should be placed on the suprapubic tube to bring the cystotomy in contact with the anterior abdominal wall in order to reduce leakage. The suprapubic tube is then secured to the skin with a permanent nylon suture.

Endoscopic realignment may be attempted by using a single flexible cystoscope from below and a wire. Other techniques include the use of two scopes looking both antegrade and retrograde, followed by catheter placement across the injury by the Seldinger technique [62].

59.2.2.5 Percutaneous Suprapubic Tube

A percutaneous cystotomy tube may need to be placed in situations where a laparotomy is not required and should only be performed in a patient with a distended bladder. The patient should be placed supine on a stretcher in as steep Trendelenburg as can be tolerated to pull the bowels away from the dome of the bladder. If ultrasound is available, this can be used to help guide the placement. A puncture incision is made three to four fingerbreadths above the symphysis pubis in the midline. One can use a finder needle in order to establish the depth needed to penetrate and obtain urine. A trocar should be placed into the dome of the bladder at a 45° angle with the tip of the finder needle directed caudally. Once urine is obtained with a puncture cystotomy tube, it is important to advance the tube 1–2 cm deeper prior to inflating the balloon in order to ensure that the balloon is within the dome of the bladder. Once placed, the balloon is inflated with 10 cc of sterile water, and tension is placed on the suprapubic tube in order to pull the dome of the bladder flush with the anterior abdominal wall. This is then secured to the skin with nylon suture.

In contrast to male urethral injuries, women with pelvic fractures and proximal urethral injuries should undergo immediate vaginal or retropubic exploration with realignment or primary anastomosis. When these injuries are managed with urinary diversion alone, these patients commonly develop urethrovaginal fistulas or obliterative strictures [63].

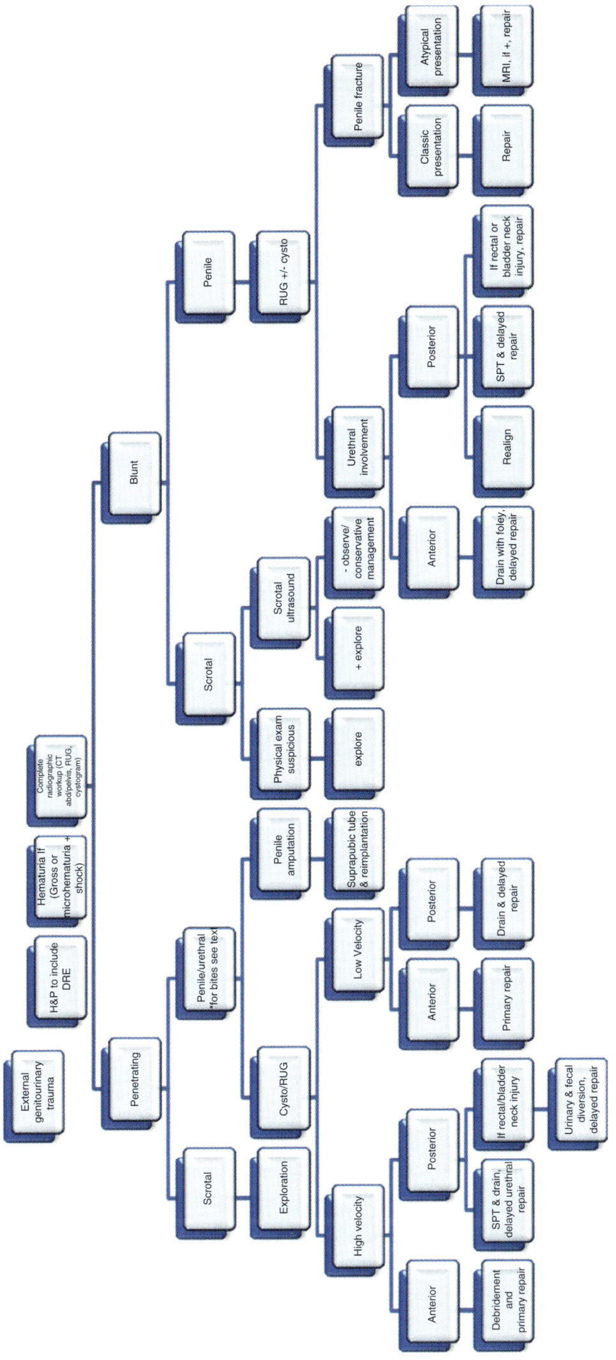
External genitourinary trauma
H&P to include DRE
Hematuria if (Gross or microhematuria + shock)
Complete radiographic workup (CT abd/pelvis, RUG, cystogram)
Penetrating
Blunt
Scrotal
Penile/urethral *for bites see tex
Exploration
Cysto/RUG
Penile amputation
Suprapubic tube & reimplantation
High velocity
Low Velocity
Anterior
Posterior
Anterior
Posterior
Debridement and primary repair
SPT & drain, delayed urethral repair
If rectal/bladder neck injury
Urinary & fecal diversion, delayed repair
Primary repair
Drain & delayed repair
Scrotal
Penile
Physical exam suspicious
explore
Scrotal ultrasound
+ explore
- observe/ conservative management
RUG +/- cysto
Urethral involvement
Anterior
Posterior
Drain with foley, delayed repair
Realign
SPT & delayed repair
If rectal or bladder neck injury, repair
Penile fracture
Classic presentation
Atypical presentation
Repair
MRI, if +, repair

59.2.2.6 Complications

A delayed or missed diagnosis of a urethral injury can have devastating consequences to include urinoma, abscess formation, infection, urethral stricture, impotence, or incontinence.

59.2.3 Scrotum and Testicular Trauma

59.2.3.1 General

The scrotal contents may be involved with penetrating, blunt, and avulsion injuries. Non-penetrating injuries resulting from crush or saddle injuries to the penis, scrotum, and perineum can cause significant damage to the internal structures without disrupting the skin; therefore again, a high index of suspicion is required in order to make the appropriate diagnosis. Up to 85 % of testicular injuries are the result of blunt trauma [47]. The scrotum is much more often involved in penetrating trauma than the penis and prompt surgical exploration is recommended in most cases (Fig. 59.4a–c).

59.2.3.2 Symptoms, Classification, and Grading

Scrotal injuries can be classified into blunt (straddle injury, sports), penetrating (stab wound, guns shot wound, bite), avulsion (machinery or motorcycle accidents), or burns. When evaluating a patient with blunt scrotal trauma, ultrasonography is the most sensitive and specific imaging modality for detecting intrascrotal injury. The most significant finding indicating injury to the testicle is the presence of heterogeneity within the testicle. Hematomas and contusions appear hypoechoic within the testicle and should be considered diagnostic of rupture [64, 65]. While scrotal ultrasound is usually reliable, easily accessible, and inexpensive, it is operator-dependent and this limitation should be considered [65]. A normal ultrasound should not delay surgical exploration if clinical suspicion for injury is high. The use of ultrasonography to rule out injury in cases of penetrating trauma should be discouraged with preference always relying upon surgical exploration (Fig. 59.5a, b).

59.2.3.3 Therapy

Whenever possible, every attempt should be made to preserve viable testicular tissue.

The scrotum is best accessed through a midline median raphe incision where both of the hemiscrotal compartments can be opened and both testicles delivered, inspected, and repaired. During this procedure, it is important to note the normal anatomy of the testicle where the lateral raphe, the crevice between the epididymis, and the testicle will always lie laterally. This is a good landmark for orientation while placing the testicles back into the scrotal compartment after exploration and avoids twisting of the testicle with possible concomitant ischemia. When the testicle is injured and the tunica albuginea has been ruptured or lacerated, the testicle should be copiously irrigated. Any extruded seminiferous tubules should be debrided and the tunica closed with running 2-0 Vicryl suture for a watertight repair. If there is

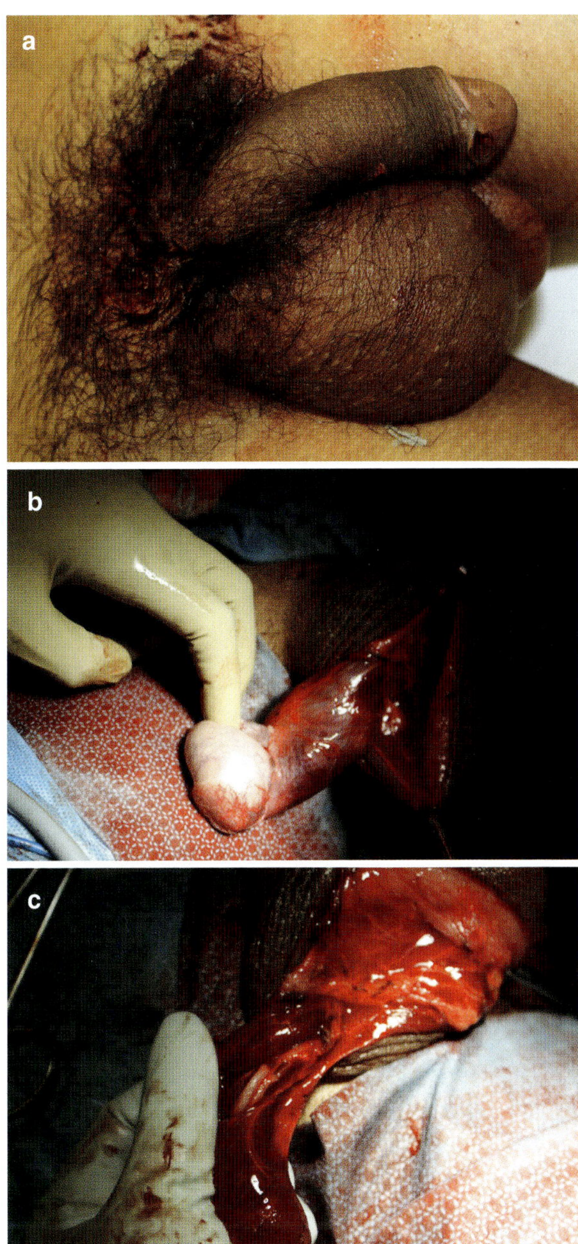

Fig. 59.4 Gunshot wound to the scrotum (**a**). The ultrasound showed a normal testicle (**b**) but on exploration a chord injury with transection of the vas deferens is found (**c**)

not enough tunica albuginea left after the injury to successfully close the testicle, consideration should be given to grafting options with the use of various biologic products that are currently available. However, sometimes the testicle must be removed in order to avoid the accumulation of necrotic debris or abscess and

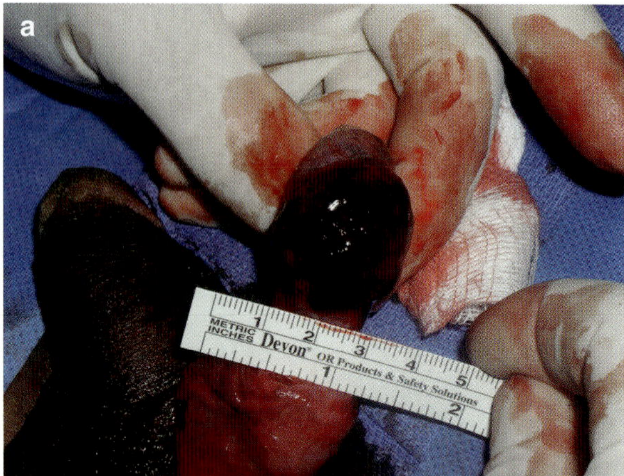

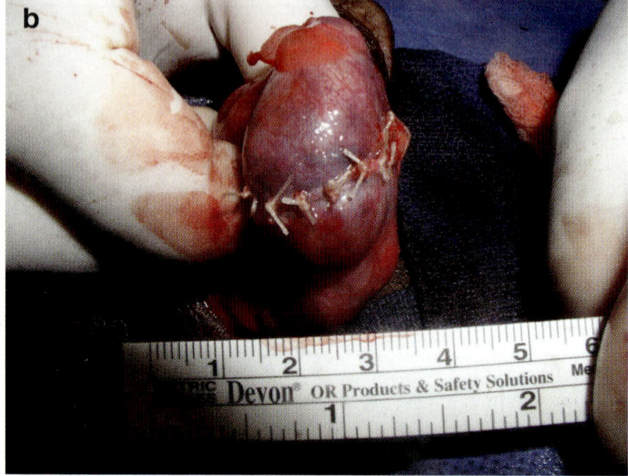

Fig. 59.5 Disruption of the testicle after blunt trauma (**a**). The seminiferous tubules are debrided and the tunica is closed in a watertight fashion with absorbable suture to preserve the remainder of the testicle (**b**)

hematoma formation. The testicles should be placed back into their respective hemiscrotal compartments in the normal anatomic alignment and the compartments closed with running 3-0 Vicryl suture; the skin can be closed with a running 4-0 absorbable suture. Leave a Penrose drain in each of the hemiscrotal compartments through a separate stab incision to allow drainage for 24–36 h.

Orchiectomy may be required in up to 90 % of penetrating trauma cases [45], and the remaining testicle will provide enough testosterone for normal sexual characteristic maintenance as well as fertility. Gunshot wounds typically disrupt the tunica albuginea and rarely involve the spermatic cord, while laceration injuries may involve a vascular component which can prevent successful reconstruction [66]. There is rarely a need to leave the scrotal wound open unless it has been severely grossly contaminated with debris, necrotic material, or abscess formation.

Avulsion injuries with an intact tunica vaginalis and no evidence of injury to the testis can be treated by copious irrigation, debridement, and hemostasis. Noninfected wounds should be closed primarily in two layers and treated with conservative management: rest, ice, NSAIDS, and scrotal elevation. Infected wounds should not be closed primarily. Consider wet to dry dressings or placement of a negative pressure wound management system and broad-spectrum antibiotics. Injuries that involve an extensive area of the scrotum may require a skin graft; however, due to the vascularity and elasticity of the scrotal skin, primary closure is possible even when up to 60 % of scrotal tissue is lost [67]. In severe avulsion injuries where the majority or the entire scrotum has been removed, consideration should be given to placing the testicles in the thigh pouches temporarily in order to allow healing in preparation for definitive reconstruction at a later date.

59.2.3.4 Complications

Complications from scrotal trauma include testicular loss, hematoma, infection, chronic pain, and psychological impact. Studies have found that testicular preservation has no negative effect on future fertility [68].

References

1. Adams JE, Davis GG, Alexander CB, Alonso JE. Pelvic trauma in rapidly fatal motor vehicle accidents. J Orthop Trauma. 2003;17(6):406–10.
2. Benoit L, Spie R, Favoulet P, Cheynel N, Kretz B, Gouy S, Dubruille T, Fraisse J, Cuisenier J. Management of ureteral injuries. Ann Chir. 2005;130(8):451–7.
3. Bosch U, Pohlemann T, Haas N, Tscherne H. Classification and management of complex pelvic trauma. Unfallchirurg. 1992;95(4):189–96.
4. Buchberger W, Penz T, Wicke K, Eberle J. Diagnosis and staging of blunt kidney trauma. A comparison of urinalysis, i.v. urography, sonography and computed tomography. Rofo. 1993;158(6):507–12.
5. Buse S, Lynch TH, Martinez-Piñeiro L, Plas E, Serafetinides E, Turkeri L, Santucci RA, Sauerland S, Hohenfellner M, German Society for Trauma Surgery. Urinary tract injuries in polytraumatized patients. Unfallchirurg. 2005;108(10):821–8.
6. Carlin BI, Resnick MI. Indications and techniques for urologic evaluation of the trauma patient with suspected urologic injury. Semin Urol. 1995;13(1):9–24.
7. Carpio F, Morey AF. Radiographic staging of renal injuries. World J Urol. 1999;17(2): 66–70.
8. Corriere Jr JN, Sandler CM. Management of the ruptured bladder: seven years of experience with 111 cases. J Trauma. 1986;26(9):830–3.
9. Deck AJ, Shaves S, Talner L, Porter JR. Computerized tomography cystography for the diagnosis of traumatic bladder rupture. J Urol. 2000;164(1):43–6.
10. Elliott SP, McAninch JW. Ureteral injuries from external violence: the 25–year experience at San Francisco General Hospital. J Urol. 2003;170(4 Pt 1):1213–6.
11. Feliciano DV. Management of traumatic retroperitoneal hematoma. Ann Surg. 1990;211(2):109–23.
12. Figler B, Hoffler CE, Reisman W, Carney KJ, Moore T, Feliciano D, Master V. Multidisciplinary update on pelvic fracture associated bladder and urethral injuries. Injury. 2012;43(8):1242–9.
13. Friese RS, Malekzadeh S, Shafi S, Gentilello LM, Starr A. Abdominal ultrasound is an unreliable modality for the detection of hemoperitoneum in patients with pelvic fracture. J Trauma. 2007;63(1):97–102.
14. Gomez RG, Ceballos L, Coburn M, Corriere Jr JN, Dixon CM, Lobel B, McAninch J. Consensus statement on bladder injuries. BJU Int. 2004;94(1):27–32.

15. Griffin XL, Pullinger R. Are diagnostic peritoneal lavage or focused abdominal sonography for trauma safe screening investigations for hemodynamically stable patients after blunt abdominal trauma? A review of the literature. J Trauma. 2007;62(3):779–84.
16. Hagiwara A, Sakaki S, Goto H, Takenega K, Fukushima H, Matuda H, Shimazaki S. The role of interventional radiology in the management of blunt renal injury: a practical protocol. J Trauma. 2001;51(3):526–31.
17. Hammer CC, Santucci RA. Effect of an institutional policy of nonoperative treatment of grades I to IV renal injuries. J Urol. 2003;169(5):1751–3.
18. Harrahill M. Bladder trauma: a review. J Emerg Nurs. 2004;30(3):287–8.
19. Helling TS, Wilson J, Augustosky K. The utility of focused abdominal ultrasound in blunt abdominal trauma: a reappraisal. Am J Surg. 2007;194(6):728–32.
20. Hsieh CH, Chen RJ, Fang JF, Lin BC, Hsu YP, Kao JL, Kao YC, Yu PC, Kang SC. Diagnosis and management of bladder injury by trauma surgeons. Am J Surg. 2002;184(2):143–7.
21. Hsu JM, Joseph AP, Tarlinton LJ, Macken L, Blome S. The accuracy of focused assessment with sonography in trauma (FAST) in blunt trauma patients: experience of an Australian major trauma service. Injury. 2007;38(1):71–5.
22. Lynch TH, Martínez-Piñeiro L, Plas E, Serafetinides E, Türkeri L, Santucci RA, Hohenfellner M, European Association of Urology. EAU guidelines on urological trauma. Eur Urol. 2005;47(1):1–15.
23. Matsui Y, Ohara H, Ichioka K, Terada N, Yoshimura K, Terai A. Traumatic bladder rupture managed successfully by laparoscopic surgery. Int J Urol. 2003;10(5):278–80.
24. Melton LJ 3rd, Sampson JM, Morrey BF, Ilstrup DM. Epidemiologic features of pelvic fractures. Clin Orthop Relat Res. 1981;155:43–7.
25. Morey AF, Hernandez J, McAninch JW. Reconstructive surgery for trauma of the lower urinary tract. Urol Clin North Am. 1999;26(1):49–60, viii.
26. Mucha Jr P, Farnell MB. Analysis of pelvic fracture management. J Trauma. 1984;24(5): 379–86.
27. Natarajan B, Gupta PK, Cemaj S, Sorensen M, Hatzoudis GI, Forse RA. FAST scan: is it worth doing in hemodynamically stable blunt trauma patients? Surgery. 2010;148(4):695–700.
28. Nicolaisen GS, McAninch JW, Marshall GA, Bluth Jr RF, Carroll PR. Renal trauma: re-evaluation of the indications for radiographic assessment. J Urol. 1985;133(2):183–7.
29. Palmer LS, Rosenbaum RR, Gershbaum MD, Kreutzer ER. Penetrating ureteral trauma at an urban trauma center: 10-year experience. Urology. 1999;54(1):34–6.
30. Prando A. Blunt renal trauma: minimally invasive management with microcatheter embolization – experience in nine patients. Int Braz J Urol. 2002;28(4):372–3.
31. Rehm CG, Mure AJ, O'Malley KF, Ross SE. Blunt traumatic bladder rupture: the role of retrograde cystogram. Ann Emerg Med. 1991;20(8):845–7.
32. Reilly KJ, Shapiro MB, Haskal ZJ. Angiographic embolization of a penetrating traumatic renal arteriovenous fistula. J Trauma. 1996;41(4):763–5.
33. Santucci RA, Bartley JM. Urologic trauma guidelines: a 21st century update. Nat Rev Urol. 2010;7(9):510–9.
34. Santucci RA, Wessells H, Bartsch G, Descotes J, Heyns CF, McAninch JW, Nash P, Schmidlin F. Evaluation and management of renal injuries: consensus statement of the renal trauma subcommittee. BJU Int. 2004;93(7):937–54.
35. Schmidlin F. Renal trauma. Treatment strategies and indications for surgical exploration. Urologe A. 2005;44(8):863–9.
36. Schmit-Neuerburg KP, Joka T. Principles of treatment and indications for surgery in severe multiple trauma. Acta Chir Belg. 1985;85(4):239–49.
37. Schroeppel TJ, Croce MA. Diagnosis and management of blunt abdominal solid organ injury. Curr Opin Crit Care. 2007;13(4):399–404.
38. Staehler M, Nuhn P, Haseke N, Tüllmann C, Bader M, Graser A, Stief CG. Clinical approach to renal trauma. Urologe A. 2010;49(7):837–41.
39. Tayal VS, Nielsen A, Jones AE, Thomason MH, Kellam J, Norton HJ. Accuracy of trauma ultrasound in major pelvic injury. J Trauma. 2006;61(6):1453–7.

40. Tezval H, Tezval M, von Klot C, Herrmann TR, Dresing K, Jonas U, Burchardt M. Urinary tract injuries in patients with multiple trauma. World J Urol. 2007;25(2):177–84.
41. Toporoff B, Sclafani S, Scalea T, Vieux E, Atweh N, Duncan A, Trooskin S. Percutaneous antegrade ureteral stenting as an adjunct for treatment of complicated ureteral injuries. J Trauma. 1992;32(4):534–8.
42. Mohr AM, Pham AM, Lavery RF, Sifri Z, Bargman V, Livingston DH. Management of trauma to the male external genitalia: the usefulness of American Association for the Surgery of Trauma organ injury scales. J Urol. 2003;170(6 Pt 1):2311–5.
43. Jankowski JT, Spirnak JP. Current recommendations for imaging in the management of urologic traumas. Urol Clin North Am. 2006;33(3):365–76.
44. Martinez-Pineiro L, Djakovic N, Plas E, et al. EAU guidelines on urethral trauma. Eur Urol. 2010;57(5):791–803.
45. Brandes SB, Buckman RF, Chelsky MJ, Hanno PM. External genitalia gunshot wounds: a ten-year experience with fifty-six cases. J Trauma. 1995;39(2):266–71.
46. Tiguert R, Harb JF, Hurley PM, et al. Management of shotgun injuries to the pelvis and lower genitourinary system. Urology. 2000;55(2):193–7.
47. Morey AF, Metro MJ, Carney KJ, Miller KS, McAninch JW. Consensus on genitourinary trauma: external genitalia. BJU Int. 2004;94(4):507–15.
48. Zargooshi J. Penile fracture in Kermanshah, Iran: report of 172 cases. J Urol. 2000;164(2): 364–6.
49. Zargooshi J. Penile fracture in Kermanshah, Iran: the long-term results of surgical treatment. BJU Int. 2002;89(9):890–4.
50. Fedel M, Venz S, Andreessen R, Sudhoff F, Loening SA. The value of magnetic resonance imaging in the diagnosis of suspected penile fracture with atypical clinical findings. J Urol. 1996;155(6):1924–7.
51. Wessells H, Long L. Penile and genital injuries. Urol Clin North Am. 2006;33(1):117–26, vii.
52. Jordan G. Lower genitourinary tract trauma and male external genital trauma (nonpenetrating injuries, penetrating injuries, and avulsion injuries). Part II. AUA Update Series. 2000;19(11):82–7.
53. Zargooshi J. Sexual function and tunica albuginea wound healing following penile fracture: an 18-year follow-up study of 352 patients from Kermanshah, Iran. J Sex Med. 2009; 6(4):1141–50.
54. Bandi G, Santucci RA. Controversies in the management of male external genitourinary trauma. J Trauma. 2004;56(6):1362–70.
55. Pantuck AJ, Lobis MR, Ciocca R, Weiss RE. Penile replantation using the leech Hirudo medicinalis. Urology. 1996;48(6):953–6.
56. Morey AF. Consensus statement on urethral trauma. J Urol. 2005;174(3):968–9.
57. Breyer BN, Cooperberg MR, McAninch JW, Master VA. Improper retrograde urethrogram technique leads to incorrect diagnosis. J Urol. 2009;182(2):716–7.
58. Webster GD, Guralnick ML. Reconstruction of posterior urethral disruption. Urol Clin North Am. 2002;29(2):429–41, viii.
59. Brandes S. Initial management of anterior and posterior urethral injuries. Urol Clin North Am. 2006;33(1):87–95, vii.
60. Kotkin L, Koch MO. Impotence and incontinence after immediate realignment of posterior urethral trauma: result of injury or management? J Urol. 1996;155(5):1600–3.
61. Cline KJ, Mata JA, Venable DD, Eastham JA. Penetrating trauma to the male external genitalia. J Trauma. 1998;44(3):492–4.
62. Mouraviev VB, Coburn M, Santucci RA. The treatment of posterior urethral disruption associated with pelvic fractures: comparative experience of early realignment versus delayed urethroplasty. J Urol. 2005;173(3):873–6.
63. Black PC, Miller EA, Porter JR, Wessells H. Urethral and bladder neck injury associated with pelvic fracture in 25 female patients. J Urol. 2006;175(6):2140–4.
64. Fournier Jr GR, Laing FC, McAninch JW. Scrotal ultrasonography and the management of testicular trauma. Urol Clin North Am. 1989;16(2):377–85.

65. Fournier Jr GR, Laing FC, Jeffrey RB, McAninch JW. High resolution scrotal ultrasonography: a highly sensitive but nonspecific diagnostic technique. J Urol. 1985;134(3):490–3.
66. Phonsombat S, Master VA, McAninch JW. Penetrating external genital trauma: a 30-year single institution experience. J Urol. 2008;180(1):192–5.
67. McAninch JW. Management of genital skin loss. Urol Clin North Am. 1989;16(2):387–97.
68. Kukadia AN, Ercole CJ, Gleich P, Hensleigh H, Pryor JL. Testicular trauma: potential impact on reproductive function. J Urol. 1996;156(5):1643–6.
69. Peiper H-J, Peitsch W. Blunt upper abdominal trauma (author's transl). Unfallheilkunde. 1976;79(8):341–7.
70. Hegelmeier C, Kozianka J. Parenchymatöse Organverletzung beim stumpfen Bauchtrauma des mehrfach verletzten Patienten. In: Kozuschek W, Reith HB (ed.) Das Polytrauma – Diagnostik, Therapie, 1993. Karger, Freiburg, S. 140–155.

Cushing's Syndrome

60

Christoph A.J. von Klot

60.1 General Facts

Cushing's syndrome describes the symptoms originating from inappropriately high cortisol exposure of any etiology [1]. The prevalence of Cushing's syndrome ranges at about 13 cases per one million people in the USA. The incidence is 2–3 new cases per one million people per year. Females are more likely than men to develop hypercortisolism from pituitary or adrenal tumors [2]. The regulatory principle of glucocorticoid regulation is shown in Fig. 60.1.

60.2 Symptoms and Classification

60.2.1 Symptoms

Signs and symptoms of Cushing's syndrome are mostly attributed to the elevated levels of serum cortisol. Most prominent changes are depicted in Fig. 60.2.

Changes in body shape include obesity (prominent at the center of the body with often thin extremities), a dorsocervical fat pad, edema, round facial shape, wide purple striae, growth retardation, infections of the skin, and myopathy.

Radiological examination may show signs of osteoporosis, adrenal mass or nodal cortical hyperplasia, or a pituitary tumor.

Metabolic changes include diabetes mellitus, hyperlipoproteinemia, hypertension, oligo- or amenorrhea and infertility, hypogonadotropic hypogonadism, and polycystic ovary syndrome.

Psychological changes may include reduced libido, depression, irritability, and anxiety.

C.A.J. von Klot
Department of Urology and Urological Oncology, Hannover University Medical School, Carl-Neuberg-Str. 1, Hannover 30625, Germany
e-mail: klot.christoph@mh-hannover.de

A.S. Merseburger et al. (eds.), *Urology at a Glance*,
DOI 10.1007/978-3-642-54859-8_60,

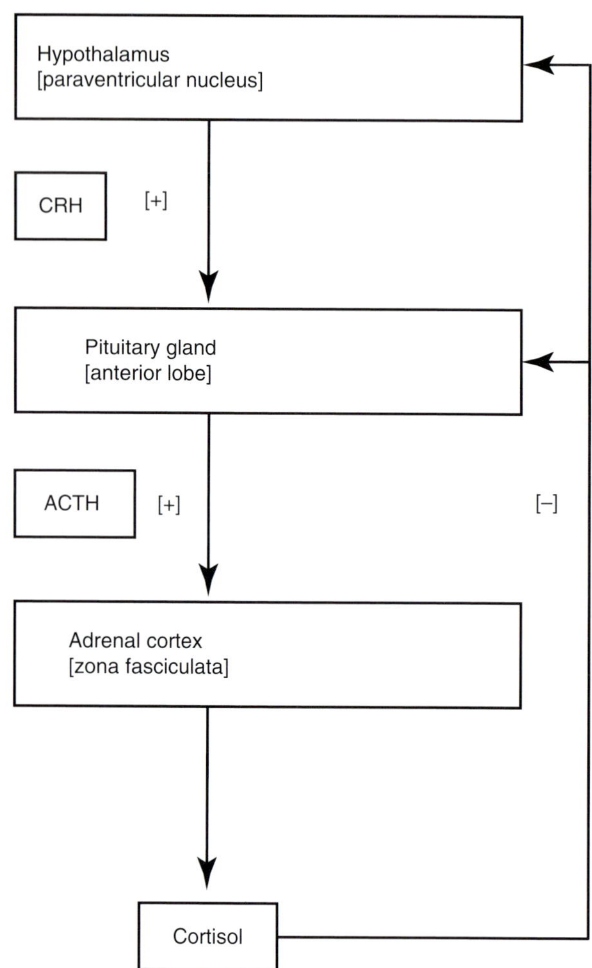

Fig. 60.1 The paraventricular nucleus in the hypothalamus releases corticotropin-releasing hormone (*CRH*). CRH stimulates adrenocorticotropin (*ACTH*) production in the anterior lobe of the pituitary gland. ACTH reaches the adrenal cortex via bloodstream where it increases cortisol release from the zona fasciculata. Rising levels of cortisol exert a negative feedback on the hypothalamus and pituitary gland

60.2.2 Classification

There are two causes of Cushing's syndrome, an exogenous and endogenous form. A typical endogenous cause is an ACTH-secreting tumor of the pituitary gland which is referred to as *Cushing's disease*. The American neurosurgeon H. Cushing published the first description of this pathology in 1932 [3]. However, not all pituitary tumors cause excessive hormone production [4].

Another cause of endogenous elevated serum cortisol can be a *cortisol-secreting adenoma of the adrenal cortex* causing primary hypercortisolism. However, only about 10 % of adrenal incidentalomas secrete cortisol [5].

The most common cause of exogenous cortisol excess is *iatrogenic administration of glucocorticosteroids*.

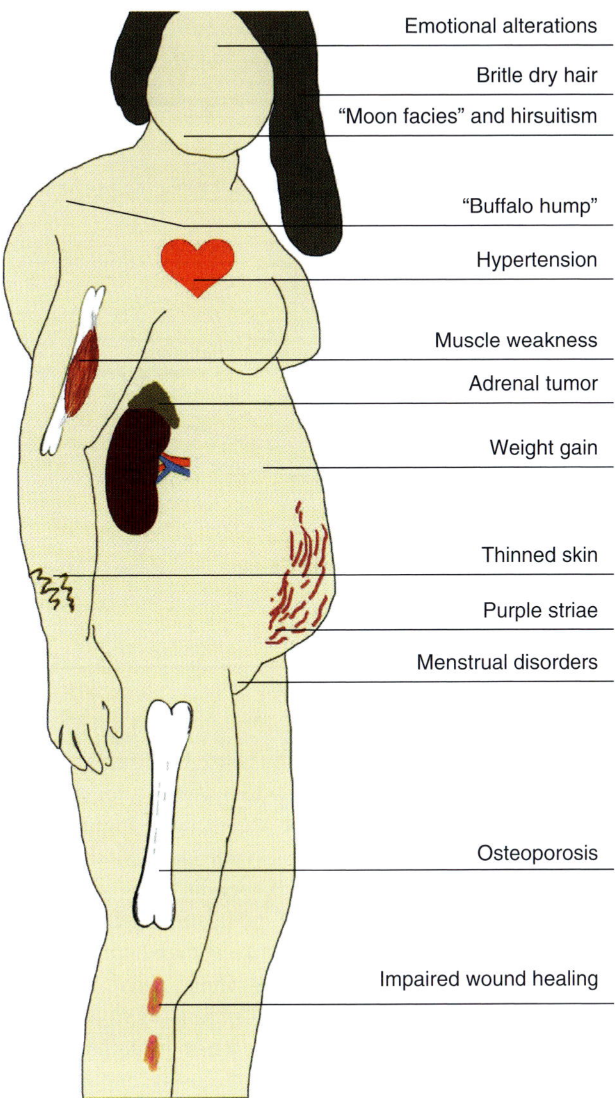

Fig. 60.2 Signs and symptoms of elevated serum cortisol levels

Rarer causes of Cushing's syndrome include paraneoplastic secretion or stimulation of cortisol secretion. Of all tumor entities, carcinoma of the lung and pancreatic neoplasia are most often associated with *paraneoplastic Cushing's syndrome* [6].

The elevation of serum cortisol levels due to excess production of corticotropin-releasing hormone (CRH) is referred to as *tertiary hypercortisolism* and is very rare [1].

Aside from Cushing's disease patients can also show the signs and symptoms of abnormally elevated levels of cortisol without a pathology in the hypothalamic-pituitary-adrenal axis. This condition is mostly alcohol induced and is referred to as *pseudo-Cushing's syndrome* [7, 8].

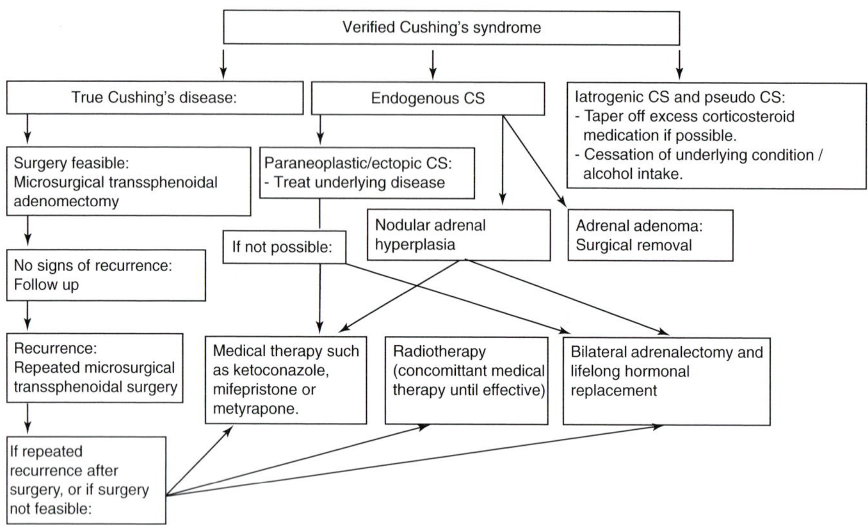

Fig. 60.3 Therapeutic pathway for Cushing's syndrome (*CS*)

60.3 Therapy

Various underlying conditions can cause Cushing's syndrome. It is therefore of outmost importance to adequately assess a variety of possible causes for elevated cortisol levels and adapt treatment accordingly. Figure 60.3 depicts clinical decision making on therapy for Cushing's syndrome.

Cushing's syndrome due to exogenous causes, as in most cases, can effectively be treated by tapering off steroid medication; this also pertains to pseudo-Cushing's where the cessation of alcohol intake is mandatory to alleviate symptoms.

Endogenous causes include a hormone-active tumor of the pituitary gland with increased ACTH levels or a cortisol-producing tumor of the adrenal cortex. Pituitary tumors should surgically be removed using microsurgical techniques. Cortisol levels after therapy should be monitored closely, and transient or permanent decreased blood levels of cortisol require corticosteroid replacement therapy. Cure rates after surgery of the pituitary gland range from 85 to 95 % [9]. In most cases return of normal adrenal hormone production occurs within 1 year. However, some patients never have a return of normal adrenal function after definitive therapy of Cushing's syndrome and need permanent replacement therapy. If unfit for surgery or in the case of recurrent disease after surgical therapy for pituitary adenoma, radiation of the pituitary gland may be necessary. The effect on cortisol levels however may take several months; thus concomitant medical therapy is administered to alleviate symptoms.

Isolated corticosteroid-producing adrenal adenomas or adrenal carcinomas are treated surgically.

Another pathological entity of the adrenal gland that can cause endogenous Cushing's syndrome is the so-called nodular adrenal hyperplasia. Micro- and macronodular changes may be observed as well as concomitant pituitary disease and even a sequence to adrenocortical adenoma or rarely carcinoma. Nodular adrenal hyperplasia is usually treated with adrenalectomy using a posterior approach. Before treatment, medical therapy such as ketoconazole or metyrapone can lower cortisol levels. Replacement therapy after bilateral adrenalectomy is mandatory [10].

Hypertension can improve after surgical removal of the adrenals, but some patients may require concomitant antihypertensive therapy. No diuretics with negative effect on potassium concentration should be administered since they may worsen hypokalemia. Angiotensin II receptor blockers and angiotensin-converting enzyme inhibitors are recommended [11].

After removal of the adrenal glands, up to 20 % of patients may develop a pituitary adenoma due to increased levels of ACTH. This medical condition is referred to as Nelson's syndrome. Mass effects due to growing adenoma of the pituitary gland may cause brain tissue compression. Elevated levels of ACTH and melanocyte-stimulating hormone (MSH) can lead to muscle weakness and skin hyperpigmentation. Therapy comprises surgery or prophylactic radiotherapy of the pituitary gland [12].

If surgical therapy is not feasible, a variety of medication regimens have been proposed such as ketoconazole, mifepristone, and metyrapone. The use of mifepristone should not be used during pregnancy since it is an abortifacient. Cabergoline and pasireotide are new agents that may normalize ACTH and thus cortisol levels in about one third of patients [13, 14].

Patients with ectopic ACTH production need treatment of the primary tumor. Medical therapy can be provided with aminoglutethimide which is an aromatase-blocking agent that also blocks the conversion of cholesterol to pregnenolone by inhibiting cholesterol side-chain cleavage enzyme (P450scc). Caution must be taken since it impairs aldosterone production and can cause hepatotoxicity and hypothyroidism [15].

60.4 Complications

Overall mortality in patients with untreated Cushing's syndrome is greatly increased; however, the life expectancy for patients with treated Cushing's syndrome resembles that or falls short of those with normal corticosteroid levels [16]. Most of the complications as well as mortality are attributed to prolonged high corticosteroid levels which induce insulin resistance and may also cause type 2 diabetes mellitus with the known cardiovascular and metabolic sequelae. Because of mineralocorticoid excess, patients may develop severe hypertension and concomitant hypokalemia. Other known complications of Cushing's syndrome include osteoporosis and impaired osteoblast function with hypercalcemia with skin necrosis in rare cases and urolithiasis. Psychological changes can range from depression and irritability to even psychotic symptoms. Excess in corticosteroid levels may also affect other endocrine organs. Patients can present with oligo- or amenorrhea or polycystic ovary syndrome and infertility [17]. High cortisol levels exert a negative feedback on the hypothalamus as depicted in Fig. 60.1 which results in impaired GnRH release. In Cushing's syndrome with elevated ACTH, symptoms may include hyperpigmentation due to the increased levels of pro-opiomelanocortin.

References

1. Arnaldi G, Angeli A, Atkinson AB, Bertagna X, Cavagnini F, Chrousos GP, et al. Diagnosis and complications of Cushing's syndrome: a consensus statement. J Clin Endocrinol Metab. 2003;88(12):5593–602.
2. Findling JW, Raff H. Screening and diagnosis of Cushing's syndrome. Endocrinol Metab Clin North Am. 2005;34(2):385–402, ix–x. Available from: http://dx.doi.org/10.1016/j.ecl.2005.02.001.
3. Cushing H. The basophil adenomas of the pituitary body and their clinical manifestations (pituitary basophilism). 1932. Obes Res. 1994;2(5):486–508.
4. Ezzat S, Asa SL, Couldwell WT, Barr CE, Dodge WE, Vance ML, et al. The prevalence of pituitary adenomas: a systematic review. Cancer. 2004;101(3):613–9. Available from: http://dx.doi.org/10.1002/cncr.20412.
5. Ross NS. Epidemiology of Cushing's syndrome and subclinical disease. Endocrinol Metab Clin North Am. 1994;23(3):539–46.
6. Alexandraki KI, Grossman AB. The ectopic ACTH syndrome. Rev Endocr Metab Disord. 2010;11(2):117–26. Available from: http://dx.doi.org/10.1007/s11154-010-9139-z.
7. Newell-Price J, Trainer P, Besser M, Grossman A. The diagnosis and differential diagnosis of Cushing's syndrome and pseudo-Cushing's states. Endocr Rev. 1998;19(5):647–72.
8. Besemer F, Pereira AM, Smit JWA. Alcohol-induced Cushing syndrome. Hypercortisolism caused by alcohol abuse. Neth J Med. 2011;69(7):318–23.
9. Lüdecke DK. Transnasal microsurgery of Cushing's disease 1990. Overview including personal experiences with 256 patients. Pathol Res Pract. 1991;187(5):608–12. Available from: http://dx.doi.org/10.1016/S0344-0338(11)80155-X.
10. Joffe SN, Brown C. Nodular adrenal hyperplasia and Cushing's syndrome. Surgery. 1983;94(6):919–25.
11. Magiakou MA, Smyrnaki P, Chrousos GP. Hypertension in Cushing's syndrome. Best Pract Res Clin Endocrinol Metab. 2006;20(3):467–82. Available from: http://dx.doi.org/10.1016/j.beem.2006.07.006.
12. Jenkins PJ, Trainer PJ, Plowman PN, Shand WS, Grossman AB, Wass JA, et al. The long-term outcome after adrenalectomy and prophylactic pituitary radiotherapy in adrenocorticotropin-dependent Cushing's syndrome. J Clin Endocrinol Metab. 1995;80(1):165–71.
13. Alexandraki KI, Grossman AB. Medical therapy of Cushing's disease: where are we now? Front Horm Res. 2010;38:165–73. Available from: http://dx.doi.org/10.1159/000318507.
14. Beal MW, Simmonds K. Clinical uses of mifepristone: an update for women's health practitioners. J Midwifery Womens Health. 2002;47(6):451–60.
15. Santen RJ, Misbin RI. Aminoglutethimide: review of pharmacology and clinical use. Pharmacotherapy. 1981;1(2):95–120.
16. Clayton RN, Raskauskiene D, Reulen RC, Jones PW. Mortality and morbidity in Cushing's disease over 50 years in Stoke-on-Trent, UK: audit and meta-analysis of literature. J Clin Endocrinol Metab. 2011;96(3):632–42. Available from: http://dx.doi.org/10.1210/jc.2010-1942.
17. Lado-Abeal J, Rodriguez-Arnao J, Newell-Price JD, Perry LA, Grossman AB, Besser GM, et al. Menstrual abnormalities in women with Cushing's disease are correlated with hypercortisolemia rather than raised circulating androgen levels. J Clin Endocrinol Metab. 1998;83(9):3083–8.

Neuroblastoma

61

Armin Pycha and Evi Comploj

61.1 General Facts

The incidence of neuroblastoma is 1:100,000 per year with a median age of approximately 2 years. It represents 7 % of all cancers and is the cause of 15 % of all childhood cancer deaths. More than 95 % of cases are diagnosed in children younger than 10 years of age and 50 % of them have metastases at diagnosis. Neuroblastoma arises from cells of the neural crest that form the adrenal medulla and sympathetic ganglia. Neuroblastoma can manifest anywhere along the sympathetic chain. The most common sites of the primary tumor are the adrenal gland (40 %), paravertebral ganglia (25 %), thorax (15 %), and pelvis 5 % [1]. Thoracic primaries are most common in children of less than 1 year of age. The most common sites of metastases are the cortical bone and bone marrow as well as both the regional and distant lymph nodes. Many neuroblastomas secrete catecholamines. These are extensively metabolized within the tumor itself so that urinary levels of vanillylmandelic acid and homovanillic acid are disproportionately elevated and hypertension is unusual [1–3]. Age still remains an important indicator of outcome. Children of 1 year or younger have better survival than others, which may be attributed to more favorable biological parameters in tumor diagnosis at this age.

The N-myc oncogene amplification is nearly always present at the time of diagnosis within the high-risk group and is connected with rapid tumor progression and a poor prognosis [2]. Amplification is found in only 5 % of low stages but in 40 % of those with advanced stages. The poor prognosis associated with N-myc amplification is independent of a patient's age or stage of disease at diagnosis. The overall 15-year survival rate achieves 79 % with a >95 % survival rate in the low-risk group but only 30–40 % [2, 3] in the high-risk group. Chromosome 1p deletions are found

A. Pycha, MD, FEBU (✉) • E. Comploj, MD, FEBU, FEAPU
Department of Urology, Central Hospital of Bozen/Bolzano,
Lorenz Böhler Street 5, Bozen/Bolzano 39100, Italy
e-mail: armin.pycha@libero.it; complojevi94@yahoo.de

A.S. Merseburger et al. (eds.), *Urology at a Glance*,
DOI 10.1007/978-3-642-54859-8_61, © Springer-Verlag Berlin Heidelberg 2014

in 70–80 % in patients with neuroblastoma mostly in advanced stages. The inactivation of a tumor suppressor gene within 1p36.3 is associated with an increased risk for disease relapse [4].

61.2 Symptoms, Classification, and Grading

The symptoms of the neuroblastoma vary widely depending on the site of manifestation. Most children have a palpable tumor, fever of unknown origin, anemia, hematuria, cord compression, and pathological fracture. Most primary tumors arise within the abdomen (65 %) [5]. The palpable mass leads to an imaging study, which plays an important role in the evaluation. Plain radiographs, bone scintigraphy, and iodine-^{131}metaiodobenzylguanidine (MIBG) scintigraphy should be performed [1], as well as two marrow aspirates and two biopsies. MIBG is incorporated in the adrenergic secretory vesicles of the tumor cells in both primary and metastatic sites. It can be used to determine the extent of the disease and also to detect recurrency during follow-up. Ultrasonography and MRI provide more details on the local extension of the disease and are mandatory for planning the therapy.

The International Neuroblastoma Staging System (INSS) [6] is based on clinical, radiographic, and surgical evaluation and is given in Table 61.1. The risk group classification which combines pathological findings, stage, and biological markers is given in Table 61.2. Nowadays, the International Neuroblastoma Response Criteria (INRC) have replaced all previous established systems and are being used worldwide [7].

Table 61.1 International neuroblastoma staging system [6]

Stage	Definition
1	Localized tumor with complete gross excision, with or without microscopic residual disease; representative ipsilateral lymph nodes negative for tumor microscopically (nodes attached to and removed with the primary tumor may be positive)
2A	Localized tumor with incomplete gross excision; representative ipsilateral nonadherent lymph nodes negative for tumor microscopically
2B	Localized tumor with or without complete gross excision, with ipsilateral nonadherent lymph nodes positive for tumor. Enlarged contralateral lymph nodes must be negative microscopically
3	Unresectable unilateral tumor infiltrating across the midline, with or without regional lymph node involvement; localized unilateral tumor with contralateral regional lymph node involvement; or midline tumor with bilateral extension by infiltration (unresectable) or by lymph node involvement
4	Any primary tumor with dissemination to the distant lymph node, bone, bone marrow, liver, skin, and/or other organs
4S	Localized primary tumor (as defined for stage 1, 2A, or 2B), with dissemination limited to the skin, liver, and/or bone marrow (less than 10 % tumor) in infants <1 year of age

Table 61.2 Risk group classification [10]

Risk group	INSS stage	Age (days)	N-myc status	DNA index	Shimada histopathology
Low	1	Any	Any	Any	Any
	2A, 2B	<365	Any	Any	Any
	2A, 2B	>365	Nonamplified	Any	Any
	2A, 2B	>365	Amplified	Any	Favorable
	4S	<365	Nonamplified	>1.0	Favorable
Intermediate	3	<365	Nonamplified	Any	Any
	3	>365	Nonamplified	Any	Favorable
	4	<365	Nonamplified	Any	Any
	4S	<365	Nonamplified	1.0	Favorable
	4S	<365	Nonamplified	Any	Unfavorable
High	2A, 2B	>365	Amplified	Any	Unfavorable
	3	<365	Amplified	Any	Any
	3	>365	Nonamplified	Any	Unfavorable
	3	>365	Amplified	Any	Any
	4	<365	Amplified	Any	Any
	4	>365	Any	Any	Any
	4S	<365	Amplified	Any	Any

61.3 Therapy

Current treatment for high-risk neuroblastoma patients involves induction chemotherapy, surgery, myeloablative chemotherapy with stem cell rescue, radiotherapy and continuing therapy with 13-cis-retinoic acid, and immunotherapy [8].

The goal of induction chemotherapy is rapid reduction of the entire tumor burden: both metastatic and primary sites, the latter to facilitate complete resection of soft tissue disease.

While most tumors respond to chemotherapy, surgery is critical to achieving complete remission (CR) in primary site for most patients, since radiotherapy alone is generally unable to destroy all soft tissue manifestations. Nevertheless, neuroblastoma is considered to be a chemosensitive tumor and radiotherapy is a critical component of local control of primary site where tumor was left behind. Chemotherapy has also been applied to metastatic sites of bulky disease post induction therapy and surgery. Patients treated with chemotherapy benefit from total body irradiation (TBI)-based myeloablative chemotherapy followed by autologous hematopoietic stem cell rescue (ASCT). Anti-GD2 monoclonal antibodies currently form the mainstay of neuroblastoma immunotherapy with the goal to maintain achieved remission. Retinoids induce differentiation and growth arrest of malignant neuroblastoma cells binding to retinoid acid receptors. These are used for frontline therapy for patients in remission. MIBG is incorporated in over 90 % of all

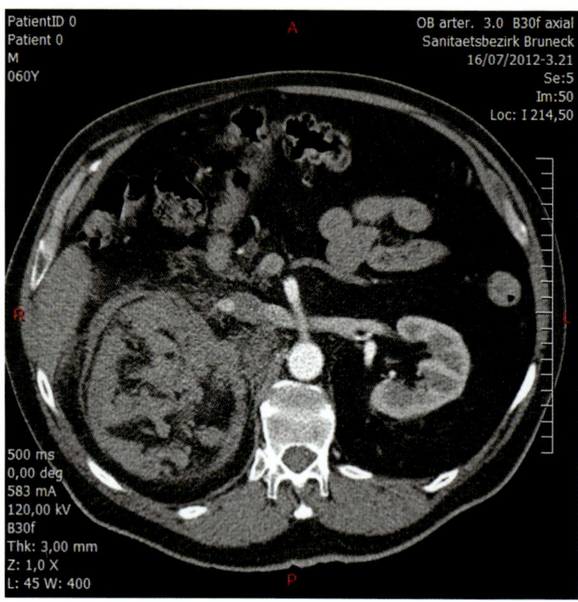

Fig. 61.1 CT scan of a 16-year-old man who presented with anemia and sudden abdominal pain and showed this suprarenal mass, histologically proved to be a neuroblastoma with intratumoral bleeding

neuroblastomas. ^{131}I-MIBG has been used to target radiation for the therapy of metastatic neuroblastoma since the 1980s. MIBG monotherapy achieves responses up to 37 % of refractory or relapsed patients, usually at doses >12 mCi/kg, but responses are normally transient [8].

61.3.1 Complications

Complications develop on the one hand primarily through the natural history of the disease and on the other hand as side effects of chemotherapy (bone marrow depression with anemia, thrombocytopenia leading to hemorrhages, as well as leucopenia to infections). Postoperative complications were observed more often with radical ablative surgery than with surgery after cytoreductive chemotherapy [9] (Figs. 61.1 and 61.2).

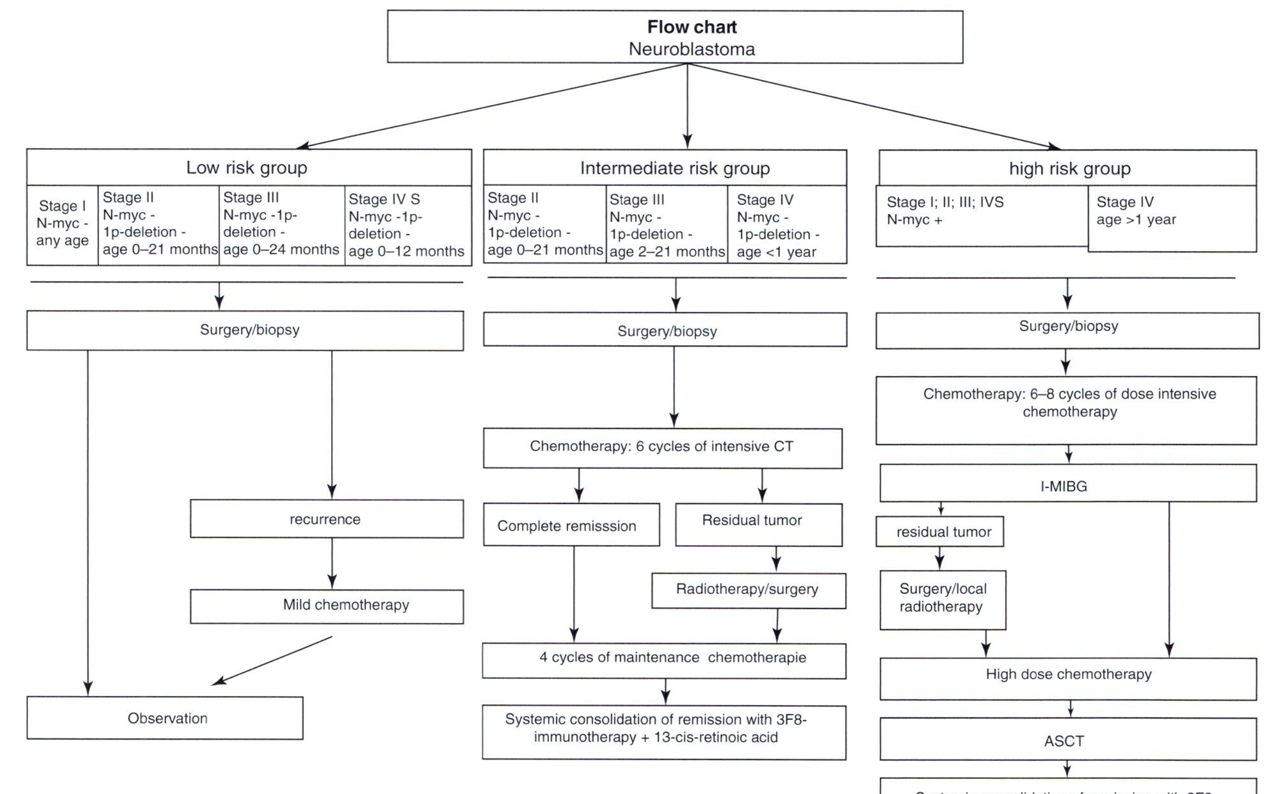

Fig. 61.2 *N-myc*– N-myc nonamplified, *N-myc*+ N-myc amplified

References

1. Charron M. Contemporary approach to diagnosis and treatment of neuroblastoma. Q J Nucl Med Mol Imaging. 2013;57:40–52.
2. Schwab M, Alitalo K, Klempnauer KH, Varmus HE, Bishop JM, Gilbert F, Brodeur G, Goldstein M, Trent J. Amplified DNA with limited homology to myc cellular oncogene is shared by human neuroblastoma cell lines and neuroblastoma tumor. Nature. 1983;305:245–8.
3. Kinderkrebsregister D. Jahresbericht des Deutschen Kinderkrebsregister. 2009. www.kinderkrebsregister.de.
4. Schwab M, Hero B, Berthold F. Neuroblastoma: biology and molecular and chromosomal pathology. Lancet Oncol. 2003;4:472–80.
5. Woods WG, Gao RN, Shuster JJ, Robinson LL, Bernstein M, Weitzman S, Bunin G, Levy I, Brossard J, Dougherty G, Tuchman M, Lemieux B. Screening of infants and mortality due to neuroblastoma. N Engl J Med. 2002;346:1041–6.
6. Brodeur GM, Berthold F, Carlsen NLT, Castel V, Castelberry RP, de Bernardi B, Evans AE, Favrot M, Hedborg H, Kaneko M, Kemshead J, Lampert F, Lee REJ, Look AT, Pearson AD, Philip T, Roals B, Sawada T, Seeger RC, Tsuchida Y, Voute PA. Revision of the international criteria for neuroblastoma diagnosis, staging and response to treatment. J Clin Oncol. 1993;11:1466–77.
7. Castel V, Garcia-miguel P, Canete A, Melero C, Navajas A, Ruiz-Jimenez JI, Navarro S, Badal MD. Prospective evaluation of the International Neuroblastoma Staging System (INSS) and the International Neuroblastoma Response Criteria (INCR) in a multicentre setting. Eur J Cancer. 1999;35(4):606–11.
8. Modak S, Cheung NK. Neuroblastoma: therapeutic strategies for a clinical enigma. Cancer Treat Rev. 2010;36:307–17.
9. Thüroff JW, Stein R, Beetz R. Kinderurologie in Klinik und Praxis. 3. Auflage. Stuttgart/New York: GeorgThieme Verlag; 2012. p. 596–600.
10. Monclair T, Brodeur GM, Ambros PF, Brisse HJ, Cechetto G, Holmes K, Kaneko M, London WB, Matthay KK, Nuchtern JG, von Schweinitz D, Simon T, Cohn SL, Pearson AD. INRG task force: the International Neuroblastoma Risk Group staging system: an INRG task force report. J Clin Oncol. 2009;27(2):298–303.

Priapism

62

Hartwig Schwaibold

62.1 General Facts

Priapism is defined as a prolonged and persistent erection of the penis that lasts for 4 h or longer and is unrelated to sexual activity [1]. Priapism, especially the ischemic form, is a urological emergency and requires immediate evaluation and therapy. Unfortunately, the literature on this subject is somewhat amorphous compromising rather case series than controlled trials. Therefore, the evidence for different treatments is not clear [2]. The main consequence of priapism if left untreated or if treatment is delayed is erectile dysfunction. Historically, priapism refers to the Greek God Priapus, the god of fertility and horticulture.

62.2 Symptoms, Classification, and Grading

Priapism affects the corpora cavernosa; the corpus spongiosum and glans remain uninvolved. There are *three subtypes* with a variety of different and common etiological factors (Table 62.1):

62.2.1 Ischemic (Venoocclusive or Low Flow) Priapism

Low-flow priapism is a painful nonsexual, persistent erection where the corpora are fully rigid due to "sludging" of blood. It is characterized by little or no cavernous blood flow and hypoxic, hypercarbic and acidotic blood gases [1]. In up to 60 % of

H. Schwaibold
Department of Urology, Klinikum am Steinenberg,
Steinenbergstraße 31, Reutlingen 72764, Germany
e-mail: schwaibold_h@klin-rt.de

A.S. Merseburger et al. (eds.), *Urology at a Glance*,
DOI 10.1007/978-3-642-54859-8_62, © Springer-Verlag Berlin Heidelberg 2014

Table 62.1 Aetiology of priapism

Idiopathic priapism (mostly ischemic priapism)	
Non-idiopathic priapism	
Haematologic dyscrasias	Sickle cell disease, thalassemia, leukaemia, haemodialysis, thalassemia
Medications	Vasoactive erectile agents (oral, intraurethral and intracorporeal) Alpha-adrenergic receptor antagonists Antianxiety agents Anticoagulants Antidepressants and antipsychotics Antihypertensives Corticosteroids IV alimentation
Recreational drug abuse	Cocaine, marijuana, alcohol
Neurological disorders	Infections, tumours, trauma spinal stenosis, spinal anaesthesia
Metabolic	Fabry disease, gout, diabetes
Traumatic	Perineal, coital injury
Vascular diseases	Pelvic thrombosis, AV fistulas
Hormones	GnRH, testosterone
Metastatic	Tumour infiltration in the corpora

cases, the aetiology is idiopathic, followed by pharmacotherapy for ED. Intracorporeal papaverine has been associated with a 5 % risk at initial testing, whereas PGE1 has a much lower risk of <1 % [3]. Haematological diseases are another common cause of ischemic priapism, usually caused by hyperviscosity syndromes. The best known is sickle cell disease, where presumably sickled erythrocytes obstruct the venous outflow from the corporal bodies [4].

62.2.2 Nonischemic (Arterial, High Flow) Priapism

High-flow priapism is caused by unregulated cavernous arterial inflow. The corpora are not painful and not fully rigid and the blood gases show no signs of hypoxia. Therefore, high-flow priapism is not a medical emergency. The aetiology is usually corporal or perineal trauma and sometimes complications of penile diagnostics or metastatic infiltration of the corpora, leading to arterial–venous "fistulas".

62.2.3 Stuttering Priapism

Stuttering priapism is a variant of ischemic priapism, characterized by multiple episodes of painful, ischemic priapism. Quite often, the men get woken up by

Table 62.2 Thresholds of blood gas values

	pO_2 (mmHG)	pCO_2 (mmHG)	pH
Normal arterial blood	40	50	7.35
High-flow priapism	>70	<40	7.4
Low-flow priapism	<30	>60	<7.25

painful erections which last up to 4 h. Causes are mostly sickle cell disease, but it is thought that any man with ischemic priapism may suffer from stuttering priapism later on [2].

62.2.4 Diagnosis of Priapism

Clinical history including drug history is important and followed by laboratory tests: haematological testing including testing for haemoglobin S, relevant urinary tests and most importantly corporal aspiration with blood gas analysis to differentiate between high- and low-flow priapism (see Table 62.2). Doppler ultrasonography and, recently, MRI examination have been shown to be very valuable in discriminating ischemic and nonischemic priapism [5].

62.3 Therapy

The treatment of priapism aims to achieve rapid detumescence and restore arterial inflow and venous outflow. General measurements include an IV access, pain medication, regional anaesthesia, sedation of the patient and local cooling using ice packs.

In *high-flow* priapism without ischemic damage to the penis, clinical observation is the standard primary intervention, because up to two-thirds of cases resolve spontaneously. However, if the priapism is permanent, radiological embolization using resorbable or non-resorbable materials has been shown to be very effective [6].

In *low-flow* priapism, corporal blood aspiration with a 19 G needle of at least 200 ml is the first step. If erection persists, intracorporeal injection of sympathomimetic drugs is considered to be the gold standard. The first choice is 0.1–0.5 mg phenylephrine (200 mcg/ml) given in 0.5–1.0 ml doses every 5–10 min. Continuous monitoring of blood pressure and pulse are crucial. Alternatively etilefrine (5–20 mg), epinephrine (0.03–0.05 mg) and methylene blue (50 mg injected intracavernosally followed by aspiration and penile compression for 5 min) have been shown to be effective [7]. These first-line treatments may be repeated as necessary according to clinician's judgement.

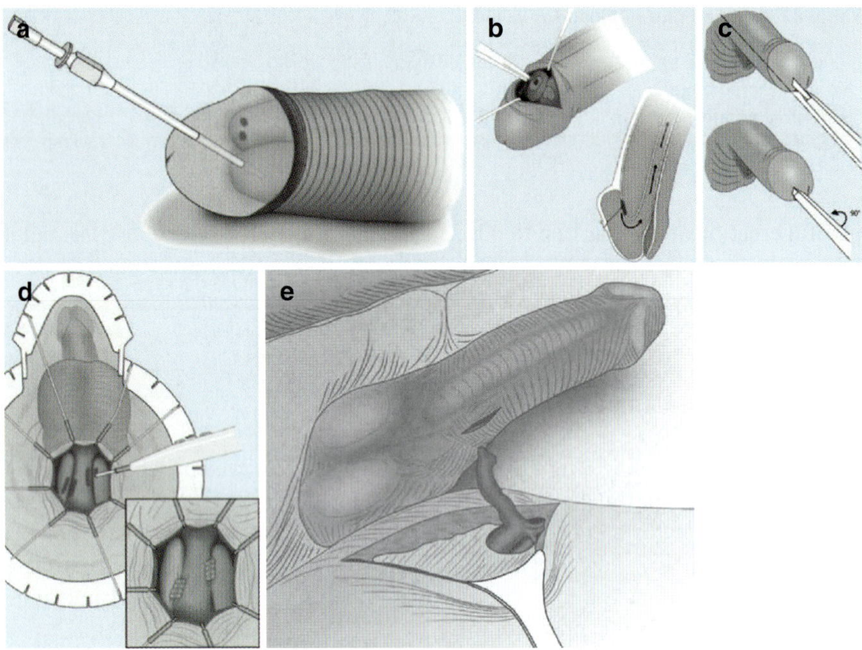

Fig. 62.1 Different shunt techniques: (**a**–**c**) distal (cavernoglanular) shunt, (**a**) Winter shunt; (**b**) Al-Ghorab; (**c**) T-shunt; (**d**–**e**) proximal shunt; (**d**) corpus cavernosum – corpus spongiosum, Quackles shunt; (**e**) corpus cavernosum – V. saphena magna, Grayhack shunt

Penile shunt surgery aims to re-establish blood circulation within the corpora cavernosa [8] by creating a communication between the corpora and either the glans (Winter, Ebbehoj, Al-Ghorab), the corpus spongiosum (Quackles) or a vein (Grayhack) (Fig. 62.1). Success rates of the different procedures vary between 66 and 77 %. Recently, some experts advocate early insertion of a penile prosthesis which is technically easier and maintains penile length [9]. Figure 62.2 shows a proposed algorithm of diagnosis and therapy.

62.4 Complications

The most feared complication of priapism is permanent erectile dysfunction. In low-flow priapism, this is caused by stagnant ischemia within the corpora cavernosa leading to fibrosis and loss of elasticity. More than 90 % of patients develop erectile dysfunction if the priapism lasts >24 h. But therapeutic measures have their own complications: Intracorporeal injection of sympathomimetics may cause headache, dizziness, hypertension, bradycardia, tachycardia and irregular cardiac

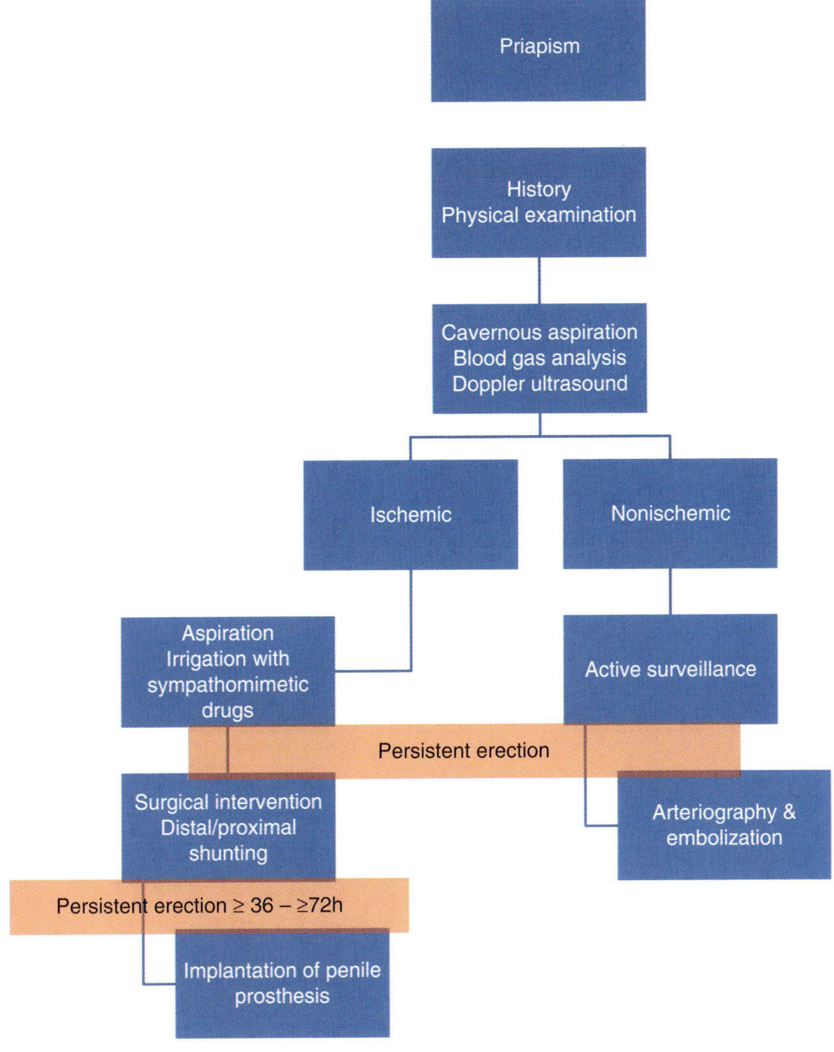

Fig. 62.2 Flow chart demonstrating the pathway from diagnosis to therapy

rhythms requiring thorough cardiovascular monitoring. Shunt surgery can cause purulent cavernositis and erectile dysfunction through venoocclusive malfunction and – if vein shunting is performed – saphenofemoral vein thrombus and pulmonary embolism. Arterial embolization in men with high-flow priapism has an up to 40 % risk of erectile dysfunction among other side effects like penile gangrene, gluteal ischemia and cavernositis.

References

1. Montague DK, Jarow J, Broderick GA, Dmochowski RR, Heaton JP, Lue TF, Nehra A. Sharlip ID and members of the erectile dysfunction guideline update panel: American Urological Association guideline on the management of priapism. J Urol. 2003;170:1318–24.
2. Broderick GA, Kadoglu A, Bivalacqua TJ, Ghanem H, Nehra A, Shamloul R. Priapism: pathogenesis, epidemiology, and management. J Sex Med. 2010;7:476–500.
3. Keoghane SR, Sullivan ME, Miller MA. The aetiology, pathogenesis and management of priapism. BJU Int. 2002;90:149–54.
4. Lue TF. Physiology of penile erection and pathophysiology of erectile dysfunction and priapism. In: Walsh PC, Retik A, Vaughan E, Wein AJ, Kavoussi AR, Novick AC, editors. Campbell's urology. Philadelphia: W.B. Saunders; 2002. p. 1610–96.
5. Ralph DJ, Borley NC, Allen C, Kirkham A, Freeman A, Minhas S, Muneer A. The use of high-resolution magnetic resonance imaging in the management of patients presenting with priapism. BJU Int. 2010;106:1714–8.
6. Kuefer R, Bartsch G, Herkommer K, Krämer SC, Kleinschmidt K, Volkmer BG. Changing diagnostic and therapeutic concepts in high-flow priapism. Int J Impot Res. 2005;17:109–13.
7. Anheuser P, Treiyer A, Steffens J. Priapism. Urologe. 2009;48:1105–12.
8. Burnett AL. Surgical management of ischemic priapism. J Sex Med. 2012;9:114–20.
9. Ralph DJ, Garaffa G, Muneer A, Freman A, Rees R, Christopher AN, Minhas S. The immediate insertion of a penile prosthesis for acute ischaemic priapism. Eur Urol. 2009;56:1033–8.

Hematuria

63

Wanjian Jia

63.1 Definition

Haematuria or hematuria is defined as the presence of erythrocytes in the urine. The causes of hematuria ranges from being negligible to lethal malignant. Generally, 1-ml blood in 1-l urine can cause visible urine discoloration and is alarming to patients, which is termed gross, frank, or macroscopic hematuria.

A small amount of blood in urine only found by light microscope is called microscopic hematuria, most microscopic hematuria cases have no symptoms, and the use of urine dipstick largely promotes the discovery of asymptomatic microscopic hematuria with a 95 % sensitivity and 75 % specificity [2], though currently there is no evidence to support opportunistic screening of the general population [1]. Since free hemoglobin, myoglobin, povidone-iodine, and bacterial peroxidase can give dipstick false-positive reading, further microscopic examination is still necessary for hematuria diagnosis.

Microscopic hematuria diagnostic standard: centrifuge 10-ml fresh, clean-catch midstream urine specimen for 10 min at 2,000 rpm, pour supernatant, and then resuspend sediment; microscopic hematuria is defined as >3 red blood cells per high-power field (rbc/hpf) on two of three specimens [1, 2].

63.2 Medical History

A complete history and physical exam (especially palpation of the abdomen and blood pressure) is required. Concomitant symptoms combining the risk factors, e.g., age, usually can provide diagnostic clue:

W. Jia
Division of Pediatric Urology, Department of Surgery,
University of Utah, Salt Lake City, UT 84108, USA
e-mail: jia73wj@hotmail.com, wanjian.jia@utah.edu

A.S. Merseburger et al. (eds.), *Urology at a Glance*,
DOI 10.1007/978-3-642-54859-8_63, © Springer-Verlag Berlin Heidelberg 2014

- Flank pain or typical renal colic often suggests the existence of urolithiasis; but notably, clot obstruction can also cause renal colic symptoms when bleeding exceeds a certain amount in a short amount of time resulting from other causes, e.g. renal or ureteral malignancy.
- For patients >40 years old, asymptomatic total gross hematuria has the likelihood of urinary tract malignancy, especially for cases with a history of smoking and industrial chemical exposure.
- Cases (many are young females) with lower urinary tract symptoms (LUTs) such as urgency, frequency, and dysuria will usually lead a urinary tract infection (UTI) diagnosis.
- A large amount of gross hematuria or just microscopic hematuria depends on the severity of abdominal or waist trauma and whether there is a rupture to the urinary tract.
- Recent pharyngitis or skin infection may suggest postinfectious glomerulonephritis. Other instances which can be suggested from medical history:
- Physical exertion can cause self-limiting hematuria (especially in youth) and have definitive exercise–hematuria relation.
- Hypertension, significantly increasing foams in urine (proteinuria) with or without peripheral edema often suggest glomerular hematuria. Known prior renal problems, renal masses, altered renal function tests could be other possible clues into the diagnosis.
- Drug-related hematuria, e.g., sulfonamides, nonsteroidal anti-inflammatory drugs use, analgesic abuse, or therapeutic anticoagulant administration.
- Hematuria after bladder catheterization, prostate biopsy, replacement of ureteral dwelling stent, etc. could be regarded as the result of urological interventions.
- Urinary schistosomiasis usually is seen in many African and Middle-Eastern countries.
- Polycystic kidney disease—often has a positive family history.
- Urinary tract invasion from the female reproductive organs or gastrointestinal tract malignancies: corresponding symptoms, physical exam, and/or imaging findings can suggest relevant diagnosis.

63.3 Diagnostic

The diagnosis of the causes of hematuria should be made based on a through medical history and physical exam followed by microscopic urinalysis to confirm the existence of hematuria and disclose the evidences of UTI (>5 white blood cells per high-power field), tube cast, crystal, etc. Sometimes, ultrasound scan, CT, and X-ray (KUB or KUB + IVP) are needed. In some cases, further cystoscopy (may + urethra, bladder biopsy), renal biopsy, MRI, etc. will be performed. Urine cytological exam has a relatively low sensitivity (especial in low-grade malignancy cases) but a high specificity [3–5, 7–9].

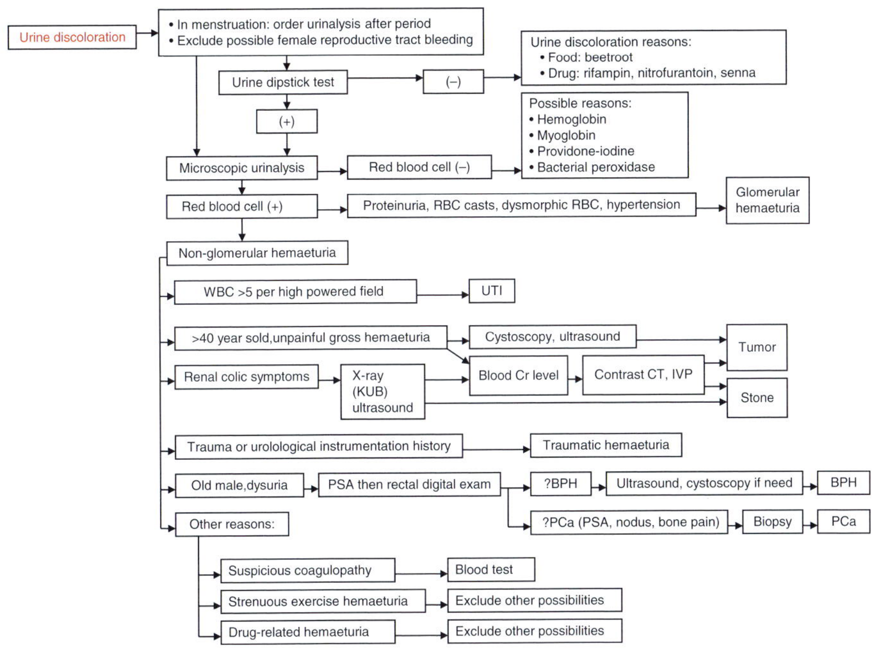

Fig. 63.1 Flow chart demonstrating the pathway from symptoms to diagnosis

Reasons of hematuria

Hematuria causes	Incidence	Diagnostics
UTI	++++	Leukocytes >5 per high-power field
Urolithiasis	++++	Imaging examination
Bladder cancer	++++	Cystoscopy + biopsy
Other urinary tumors	+++	Imaging, endoscopy
Glomerular disease	+++	Nephrology consultation, renal biopsy
BPH	+++	Medical history, digital rectum exam, PSA
Trauma	++	Medical history, imaging
Drug side effects	+	Medical history
Strenuous exercise	+	Medical history
Other systematic urinary tract invasion	+	Medical history, imaging
Prostate cancer	+	PSA, biopsy
Coagulopathy	+	Medical history, blood test

If after undertaking recommended procedures a definite diagnosis still cannot be made, long-term monitoring for patients with hematuria should be taken [3–5, 7–9]. For gross hematuria cases, investigations should be repeated whenever gross hematuria occurs or after 4–6 months. Occult cancer will usually become evident within 1 year [1, 6] (Fig. 63.1).

63.4 Differential Diagnosis

- Drugs that cause urine color change, such as rifampin, nitrofurantoin, and senna
- Food that causes urine color change, e.g., beetroot
- Pseudohematuria from the menses and adjacent organ blooding, e.g., vagina

References

1. The National Collaborating Centre for Chronic Conditions (UK). Chronic kidney disease, NICE clinical guideline. Early identification and management of chronic kidney disease in adults in primary and secondary care. London: Royal College of Physicians (UK); 2008.
2. American urological associate, national medical student curriculum- hematuria. Updated June 2012. http://www.auanet.org/common/pdf/education/Hematuria.pdf.
3. Renal Association and British Association of Urological Surgeons. Joint consensus statement on the initial assessment of haematuria. 2008. http://www.baus.org.uk/AboutBAUS/publications/haematuria-guidelines
4. Loo R, Whittaker J, Rabrenivich V. National practice recommendations for hematuria: how to evaluate in the absence of strong evidence? Perm J. 2009;13(1):37–46.
5. Yun EJ, Meng MV, Carroll PR. Evaluation of the patient with haematuria. Med Clin North Am. 2004;88(2):329–43.
6. Wein AJ, et al. Campbell-Walsh urology. 9th ed. Philadelphia: WB Saunders; 2007. p. 97–100.
7. Wollin T, Laroche B, Psooy K. Canadian guidelines for the management of asymptomatic microscopic hematuria in adults. Can Urol Assoc J. 2009;3(1):77–80.
8. Rodgers M, Nixon J, Hempel S, Aho T, Kelly J, Neal D, Duffy S, Ritchie G, Kleijnen J, Westwood M. Diagnostic tests and algorithms used in the investigation of haematuria: systematic reviews and economic evaluation. Health Technol Assess. 2006;10(18):iii–iv, xi–259.
9. Mazhari R, Kimmel PL. Hematuria: an algorithmic approach to finding the cause. Cleve Clin J Med. 2002;69(11):870, 872–4, 876 passim.

Testicular Torsion

64

Abdul-Rahman Kabbani

64.1 General Facts

Testicular torsion is defined as an acute rotation of testis and spermatic cord with subsequent reduction or interruption of the blood flow. Left untreated a hemorrhagic infarction and necrosis of testicular tissue can be anticipated within 6–8 h depending on the extent of the ischemia. Although testicular torsion can occur at any age, there is peak incidence in the first age and in the puberty. The estimated yearly incidence of testicular torsion for males younger than 18 years old is 3.8 per 100,000 with a 22–41.9 % rate of orchiectomy [1, 2]. The morbidity rate for testicular torsion is usually reported as 1 per 4,000 males until the age of 25 [1]. While the majority of the torsed testes are medially rotated, one-third are laterally rotated [3]. Trauma is not a common cause for testicular torsion as it often occurs without any precipitating events. Etiologically risk factors seem to be cold temperature, increased testicular volume or tumour, a history of cryptorchidism or late descent, a spermatic cord with a long intrascrotal portion and testicles with horizontal lie (e.g., bell-clap anomaly with its extremely wide movement radius within the testicular sheet) [4].

A.-R. Kabbani
Department of Urology and Urological Oncology, Hannover University Medical School, Carl-Neuberg-Str. 1, Hannover 30625, Germany
e-mail: kabbaniar@gmail.com

A.S. Merseburger et al. (eds.), *Urology at a Glance*,
DOI 10.1007/978-3-642-54859-8_64, © Springer-Verlag Berlin Heidelberg 2014

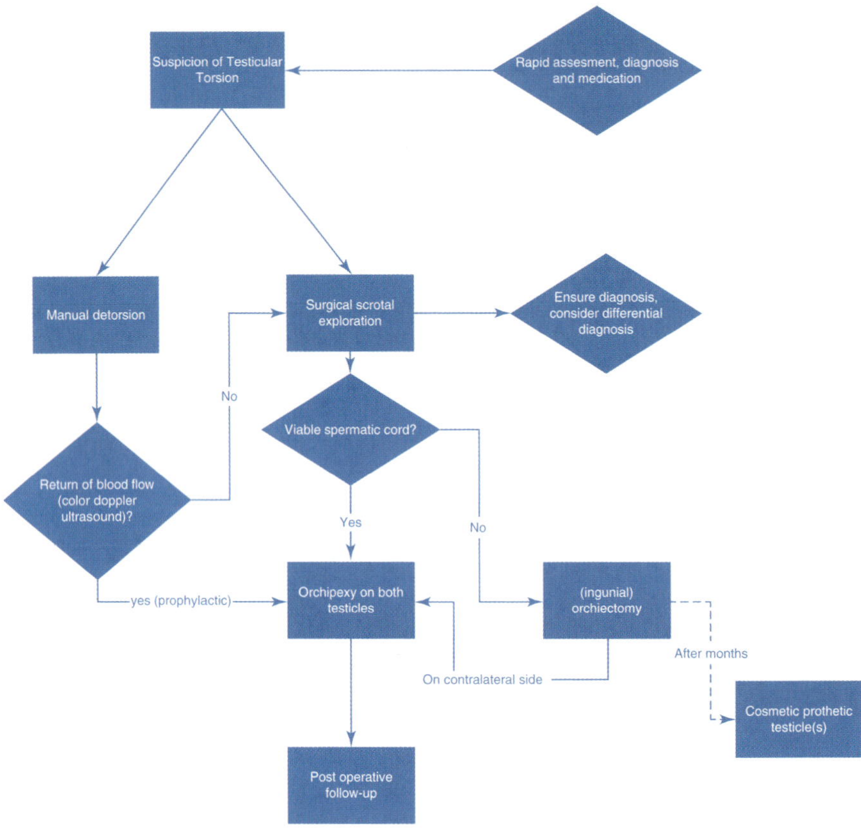

64.2 Symptoms, Classification, and Grading

The cardinal symptom for testicular torsion is acute pain of one scrotal half with possible initial tenderness of the epididymis and pyuria. The pain amplified by the swollen scrotum may extend to the lower abdomen or the inguinal canal and induce nausea, emesis, sweating and tachycardia. Infants, however, could present completely symptomless. Important differential diagnoses include epididymitis, torsion of the appendix testis or epididymis, varicocele, hydrocele, spermatocele, (incarcerated) hernia, orchitis/mumps and acute appendicitis. Depending on the rotation of the spermatic cord in relation to the tunica vaginalis, one differentiates between intravaginal and extravaginal forms. These can be further classified as partial or complete torsions in dependence of the remaining blood flow: Partial torsion twists more than 90°, only compromising the blood vessels and having a delayed ischemia in contrast to complete testicular torsion (≥360°), which cut off the vessels, prompting a rapid necrosis. Only the evidence of a normal arterial *AND* venous blood flow justifies in assuming to exclude a torsion with a high probability. Thus, if a low suspicion of testicular torsion exists, color Doppler ultrasound seems to be suitable in regard to sensitivity and specificity and in addition to not being time-consuming (unlike MRI or scintigraphy) [5].

64.3 Therapy

Regardless of the subsequent therapy, a rapid diagnosis and assessment in combination with an analgetic and/or antiemetic therapy should be initiated; spontaneous detorsion can develop thereby. Suspicion of a testicular torsion needs an immediate surgery, as this is the only method providing definite resolution and above may be needed for definitive diagnosis. In nonclinical emergencies, at time delays or as the first attempt, manual detorsion can provide a quick and noninvasive treatment. By manually untwisting the testicles, the pain should be dramatically relieved. Manual detorsion is successful by the return of blood flow (confirmed via color Doppler US) [5] and a prophylaxis should be attached timely by surgical fixation of both testicles within the scrotal wall so they can no longer twist (orchiopexy). In a clinical setting, in non-successful manual treatment and/or in all patients with a positive history, a surgical scrotal exploration should be performed instantaneously. After untwisting the spermatic cord, the testicles are to be evaluated regarding their viability. If the testis is necrotic, an orchiectomy should be performed to avoid prolonged pain, tenderness, gangrenes and furthermore a potential autoimmune process on the contralateral side [6]. In doubtful cases, the damaged testicle could be left under the idea that the less sensitive hormone-producing Leydig cells still retain a partial function of the testis (ischemia time approx. 12 h) [7]. Whether the testicles are saved or not, the patient should undergo an orchiopexy on both sides, as a prevention for subsequent torsions. After months/weeks patients passing orchiectomy may benefit from the placement of a testicular prosthesis for cosmetic reasons.

64.4 Complications

The most significant complication of testicular torsion is the loss of testis with a possible loss of fertility if both testicles are affected. With only one affected testis, it seems that the endocrine and exocrine functions may be substandard, but this has no impact on the fertility. Actually, fertility depends more to the duration of torsion if the ischemic testis is retained in the scrotum after untwisting [8]. In prepubertal ages, torsion does not appear to affect fertility with normal testicular growth and inconspicuous semen analysis [9].

References

1. Zhao LC, Lautz TB, Meeks JJ, Maizels M. Pediatric testicular torsion epidemiology using a national database: incidence, risk of orchiectomy and possible measures toward improving the quality of care. J Urol. 2011;186(5):2009–13.
2. Watkin N, Reiger N, Moisey C. Is the conservative management of the acute scrotum justified on clinical grounds? Br J Urol. 1996;78(4):623–7.
3. Sessions AE, et al. Testicular torsion: direction, degree, duration and disinformation. J Urol. 2003;169(2):663–5.
4. Ringdahl E, Teague L. Testicular torsion. Am Fam Physician. 2006;74(10):1739–43.

5. Almufti R, Ogedegbe A, Lafferty K. The use of Doppler ultrasound in the clinical management of acute testicular pain. Br J Urol. 1995;76(5):625–7.
6. Merimsky E, Orni-Wasserlauf R, Yust I. Assessment of immunological mechanism in infertility of the rat after experimental testicular torsion. Urol Res. 1984;12(3):179–82.
7. Baker LA, Turner TT. Leydig cell function after experimental testicular torsion despite loss of spermatogenesis. J Androl. 1995;16(1):12–7.
8. Bartsch G, Frank S, Marberger H, Mikuz G. Testicular torsion: late results with special regard to fertility and endocrine function. J Urol. 1980;124(3):375.
9. Rabinowitz R, Nagler H, Kogan S, Consentino M. Experimental aspects of testicular torsion. Dialog Paediatr Urol. 1985;8:1–8.

Paraphimosis

65

Kathrin Simonis and Michael Rink

65.1 General Facts

Paraphimosis can occur when the foreskin of an uncircumcised male is left retracted behind the glans penis (Fig. 65.1). As a result a tight constrictive band of tissue causes edema and swelling of the glans due to lymphatic and venous congestion, which makes it unable to pull back the foreskin easily to its anatomic position [1]. This can happen when the foreskin is retracted in male with relative phimosis or because of the failure to return the foreskin to its normal position after urination, washing, or inserting a transurethral catheter. Besides, it can occur after direct trauma to the area, postcoital, or due to infection.

Paraphimosis is a urologic emergency and can cause serious injury including gangrene and tissue necrosis after a period of time [2].

It can occur at any age, but it is most common among adolescents and has been reported to occur in 0.7 % of uncircumcised boys [3].

Postnatal phimosis is physiologic due to natural adhesions between the foreskin and the glans. During the first 3–4 years of life, epithelial debris (smegma) accumulates under the prepuce, separating the foreskin from the glans. Intermittent penile erections make the foreskin completely retractable [4]. Recurrent infections, obstructive micturition, or paraphimosis are indications for circumcision.

65.2 Diagnosis and Symptoms

Physical examination confirms the diagnosis: The foreskin is retracted and cannot be pulled back over the glans penis.

Conflict of Interest The authors have nothing to disclose.

K. Simonis • M. Rink, MD, FEBU (✉)
Department of Urology, University Medical Center Hamburg-Eppendorf,
Martinistrasse 52, Hamburg D-20246, Germany
e-mail: k.simonis@uke.de; m.rink@uke.uni-hamburg.de

A.S. Merseburger et al. (eds.), *Urology at a Glance*,
DOI 10.1007/978-3-642-54859-8_65, © Springer-Verlag Berlin Heidelberg 2014

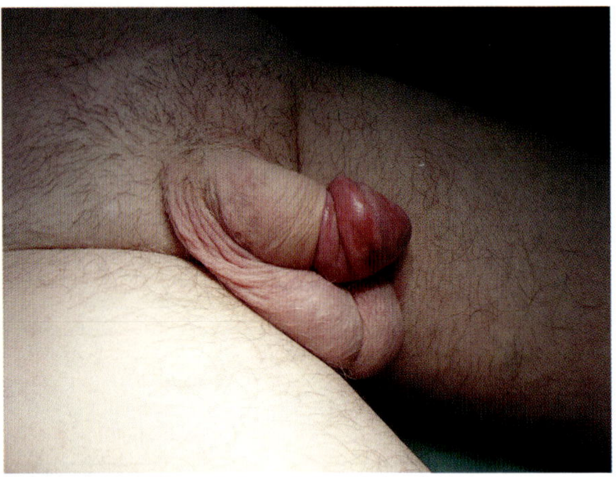

Fig. 65.1 Paraphimosis of 4-day duration in a 45-year-old diabetic patient (Permission of free use by: © http://commons.wikimedia.org/wiki/File:Paraphimosis.jpg)

Paraphimosis presents with a painful edema of the glans penis and the foreskin and livid discoloration of the glans, while the proximal part of the penis is not affected (Fig. 65.2).

65.3 Therapy

Treatment includes reducing penile and glans edema followed by retracting the foreskin over the glans. Prior to manual reduction of paraphimosis, pain control is recommended. Topical medications used are 2 % lidocaine gel or EMLA cream which can be applied directly to the skin before therapy [5]. If more invasive procedures are needed, a dorsal penile block and/or local infiltration into the foreskin can be performed [6]. A reduced or delayed allocation of local anesthetics after dorsal penile blocks has to be considered due to edema in patients with paraphimosis. Local infiltration therefore may be more effective in case of surgical intervention.

Circumferential manual compression of the distal penis can reduce edema and allow a successful reduction of the foreskin. The forefinger and the middle finger of both hands are placed on the sulcus coronarius proximal to the tight constrictive band, while both thumbs press out the edema from the glans penis [1]. The use of Babcock clamps to grasp the retracted foreskin has also been described [7].

If manual reposition of the foreskin is unsuccessful, a dorsal longitudinal incision of the preputial tight constrictive band should be done. Because of the edema and a greater risk of postoperative infections, circumcision should not be performed as an emergency procedure, but after reduction of swelling and healing [4].

In literature several other techniques are described, e.g., injecting hyaluronidase beneath the narrow band, puncturing the edematous skin before compression, or

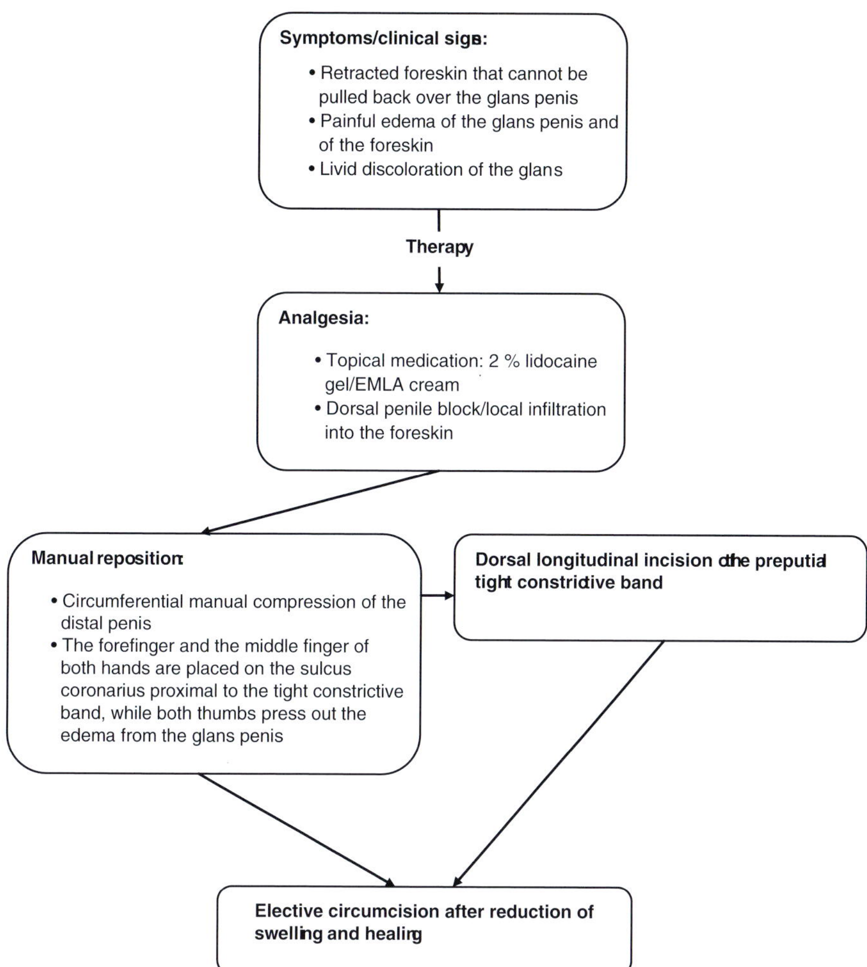

Fig. 65.2 Flowchart displaying the pathway from diagnosis to therapy in paraphimosis

applying granulated sugar to the penis [4]. However, there are no randomized studies comparing the various procedures [8]. Before invasive techniques are used (dorsal slit procedure), the attempt of manual reposition is mandatory.

65.4 Complications

Paraphimosis is a urological emergency. If left untreated, the disrupted blood flow can cause serious injury including gangrene and tissue necrosis after of the distal penis.

References

1. Pohlmann GD, Phillips JM, Wilcox DT. Simple method of paraphimosis reduction revisited: point of technique and review of the literature. J Pediatr Urol. 2013;9:104–9.
2. Hollowood AD, Sibley GN. Non-painful paraphimosis causing partial amputation. Br J Urol. 1997;80:958.
3. Herzog LW, Alvarez SR. The frequency of foreskin problems in uncircumcised children. Am J Dis Children. 1986;140:254–6.
4. Hayashi Y, Kojima Y, Mizuno K, Kohri K. Phimosis, paraphimosis, and circumcision. The Sci World J. 2011;11:289–301.
5. Choe JM. Paraphimosis: current treatment options. Am Fam Physician. 2000;62:2623–6.
6. Little B, White M. Treatment options for paraphimosis. Int J Clin Pract. 2005;59:591–3.
7. Skoglund R, Chapman WH. Reduction of paraphimosis. J Urol. 1970;104:137.
8. Mackway-Jones K, Teece S. Best evidence topic reports. Ice, pins, or sugar to reduce paraphimosis. Emerg Med J. 2004;21:77–8.

Fournier's Gangrene

66

Stephan Kruck and Jens Bedke

66.1 General Facts

The French venereologist Jean Alfred Fournier reported the first small series of a rapidly progressive gangrene of the penis and scrotum in five young men in 1883. The underlying polymicrobial necrotizing fasciitis starts in the perineal, perianal, or genital areas and can extend up to the abdominal and lumbar wall. It is most common in older men in the 5th–6th decades and associated with diseases which precondition an immunodeficiency status like diabetes mellitus, malnutrition, chronic alcoholism, and malignant or infectious diseases. Although the incidence is low and accounts for less than 0.5 % of all admissions to urologic clinics, the incidence is rising due to an increase of older people with higher comorbidities and limited immunologic status [1]. The restricted immunity together with an anorectal, urogenital, or perineal trauma is often associated with recent instrumentation and enables microorganisms, such as Enterobacteriaceae; anaerobic, streptococcal, and staphylococcal species; or fungi, to promote the fulminant infection of a Fournier's gangrene [2]. Especially, synergistic polymicrobial effects lead to a rapid spread along the superficial and deep fascial planes. Gangrenous necrosis of the fascia is followed by the involvement of adjacent subcutaneous and skin tissue [3]. Delayed treatment leads to a rapid systemic progression with fulminant sepsis, multiorgan failure, and high mortality of up to 70 % despite rapid operation and modern intensive care therapy [4].

S. Kruck (✉) • J. Bedke
Department of Urology, Eberhard-Karls-University,
Hoppe-Seyler-Str. 3, 72076 Tuebingen, Germany
e-mail: stephan.kruck@gmail.com; bedke@live.com

A.S. Merseburger et al. (eds.), *Urology at a Glance*,
DOI 10.1007/978-3-642-54859-8_66, © Springer-Verlag Berlin Heidelberg 2014

Diagnosis/resuscitation

- Vital signs/stabilization/critical care
- Extent of gangrene
- History/risk factors/tetanus prophylaxis
- Parentertal antimicrobial therapy
- Laboratory/imaging/cultures

Surgical treatment

- Multidisciplinary management
- Complete surgical debridement
- +/– Urinary/fecal diversion
- Early second-look procedure

+/– stable

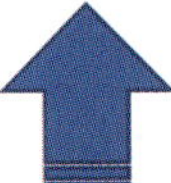

Postoperative care

- Monitoring and wound care
- Organ support
- +/–Hyperbaric oxygen
- +/–Topical agents

Diagnosis/resuscitation

- Skin graft/muscle flap
- Undiversion
- Advanced reconstruction
- Rehabilitation (functional/social)

66.2 Symptoms, Classification, and Grading

The diagnosis is made on clinical grounds and requires careful assessment, in particular in patients with reduced general health conditions. In many cases, the initial examination only shows a small necrotic area of the skin with slight perineal discomfort which might be present for up to 1 week before presentation. The underlying extensive necrosis is often invisible in early stages, while in later stages a painful edema of the scrotum and perineum with crepitus due to the presence of gas-forming organisms is seen together with a repulsive fetid odor. Especially, scrotal involvement is most frequently found and is followed by a rapid bacterial spread to the perineum and abdominal wall along the facial planes. Systemic symptoms, such as fever, tachycardia, or hypotension, may be present as harbingers of an imminent septic shock. Several disease-specific (Laboratory Risk Indicator for Necrotizing Fasciitis, Fournier Gangrene Severity Index and its update) and general prognostic scoring systems (Charlson Comorbidity Index, APACHE, or the surgical APGAR score) can be used for risk stratifications and prediction of treatment outcome [5]. In clinical practice, especially the assessment of gangrene extent, general health status, comorbidities, vital signs, and laboratory findings should be used for an initial estimation of prognosis.

66.3 Therapy

The initial management includes the early stabilization of septic conditions (fluid management, oxygen resuscitation, correction of electrolyte imbalance, anemia, coagulopathy, or diabetic metabolic state), tetanus prophylaxis, and parenteral broad-spectrum antibiotic/antimycotic therapy. Due to low antimicrobiotic tissue levels in ischemic conditions, an immediate definitive multidisciplinary surgical management is of critical importance and should not be significantly delayed by further imaging (conventional radiography, ultrasonography, or computed tomography) and laboratory procedures. Nevertheless, a rapid initial CT scan can be useful to detect the extent of abdominal spread. For surgery, the patient is placed in lithotomy position under general anesthesia after the placement of a transurethral or suprapubic catheter (in case of suspected urethral or prostatic focus). The aim of surgery is the complete removal of all devitalized skin, subcutaneous tissue, fascia, and muscle, regardless of any additional need for urinary and/or fecal diversion. Often the testicles are uninvolved and can be placed in a subcutaneous pocket to prevent desiccation. After primary debridement, an early second-look surgery is recommended to detect any residuals or recurring necrosis. The continuous monitoring and wound care are mandatory and can be supported by topical application of additional agents (hydrogen peroxide, povidone-iodine, or sodium hypochlorite). In case of any suspected or confirmed exacerbation, an early reexploration is additionally recommended. If available hyperbaric oxygen can be used as adjuvant treatment to increase tissue oxygen levels and wound healing, but cannot replace surgery. In case of disease stabilization and sufficient wound granulation, reconstructive surgery shall be performed. Depending on the skin defect extent, vacuum-assisted closure, primary closure, grafting, or muscular vascularized flaps can be used.

66.4 Complications

The major early complications of a Fournier's gangrene are closely linked to a non-resolving sepsis with multiple organ failure (respiratory failure, renal failure, septic shock, hepatic failure, and DIC) with a high mortality rate. Late complications include those due to extensive tissue loss, such as scars and contractures; lymphedema; erectile dysfunction; infertility; problems with urinary or rectal diversion; and in rare cases scar-associated squamous cell carcinoma. These complications can not only lead to cosmetic and functional impairments but can also be followed by significant psychological and social distress.

References

1. Altarac S, Katusin D, Crnica S, Papes D, Rajkovic Z, Arslani N. Fournier's gangrene: etiology and outcome analysis of 41 patients. Urol Int. 2012;88:289–93.
2. Yanar H, Taviloglu K, Ertekin C, Guloglu R, Zorba U, Cabioglu N, Baspinar I. Fournier's gangrene: risk factors and strategies for management. World J Surg. 2006;30:1750–4.
3. Mallikarjuna MN, Vijayakumar A, Patil VS, Shivswamy BS. Fournier's gangrene: current practices. ISRN Surg. 2012;2012:942437.
4. Sugihara T, Yasunaga H, Horiguchi H, Fujimura T, Ohe K, Matsuda S, Fushimi K, Homma Y. Impact of surgical intervention timing on the case fatality rate for Fournier's gangrene: an analysis of 379 cases. BJU Int. 2012;110:E1096–100.
5. Roghmann F, von Bodman C, Loppenberg B, Hinkel A, Palisaar J, Noldus J. Is there a need for the Fournier's gangrene severity index? Comparison of scoring systems for outcome prediction in patients with Fournier's gangrene. BJU Int. 2012;110:1359–65.

M. Ormond

67

Abdul-Rahman Kabbani

67.1 General Facts

Morbus Ormond, also known as Gerota's disease/fasciitis or retroperitoneal fibrosis (RF), is a rare disease (estimated incidence 1:200,000 [1]) with increasing fibrosis of the retroperitoneum and encasement of the containing vessels, nerves and ureters. RF appears most commonly in 40–60-year-olds, with males two to three times more likely to be affected than females. Approximately two third of the patients are assigned to the idiopathic primary form, which is associated with increased inflammation and is connected to autoimmune disorders. Etiologically this form is to be delineated from the secondary form that is caused by factors triggering a reactive fibrosis such as radiation, chronic inflammation, scarring after surgery, drugs, tumors, and trauma. Here again, no specific triggers are known, whereas in addition to the above stated causes, certain vasoactive drugs (alkaloids, β-blockers, phenacetin) or autoimmune diseases such as Crohn's disease, primary biliary cirrhosis, Wegener's disease, Sjogren's syndrome and Erdheim-Chester disease are known risk factors [2].

67.2 Symptoms, Classification, and Grading

RF often begins with nonspecific symptoms such as weight loss, malaise, nausea, and vomiting but without lymphadenopathy. Upon further ectasia and medial displacement of the affected ureter and kidney pelvis unit, the first compression

A.-R. Kabbani
Department of Urology and Urological Oncology, Hannover University Medical School, Carl-Neuberg-Str. 1, Hannover 30625, Germany
e-mail: kabbaniar@gmail.com

A.S. Merseburger et al. (eds.), *Urology at a Glance*,
DOI 10.1007/978-3-642-54859-8_67, © Springer-Verlag Berlin Heidelberg 2014

symptoms appear, which may present in a varied clinical picture depending on the compressed structures. In the majority of the cases, there is an involvement of the ureter thus potentially associated with pain in the back, flank, and lower abdomen area; an oliguria/anuria; and/or a hematuria. In addition, the compression of the vena cava can result in leg edema and DVT, the encasement of the aorta can led to a intermittent claudication as well as gangrenes in the lower extremities and the involvement of the mesenterial arteries may end in a mesenteric ischemia. Renal compression with uremia-connected symptoms may appear in the late course. Diagnostic tests should contain basic lab tests (including inflammatory markers, electrolytes and blood count), sonography and urography for suspected hydronephrosis. The modality of choice for the diagnosis and follow-up is cross-sectional imaging (MRI, CT), which is well suited for the detection of RF-associated changes [3]. The diagnosis is only confirmed by histology, which however represents a high-risk sampling and is only necessary when exclusion of malignancy (especially lymphoma, multiple myeloma and carcinoids) is on the foreground.

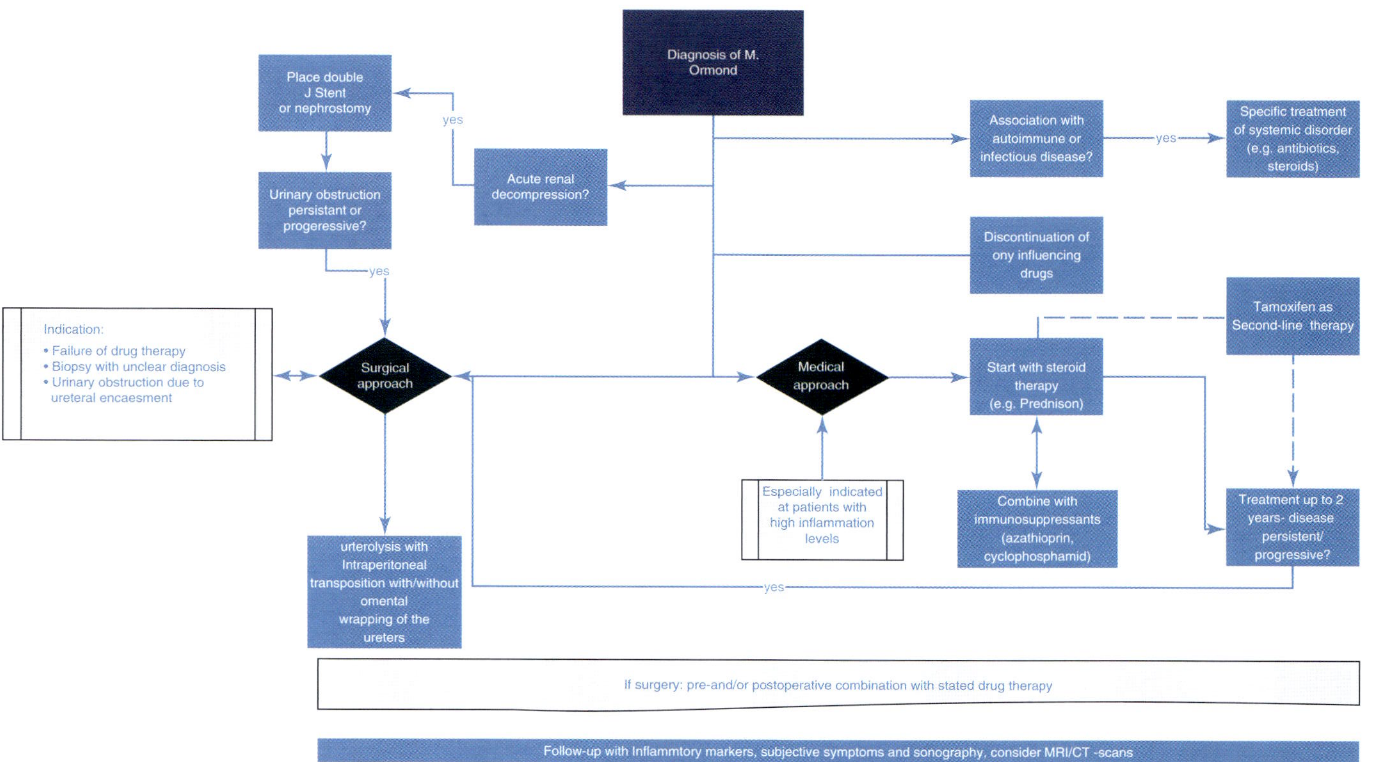
Diagnosis of M. Ormond
Place double J Stent or nephrostomy
yes
Acute renal decompression?
Urinary obstruction persistant or progeressive?
yes
Association with autoimmune or infectious disease?
yes
Specific treatment of systemic disorder (e.g. antibiotics, steroids)
Discontinuation of ony influencing drugs
Tamoxifen as Second-line therapy
Indication:
• Failure of drug therapy
• Biopsy with unclear diagnosis
• Urinary obstruction due to ureteral encaesment
Surgical approach
Medical approach
Start with steroid therapy (e.g. Prednison)
Especially indicated at patients with high inflammation levels
Combine with immunosuppressants (azathioprin, cyclophosphamid)
Treatment up to 2 years- disease persistent/ progressive?
urterolysis with Intraperitoneal transposition with/without omental wrapping of the ureters
yes
If surgery: pre-and/or postoperative combination with stated drug therapy
Follow-up with Inflammtory markers, subjective symptoms and sonography, consider MRI/CT -scans

67.3 Therapy

Regarding the therapeutic approach, there are only insufficient and nonuniform methods available in the literature. Each source describes, however, that before any initiation of therapy, secondary reversible causes should be excluded. This includes the discontinuation of all potentially influencing medication. The goal of therapy in M. Ormond involves halting the progression, regression of the fibrotic changes, preventing recurrences and removal of any obstruction. In acute renal decompression and after retrograde pyelography, the placement of DJ stents or alternatively a nephrostomy could be indicated. For patients with high inflammation levels, a steroid therapy should be initiated. This could be combined with other immunosuppressants (e.g. azathioprine or cyclophosphamide) or tamoxifen as a second-line therapy [4]. In addition there are successful trials with methotrexate, cyclosporin and mycophenolate mofetil as well [5]. Drug treatment is recommended for up to 2 years [6] and its failure should be met with a surgical approach. Surgery can be both pre- and postoperatively accompanied by steroid treatment and should always be indicated in biopsies with unclear diagnosis and to relieve urinary obstruction due to ureteral encasement. In most cases, an open ureterolysis with intraperitoneal transposition and omental wrapping of the ureters is performed. Alternatively a transposition without omental wrapping at low infestations or a laparoscopic surgical approach may be carried out [7]. After treatment, follow-ups are usually monitored by subjective symptoms, regular assessment of inflammatory markers and sonography for detecting of ureteral obstructions, and they may include CT/MRI scans for evaluating the retroperitoneal tissue as well.

67.4 Complications

Important complications include the development of a renal dysfunction up to a progredient chronic renal failure (incidence 5 % [8]). Due to surgery, the ureter can be damaged or the patient can develop a postoperative ureteral stenosis.

References

1. Kottra JJ, Dunnick NR. Retroperitoneal fibrosis. Radiol Clin North Am. 1996;34(6):1259–75. ISSN 0033-8389; 0033-8389.
2. Vaglio A, Salvarani C, Buzio C. Retroperitoneal fibrosis. Lancet. 2006;367(9506):241–51.
3. Vivas I, et al. Retroperitoneal fibrosis: typical and atypical manifestations. Br J Radiol. 2000; 73(866):214–22.
4. Loffeld R, Van Weel T. Tamoxifen for retroperitoneal fibrosis. Lancet. 1993;341(8841):382.
5. Scheel Jr PJ, Feeley N. Retroperitoneal fibrosis. Rheum Dis Clin North Am. 2013;39(2):365–81.
6. Kardar A, Kattan S, Lindstedt E, Hanash K. Steroid therapy for idiopathic retroperitoneal fibrosis: dose and duration. J Urol. 2002;168(2):550–5.
7. Elashry OM, et al. Ureterolysis for extrinsic ureteral obstruction: a comparison of laparoscopic and open surgical techniques. J Urol. 1996;156(4):1403–10.
8. Swartz RD. Idiopathic retroperitoneal fibrosis: a review of the pathogenesis and approaches to treatment. Am J Kidney Dis. 2009;54(3):546–53.

Index

DOI 10.1007/978-3-642-54859-8, © Springer-Verlag Berlin Heidelberg 2014

H

Printing: Ten Brink, Meppel, The Netherlands
Binding: Ten Brink, Meppel, The Netherlands